Principles of Biomedical Ethics

Principles of Biomedical Ethics

SIXTH EDITION

Tom L. Beauchamp

Kennedy Institute of Ethics and Department of Philosophy
Georgetown University

James F. Childress

Department of Religious Studies
University of Virginia

New York   Oxford

Oxford University Press

2009

Oxford University Press, Inc., publishes works that further Oxford University's
objective of excellence in research, scholarship, and education.

Oxford New York
Auckland Cape Town Dar es Salaam Hong Kong Karachi
Kuala Lumpur Madrid Melbourne Mexico City Nairobi
New Delhi Shanghai Taipei Toronto

With offices in
Argentina Austria Brazil Chile Czech Republic France Greece
Guatemala Hungary Italy Japan Poland Portugal Singapore
South Korea Switzerland Thailand Turkey Ukraine Vietnam

Published by Oxford University Press, Inc.
198 Madison Avenue, New York, New York 10016
http://www.oup.com

Oxford is a registered trademark of Oxford University Press

Library of Congress Cataloging-in-Publication Data

Beauchamp, Tom L.
    Principles of biomedical ethics / Tom L. Beauchamp, James F.
Childress.—6th ed.
        p. ; cm.
    Includes bibliographical references and index.
    ISBN-13: 978-0-19-533570-5 (pbk. : alk. paper) 1. Medical ethics.
    [DNLM: 1. Ethics, Medical. W 50 B372p 2009] I. Childress, James F.
II. Title.
    R724.B36 2009
    174.2—dc22   2008000233

Printing number: 9 8 7 6 5 4 3 2 1

Printed in the United States of America
on acid-free paper

To
Georgia, Ruth, and Don

I can no other answer make but thanks,
And thanks, and ever thanks.

Twelfth Night

PREFACE

Biomedical ethics was a young field when the first edition of this book went to press in late 1977—exactly thirty years ago. Immense changes have occurred in the field's literature between our first edition and this, the sixth edition. In these three decades bioethics has transitioned from having no systematic work and no meta-reflection to an enormous literature on the subject. For all who have traveled this road with us, we express our thanks for your many constructive and critical suggestions.

Although major changes have appeared in all editions after the first, this sixth edition includes as large a volume of significant changes as occurred in any previous edition. Chapter 3, on the subject of moral status, is entirely new. Major changes and expansions have been made in the theory of the common morality in Chapters 1 and 10. In Chapter 7 (on justice), globalization and new philosophical thinking about the global order have stimulated us to expand our treatment of obligations of justice at the international level. Also in Chapter 7, we have added a new section on vulnerability and exploitation, two subjects that are now introduced in the new Chapter 3. Other significant changes are these: In Chapter 2 (on moral character), our account of the ethics of care has been revised as a form of virtue ethics. In Chapter 5 (on nonmaleficence), we have heavily modified the later sections on intentionally arranged deaths to come to grips with recent legal and philosophical discussion. Similarly in Chapter 6 (on beneficence), we have adjusted the discussion of paternalism to accommodate recent literature, especially on hard and soft paternalism, and have paid closer attention to the precautionary principle. Despite these changes, the book preserves in this edition its previous chapter structure (except for the new Chapter 3) and characteristic perspectives on major issues. Most of the chapter and sectional headings have been retained from the fifth edition. The part divisions remain and have now been given brief descriptive headings. Every chapter has been shortened and tightened.

We wish to highlight one misguided interpretation of the theory in this book—an interpretation we have encountered many times in the past thirty years. Many commentators have said that the principle of respect for autonomy overrides all other moral considerations in our work, reflecting a distinctly American bias weighting autonomy higher than other principles. This interpretation is profoundly mistaken. In a properly structured theory, respect for autonomy is not an excessively individualistic, absolutistic, or overriding notion that emphasizes individual rights to the neglect or exclusion of social responsibilities. The principle of respect for autonomy is not so treated in this book and has not been so treated from the first edition to the present. We have always argued that competing moral considerations validly override this principle under many conditions. Examples include the following: If our choices endanger the public health, potentially harm innocent others, or require a scarce resource for which no funds are available, others can justifiably restrict exercises of autonomy. The principle of respect for autonomy does not by itself determine what, on balance, a person ought to be free to know or do or what counts as a valid justification for constraining autonomy.

More generally, it is usually a mistake in bioethics to frame the issues as giving an overriding status to one principle over another, as if we must prioritize principles or choose one principle over another. Framing the issues in this way can be seriously misleading. A better strategy is to appreciate the limits of principles as well as the need to give them additional content, while attempting to render consequent rules and judgments as coherent with other commitments as possible. The problems of bioethics are often problems of getting just the right specification or balance of principles. Principles should never be conceived as trumps that allow them alone to determine a right outcome.

Although we have not altered the basic structure of the book in this edition, we have developed, refined, and modified our views as a result of many conversations with readers—some oral, some written; some informal, some published; some friendly, and others adversarial. To our abiding critics for many, many years—notably Bernard Gert, John Arras, Edmund Pellegrino, Franklin Miller, David DeGrazia, Ronald Lindsay, Carson Strong, Robert Baker, and Tris Engelhardt—we express appreciation for the civility of the discourse and for their contributions to the correction and improvement of our work. We also again wish to remember the late Dan Clouser, a very wise man who seems to have been our first—and certainly one of our strongest—critics.

We have continued to receive many helpful suggestions for improvements in our work from students, colleagues, health professionals, and teachers who use the book. Jim Childress is particularly grateful to Ruth Gaare Bernheim, Richard Bonnie, and the late John Fletcher for many illuminating discussions in team-taught courses and in other contexts. He also expresses his deep gratitude to Marcia Day Childress, his wife of ten years, for many valuable suggestions and other important support. Tom Beauchamp wishes to acknowledge the many years of support, encouragement, and engaging discussion of Jeff Kahn and Ruth Faden, as well as the many years of support and encouragement of the Oxford University Press, in both the United States and the United Kingdom. We both again express our gratitude to Jeffrey House, our editor at Oxford for thirty years, for believing in this book and seeing it through the five previous editions.

We owe special thanks, in preparing the sixth edition, to Avi Craimer, who read and perceptively criticized six chapters, and to Oliver Rauprich, who critiqued in incredible detail four chapters. Tom Beauchamp also wishes to express appreciation to three dedicated undergraduate research assistants: Patrick Connolly, Stacylyn Dewey, and Traviss Cassidy. Their research in the literature and their editing of copy have made this book more comprehensive and far more readable. Likewise, Jim Childress wishes to thank two superb research assistants: Jennifer Candis-Shane Arrington and Priya Curtis. We are indebted for the office assistance of Moheba Hanif, as in previous editions. We also acknowledge with due appreciation the support provided by the Kennedy Institute's library and information retrieval systems, which kept us in touch with new literature and reduced the burdens of library research.

We dedicate this edition, just as we have dedicated each of the previous five editions, to Georgia, Ruth, and Don. Georgia, Jim's wife of thirty-five years, died in 1994, just after the fourth edition appeared. Our dedication honors her wonderful memory and pays tribute to the extraordinary influence and devotion of Ruth Faden and Donald Seldin.

Washington, D.C. and *Chilmark, Massachussets*   T.L.B.
Charlottesville, Virginia   J.F.C.
September 2007

CONTENTS

PART I

MORAL FOUNDATIONS

1

Moral Norms

Medical ethics enjoyed remarkable continuity from the time of Hippocrates until the middle of the twentieth century, when developments in the biological and health sciences created concerns about the adequacy of traditional moral guidelines.[1] The Hippocratic tradition had neglected ethical problems of truthfulness, privacy, the distribution of health care resources, communal responsibility, the use of research subjects, and the like. To avoid a similar narrowness, we primarily use philosophical reflection on morality that is distanced from the history of professional medical ethics. This philosophical reflection is not a fully adequate basis for professional ethics, but it allows us to examine and, where appropriate, depart from dominant assumptions in approaches to the biomedical sciences and health care.

NORMATIVE AND NONNORMATIVE ETHICS

The term *ethics* needs attention before we turn to the meanings of *morality* and *professional ethics*. *Ethics* is a generic term covering several different ways of examining and understanding the moral life. Some approaches to ethics are normative, others nonnormative.

Normative Ethics

General normative ethics attempts to answer the question, "Which general moral norms for the guidance and evaluation of conduct should we accept, and why?" Ethical theories attempt to identify and justify these norms, which are often called principles. In Chapter 9 we examine several theories and offer criteria for assessing them.

Many practical questions would remain unanswered even if a fully satisfactory general ethical theory were available. *Practical ethics* (used here as synonymous with *applied ethics,* and by contrast to *theoretical ethics*) is the attempt to interpret general norms for the purpose of addressing particular problems and contexts. The term *practical* refers to the use of norms in the course of deliberating about moral problems, practices, and policies in professions, institutions, and government. Often no straightforward movement from norms—in the form of theories, principles, or precedents—to particular judgments is available. General norms are usually only starting points for the development of concrete norms of conduct.

Nonnormative Ethics

There are two types of nonnormative ethics. The first type is *descriptive ethics,* which is the factual investigation of moral beliefs and conduct. It uses scientific techniques to study how people reason and act. For example, anthropologists, sociologists, psychologists, and historians determine which moral norms and attitudes are expressed in professional practice, in professional codes, in institutional mission statements and rules, and in public policies. They study phenomena such as surrogate decision making, treatment of the dying, and the nature of consent obtained from patients.

The second type is *metaethics,* which involves analysis of the language, concepts, and methods of reasoning in normative ethics. For example, metaethics addresses the meanings of terms such as *right, obligation, virtue, justification, morality,* and *responsibility.* It is also concerned with moral epistemology (the theory of moral knowledge), the logic and patterns of moral reasoning and justification, and the possibility and nature of moral truth. Whether morality is objective or subjective, relative or nonrelative, and rational or nonrational are all important topics in metaethics.

Descriptive ethics and metaethics are nonnormative because their objective is to establish what factually or conceptually *is* the case, not what ethically *ought to be* the case or what is ethically *valuable.* Often in this book we rely on reports in descriptive ethics, for example, when discussing the nature of professional codes of ethics. However, our underlying interest is usually in whether the prescriptions found in such codes are *justifiable,* which is a normative issue.[2]

THE COMMON MORALITY AS UNIVERSAL MORALITY

In its most familiar sense, *morality* refers to norms about right and wrong human conduct that are so widely shared that they form a stable (although incomplete) social agreement. As a social institution, morality encompasses many standards of conduct, including moral principles, rules, rights, and virtues. We learn about morality as we grow up, and we also learn to distinguish the universal morality that holds for everyone from norms that bind only members of special groups, such as physicians, nurses, or public health officials. All persons living a moral life grasp the core dimensions of morality. They know not to lie, not to steal others' property, to keep promises, to respect the rights of others, not to kill or cause harm to innocent persons, and the like. All persons committed to morality do not doubt the relevance and importance of these rules. They know that violating these norms is unethical and will likely generate feelings of remorse and provoke the moral censure of others. Because we are already convinced about these matters, the literature of ethics does not usually debate the merit or acceptability of these basic moral commitments. However, debates do occur about their precise meaning, scope, weight, and strength, often in relation to hard cases.

The Nature of the Common Morality

The common morality is the set of norms shared by all persons committed to morality. The common morality is not merely *a* morality, in contrast to other moralities.[3] The common morality is applicable to all persons in all places, and we rightly judge all human conduct by its standards. The following are norms that are examples (though not a complete list) of *standards of action* (rules of obligation) found in the common morality: (1) Do not kill, (2) Do not cause pain or suffering to others, (3) Prevent evil or harm from occurring, (4) Rescue persons in danger, (5) Tell the truth, (6) Nurture the young and dependent, (7) Keep your promises, (8) Do not steal, (9) Do not punish the innocent, and (10) Obey the law.

The common morality contains, in addition, standards other than rules of obligation. Here are ten examples (again, not a complete list) of *moral character traits,* or virtues, recognized in the common morality: (1) nonmalevolence, (2) honesty, (3) integrity, (4) conscientiousness, (5) trustworthiness, (6) fidelity, (7) gratitude, (8) truthfulness, (9) lovingness, and (10) kindness. These virtues are universally admired traits of character.[4] A person is deficient in moral character if he or she lacks such traits. Negative traits that are the opposite of these virtues are *vices* (malevolence, dishonesty, lack of integrity, cruelty, etc.). They are universally recognized as substantial moral defects. In this chapter we say no more about character and the virtues and vices, reserving this area of investigation for Chapter 2.

It should not be thought that our account of universal morality (in the remainder of this chapter and in Chapter 10) conceives of the common morality as ahistorical or as a priori, whereas other parts of morality are historical products relative to cultures.[5] We do not embrace an ahistorical conception, but can we demonstrate that there is a nonrelativist, or universalist, way of avoiding ahistoricism? This is an important and complicated problem in moral theory that we cannot engage in depth here. We offer only four simple clarifications of our position: First, we hold that the common morality is a product of human experience and history and is a universally shared product. The origin of the norms of the common morality is no different in principle from the origin of the norms of a particular morality in that both are learned and transmitted in communities. The primary difference is that the common morality is found in all cultures,[6] whereas particular moralities are found only in one or more cultures forming a subset of all cultures. Second, we accept moral pluralism (some would say relativism) in *particular* moralities (see pp. 5–8), but we reject a historical moral pluralism (or relativism) in the *common* morality. The common morality is not relative to cultures or individuals, because it transcends both. Third, the common morality comprises moral beliefs (what all morally committed persons believe), not standards prior to moral belief. Fourth, explications of the common morality—in books such as this one—are historical products, and every *theory* of the common morality has a history of development by the authors of the theory. (See, further, Chapter 10, pp. 387–88, 391.)

Theses about the Common Morality

The appeals that we make to the common morality might be understood as normative, nonnormative, or both. If the appeals are *normative,* the claim is that the common morality has normative force: It establishes moral standards for everyone, and failing to abide by these standards is unethical. If the appeals are *nonnormative,* the claim is that we can empirically study whether the common morality is present in all cultures. We accept both the normative force of the common morality and the possibility of studying it empirically.

Some critics of our account in this book assert that scant anthropological or historical evidence supports the empirical hypothesis that a universal common morality exists.[7] In light of this criticism, we need to consider how good the evidence is both for and against the existence of a universal common morality. This is a nuanced problem. In principle, scientific research could either confirm or falsify the hypothesis of a universal morality. However, as with all empirical research, it is essential to be clear about the hypothesis being tested. Our hypothesis is simply that all persons *committed to morality* adhere to the standards that we are calling the common morality. It would, of course, be absurd to assert that all persons do, in fact, accept the norms of the common morality. Clearly many amoral, immoral, or selectively moral persons do not care about or identify with moral demands.

We explore this hypothesis in Chapter 10 rather than here in Chapter 1 (see pp. 387–88). For now we say only that when we claim that the normative judgments found in many parts of this book are derived from the common morality, we do not mean that our *theory* of the common morality gets this morality just right or that it extends the common morality in just the right ways. There may be dimensions of the common morality that we do not correctly capture or depict. Moreover, to say that we attempt to *build* on the common morality in this book by extending it into new areas is not to say that we can validly claim its authority at every level of our account.

PARTICULAR MORALITIES AS NONUNIVERSAL

The Nature of Particular Moralities

We shift now from *universal morality* (the common morality) to *particular moralities*. Many moral norms are not shared by all cultures, groups, and individuals. Whereas the common morality contains general moral norms that are abstract, universal, and content-thin, particular moralities present concrete, nonuniversal, and content-rich norms. (More precisely, particular moralities accept norms at all levels of generality, whereas common morality is comprised only of abstract, universal, and content-thin norms. Particular moralities are distinguished by their particular norms, but share the common morality with all other particular moralities.) These specific moralities include the many responsibilities, aspirations, ideals, sympathies, attitudes, and sensitivities found in diverse cultural traditions, religious traditions, professional practice standards, institutional expectations, and the like. In some cases explication of the values in these moralities requires a special knowledge and may involve refinement by experts or scholars—as, for example, in the body of Jewish religious, legal, and moral norms in the Talmudic tradition. There may also be well-structured moral systems to adjudicate conflicts and provide methods for judgments in borderline cases—as, for example, within the norms and methods in Roman Catholic casuistry.

Professional moralities, which include moral codes and standards of practice, are one form of particular morality. These moralities often legitimately vary from other moralities in the way in which they handle conflicts of interest, protocol review, advance directives, and other subjects. (See the next section, "Professional and Public Moralities.") *Moral ideals* such as charitable goals and aspirations that exceed obligations provide a second instructive example of particular moralities. Moral ideals such as charitable beneficence, by definition, are not required of all persons; indeed they are not *required* of any person.[8] Actions performed from these ideals are morally praiseworthy, but persons who fail to fulfill their ideals cannot be blamed or criticized by others. Moral ideals can be universally praised even though they are not universally required. It is reasonable to presume that all morally committed persons share an admiration of and endorsement of *some* moral ideals, and in this respect those ideals can be said to be shared moral beliefs in the common morality. However, they are not universally shared as *demands* of the moral life. When they become requirements of conduct (e.g., in a monastic tradition), such beliefs are part of a particular morality, not part of universal morality. These ideals and their supererogatory nature are discussed in Chapter 2.

Morality, then, consists of more than principles and rules of the common morality. Morality includes nonbinding moral ideals that individuals and groups accept and act on, communal norms that bind only members of specific moral communities, extraordinary virtues, and the like.

Persons who accept a particular morality often suppose that they speak with an authoritative moral voice for all persons. They operate under the false belief that they have the force of the common morality (that is, universal morality) behind them. The particular moral viewpoints that these persons hold may be morally acceptable and even praiseworthy, but they do not bind other persons or communities. For example, persons who believe intensely that scarce medical resources, such as transplantable organs, should be distributed only by lottery rather than by medical need may have very good moral reasons for their views, but they cannot claim the support of the common morality for those views.

Professional and Public Moralities

Just as the common morality is accepted by all morally committed persons, most professions have, at least implicitly, a professional morality with standards of conduct that are generally acknowledged by those in the profession who are serious about their moral responsibilities. In medicine, professional morality specifies general moral norms for the institutions and practices of medicine. Special roles and relationships in medicine require rules that other professions may not need. For example, as we argue in Chapters 4 and 8, rules of informed consent and medical confidentiality are rooted in the more general moral requirements of respecting the autonomy of persons and protecting them from harm. These rules may not be serviceable or appropriate outside of medicine and research.

Members of professions often *informally* adhere to widely accepted moral guidelines—such as rules prohibiting discrimination against colleagues on the basis of gender, race, religion, or national origin. In recent years *formal* codifications of and instruction in professional morality have increased through codes of medical and nursing ethics, codes of research ethics, and the reports and recommendations of public commissions. Before we assess these developments, the nature of professions needs brief discussion.

According to Talcott Parsons, a profession is "a cluster of occupational roles, that is, roles in which the incumbents perform certain functions valued in the society in general, and, by these activities, typically earn a living at a full-time job."[9] Under this definition, circus performers, exterminators, and garbage collectors are professionals; prostitutes probably are not (because their function is not "valued in the society in general"), despite prostitution's reputation as "the world's oldest profession." Today, it is not surprising to find all such activities characterized as professions, inasmuch as the word *profession* has come, in common use, to mean almost any occupation by which a person earns a living. The once honorific sense of *profession* is now better reflected in the term *learned profession,* which assumes an extensive education in the arts, sciences, technologies, and the like.

Professionals in the relevant sense are usually distinguished by their specialized knowledge and training as well as by their commitment to provide important services to patients, clients, or consumers. Professions maintain self-regulating organizations that control entry into occupational roles by formally certifying that candidates have acquired the necessary knowledge and skills. In learned professions, such as medicine, nursing, and public health, the professional's background knowledge is partly acquired through closely supervised training, and the professional is committed to providing a service to others.

Health care professions specify and enforce obligations for their members, thereby seeking to ensure that persons who enter into relationships with these professionals will find them competent and trustworthy. The obligations that professions attempt to enforce are determined by an accepted role. These obligations comprise the "ethics" of the profession, although there may also be role-specific ideals such as self-effacement that are not obligatory. Problems of professional ethics usually arise either from conflicts over appropriate professional standards or conflicts between professional commitments and the commitments professionals have to activities outside the profession. Because the traditional rules of professional morality are often vague, some professions codify their standards in detailed statements aimed at reducing the vagueness.

Codes often specify rules of etiquette in addition to rules of ethics. For example, one historically significant version of the code of the American Medical Association (AMA) instructed physicians not to criticize fellow physicians who have previously been in charge of a case.[10] Such professional codes tend to foster and reinforce member identification with the prevailing values of the profession. These codes are beneficial when they effectively incorporate defensible moral norms, but some professional codes oversimplify moral requirements, make them indefensibly rigid, or make excessive and unwarranted claims about their completeness and authoritativeness. As a consequence, professionals may mistakenly suppose that they are satisfying all relevant moral requirements by strictly following the rules of the code, just as many people believe that they fully discharge their moral obligations when they meet all relevant legal requirements.

We can and should ask whether the codes specific to areas of science, medicine, and health care are coherent, defensible, and comprehensive within their domain. Historically, few codes have had much to say about the implications of several moral principles and rules such as veracity, respect for autonomy, and justice that have been the subjects of intense discussion in contemporary biomedical ethics. From ancient medicine to the present, physicians have often generated codes for themselves without subjecting them to the scrutiny or acceptance of patients and the public. These codes have rarely appealed to more general ethical standards or to a source of moral authority beyond the traditions and judgments of physicians. The articulation of professional norms in these circumstances has often appeared to protect the profession's interests more than to offer a broad and impartial moral viewpoint or to address issues of importance to patients and society.[11]

Psychiatrist Jay Katz once poignantly expressed his reservations about such codes of medical ethics. Initially inspired by his outrage over the fate of Holocaust victims, Katz became convinced that only a persistent improvement in professional ethics and an educational effort that reaches beyond traditional codes could provide meaningful guidance for research involving human subjects:

> As I became increasingly involved in the world of law, I learned much
> that was new to me from my colleagues and students about such complex
> issues as the right to self-determination and privacy and the extent of the
> authority of governmental, professional, and other institutions to intrude
> into private life.... These issues... had rarely been discussed in my medical
> education. Instead it had been all too uncritically assumed that they could
> be resolved by fidelity to such undefined principles as *primum non nocere*
> ["First, do no harm"] or to visionary codes of ethics.[12]

Public Regulation of Professional Conduct

Additional moral direction for health professionals and scientists comes through the public policy process, which includes regulations and guidelines promulgated by governmental bodies. The term *public policy* is used here to refer to a set of normative, enforceable guidelines accepted by an official public body, such as an agency of government or a legislature, to govern a particular area of conduct. The policies of corporations, hospitals, trade groups, and professional societies sometimes have a deep impact on public policy, but these policies are private, not public—though these bodies are frequently regulated by public policies. A close connection exists between law and public policy: All laws constitute public policies, but not all public policies are, in the conventional sense, laws. In contrast to laws, public policies need not be explicitly formulated or codified. For example, an official who decides not to fund a newly recommended government program with no prior history of funding is formulating a public policy. Decisions not to act, as well as decisions to act, can constitute public policies.

Public policies, such as those that fund health care for the indigent or protect subjects of biomedical research, usually incorporate moral considerations. Moral analysis is part of good policy *formation,* not merely a method for evaluating *existing* policy. Efforts to protect the rights of patients and research subjects provide instructive examples. Over the past thirty-five years the U.S. government has created several national commissions, advisory committees, and councils to formulate guidelines for research involving human subjects, as well as for other areas of biomedical ethics. Morally informed policies have guided decision making about the choice of treatments as well. For example, the U.S. Congress passed the Patient Self-Determination Act (PSDA) as the first federal legislation to ensure that health care institutions inform patients about institutional policies that allow them to accept or refuse medical treatment and about their rights under state law, including a right to formulate advance directives.[13] The relevance of bioethics to public policy is now recognized in most developed countries, several of which have influential national bioethics committees.

Many courts have been active in developing case law that sets standards for science, medicine, and health care. Legal decisions often express communal moral norms and stimulate ethical reflection that over time alters those norms. For example, the line of court decisions in the U.S. starting with the Karen Ann Quinlan case in the mid-1970s has constituted a nascent tradition of moral reflection that has been influenced by, and has influenced, literature in ethics on topics such as whether life-saving medical technologies should be viewed as medical treatments that are subject to the same standards of decision making as other forms of treatment.

Policy formation and criticism involve more complex forms of moral judgment than ethical theories, principles, and rules can handle on their own.[14] Public policy is often formulated in contexts that are marked by profound social disagreements, uncertainties, and differing interpretations of history. No body of abstract moral principles and rules can fix policy in such circumstances, because abstract norms do not contain enough specific information to provide direct and discerning guidance. The implementation of moral principles and rules must take into account factors such as feasibility, efficiency, cultural pluralism, political procedures, pertinent legal requirements, uncertainty about risk, and noncompliance by patients. Principles and rules provide the moral background for policy formation and evaluation, but a policy must also be shaped by empirical data and by information available in fields such as medicine, nursing, public health, economics, law, biotechnology, and psychology.

When using moral norms to formulate or criticize public policies, we cannot move with assurance from a judgment that an *act* is morally right (or wrong) to a judgment that a corresponding *law* or *policy* is morally right (or wrong). The judgment that an act is morally wrong does not necessarily lead to the judgment that the government should prohibit it or refuse to allocate funds to support it. For example, one can argue, without inconsistency, that sterilization and abortion are morally wrong but that the law should not prohibit them, because they are fundamentally matters of personal choice beyond the authority of government (or, alternatively, because many persons would seek dangerous and unsanitary procedures from unlicensed practitioners). Similarly, the judgment that an act is morally acceptable does not imply that the law should permit it. For example, the belief that active euthanasia is morally justified for terminally ill infants who face uncontrollable pain and suffering is consistent with the belief that the government should legally prohibit such active euthanasia because it would not be possible to control abuses if it were legalized.

We are not defending any of these moral judgments. We are maintaining that the connections between moral norms and judgments about policy or law are complicated and that a judgment about the morality of *acts* does not entail a corresponding judgment about *law* and *policy*. Factors such as the symbolic value of law, the costs of a program and its enforcement, and the demands of competing programs often must be considered.

MORAL DILEMMAS

Reasoning through dilemmas to conclusions and choices is a familiar feature of decision making. Consider a particular case.[15] Some years ago, the judges on the California Supreme Court had to reach a decision about the legal force and limits of medical confidentiality. A man killed a woman after confiding to a therapist his intention to commit the act. The therapist had attempted unsuccessfully to have the man committed but, in accordance with his duty of medical confidentiality to the patient, did not communicate the threat to the woman when the commitment attempt failed.

The majority opinion of the Court held that "When a therapist determines, or pursuant to the standards of his profession should determine, that his patient presents a serious danger of violence to another, he incurs an obligation to use reasonable care to protect the intended victim against such danger." This obligation extends to notifying the police and directly warning the intended victim. The justices in the majority opinion argued that therapists generally ought to observe the rule of medical confidentiality, but that this rule must yield in this case to the "public interest in safety from violent assault." Although these justices recognized that rules of professional ethics have substantial public value, they held that matters of greater importance, such as protecting others against violent assault, can override these rules.

In a minority opinion, one judge disagreed and argued that doctors violate patients' rights if they fail to observe standard rules of confidentiality. If it were common practice to break these rules, he reasoned, the fiduciary nature of the relationship between physicians and patients would erode. The mentally ill would refrain from seeking aid or divulging critical information because of the loss of trust that is essential for effective treatment. As a result, violent assaults would increase.

This case presents straightforward moral and legal dilemmas in which both judges cite relevant reasons to support their conflicting judgments. Moral dilemmas are circumstances in which moral obligations demand or appear to demand that a person adopt each of two (or more) alternative but incompatible actions, such that the person cannot perform all the required actions. These dilemmas occur in at least two forms.[16] (1) Some evidence or argument indicates that an act is morally permissible and some evidence or argument indicates that it is morally wrong, but the evidence or strength of argument on both sides is inconclusive. Abortion, for example, is sometimes said to be a terrible dilemma for women who see the evidence in this way. (2) An agent believes that, on moral grounds, he or she is obligated to perform two or more mutually exclusive actions. In a moral dilemma of this form, one or more moral norms obligate an agent to do x and one or more moral norms obligate the agent to do y, but the agent cannot do both in the circumstance. The reasons behind alternatives x and y are weighty and neither set of reasons is overriding. If one acts on either set of reasons, one's actions will be morally acceptable in some respects and morally unacceptable in others. Some have viewed the intentional cessation of life-prolonging therapies in the case of patients in a persistent vegetative state, such as Karen Ann Quinlan, Nancy Cruzan, and Terri Schiavo, as dilemmatic in this second way.

Conflicting moral principles and rules may create difficult dilemmas, as popular literature, novels, and films often illustrate. For example, an impoverished person who steals to save a family from starvation or a person who lies to protect a confidential family document confronts such a dilemma. The only way to comply with one obligation in such situations is to contravene another obligation. No matter which course is chosen, some obligation must be overridden or compromised. It is misleading to say that we are obligated to perform both actions in these dilemmatic circumstances. We should discharge the obligation that, in the circumstances, we judge to override or to compromise what we would have been firmly obligated to perform were it not for the conflict.

Conflicts between moral requirements and self-interest sometimes create a *practical* dilemma, but not, strictly speaking, a *moral* dilemma. If moral reasons compete with nonmoral reasons, questions about priority can still arise even though no moral dilemma is present. Examples appear in the work of anthropologist William R. Bascom, who collected hundreds of "African dilemma tales" transmitted for decades and sometimes centuries in African tribal societies. One traditional dilemma posed by the Hausa tribe of Nigeria is called *cure for impotence:*

> A friend gave a man a magical armlet that cured his impotence. Later he [the man with the armlet] saw his mother, who had been lost in a slave raid, in a gang of prisoners. He begged his friend to use his magic to release her. The friend agreed on one condition—that the armlet be returned. What shall his choice be?[17]

Hard choice? Perhaps, but presumably not a hard *moral* choice. The obligation to the mother is moral in character, whereas retaining the armlet is a matter of self-interest. We are assuming that no moral obligation exists to a sexual partner; in some circumstances, such an obligation would produce a moral dilemma. In any event, it is not clear that a moral reason in conflict with a personal reason entails that the moral reason is overriding. If a physician, in a situation of scarcity of available drugs, must choose between saving his own life or that of a patient, the moral obligation to take care of the patient may not be overriding.

Some moral philosophers and theologians have argued that although many practical dilemmas involving moral reasons exist, no irresolvable moral dilemmas exist. They do not deny that agents experience moral perplexity, conflict, and disagreement in difficult cases, but they insist that the purpose of a moral theory is to provide a principled procedure for resolving all deep conflicts. Some major figures in the history of ethics have defended this conclusion, because they accept one supreme moral value as overriding all other conflicting values (moral and nonmoral) and because they regard it as incoherent to allow contradictory obligations in a properly structured moral theory. The only *ought,* they maintain, is the *ought* generated by the supreme value.[18] We examine such theories (e.g., utilitarian and Kantian theories) in Chapter 9.

In contrast to the account of moral obligation found in these theories, we maintain throughout this book that various moral principles can and do conflict in the moral life. These conflicts sometimes produce irresolvable moral dilemmas. When forced to a choice, we may "resolve" the situation by choosing one option over another, but we still may believe that neither option is morally preferable to the competing option. A physician with a limited supply of medicine may have to choose to save the life of one patient rather than another and still find her moral dilemma irresolvable. Explicit acknowledgment of such dilemmas helps deflate unwarranted expectations of moral principles and theories. Although we often find ways of reasoning about what we should do, we may not be able to reach a reasoned resolution in many instances. In some cases, the dilemma may only become more difficult and remain unresolved even after the most careful reflection.

A Framework of Moral Norms

The common morality contains moral norms that are basic for biomedical ethics. These norms are treated individually in four chapters in Part 2 of this book (Chapters 4–7). Most classical ethical theories include these principles in some form,[19] and traditional medical codes presuppose at least some of them.

Basic Principles

The set of moral principles defended in this book functions as an analytical framework intended to express general norms of the common morality that are a suitable starting point for biomedical ethics. These principles should function as general guidelines for the formulation of the more specific rules. In Chapters 4 through 7 we defend four clusters of moral principles: (1) *respect for autonomy* (a norm of respecting and supporting autonomous decisions), (2) *nonmaleficence* (a norm of avoiding the causation of harm), (3) *beneficence* (a group of norms pertaining to relieving, lessening, or preventing harm and providing benefits and balancing benefits against risks and costs), and (4) *justice* (a group of norms for fairly distributing benefits, risks, and costs).

Nonmaleficence and beneficence have played a central historical role in medical ethics. By contrast, respect for autonomy and justice were neglected in traditional medical ethics and have risen to prominence only recently. As an example, consider the work of British physician Thomas Percival. In 1803, he published *Medical Ethics,* the first comprehensive account of medical ethics in the long history of the subject. This book served as the prototype for the AMA's first code of ethics in 1847. Percival argued (using somewhat different language) that nonmaleficence and beneficence fix the physician's primary obligations and triumph over the patient's preferences and decision-making rights in circumstances of serious conflict.[20] Percival failed to appreciate the depth of the importance of principles of respect for autonomy and distributive justice for physician conduct (despite their presence in the common morality, which he arguably did recognize as relevant for medical practice). However, in fairness to him, these considerations are now prominent in discussions of biomedical ethics in a way they were not when he wrote at the turn of the nineteenth century.

That four clusters of moral "principles" or "general norms" are central to biomedical ethics is a conclusion the authors of this work have reached by examining *considered moral judgments* and the way *moral beliefs cohere,* two notions we discuss in Chapter 10. The selection of these four principles, rather than some other cluster of principles, does not receive an argued defense in Chapters 1 through 3. However, in Chapters 4 through 7, we do defend the vital role of each principle in biomedical ethics.

Rules

Our framework encompasses several types of moral norms, including principles, rules, obligations, and rights. We treat principles as the most general and comprehensive norms, but we draw only a loose distinction between rules and principles. Both are general norms of obligation. The difference is that rules are more specific in content and more restricted in scope than principles. Principles do not function as precise guides to action that direct us in each circumstance in the way that more detailed rules and judgments do. Finally, principles and rules usually establish rights as well as obligations, as we explain in Chapter 9.

We defend several types of rules that specify principles: substantive rules, authority rules, and procedural rules.

Substantive rules. Rules of truth telling, confidentiality, privacy, forgoing treatment, informed consent, and rationing health care provide more specific guides to action than do abstract principles. An example of a rule that sharpens the requirements of the principle of respect for autonomy in certain contexts is, "Follow an incompetent patient's advance directive whenever it is clear and relevant." To indicate how this rule specifies the principle of respect for autonomy, we may state it more fully as, "Respect the autonomy of incompetent patients by following all clear and relevant formulations in their advance directives." This formulation shows how the initial norm of respect for autonomy endures while becoming specified. (See, further, the section "Specifying Principles and Rules" later in this chapter.)

Authority rules. We also defend rules about decisional authority—that is, rules regarding who may and should make decisions and perform actions. For example, *rules of surrogate authority* determine who should serve as surrogate agents when making decisions for incompetent persons, while *rules of professional authority* determine who in professional ranks should make decisions to override or to accept a patient's decisions. Another example appears in *rules of distributional authority* that determine who should make decisions about allocating scarce medical resources.

Authority rules do not delineate substantive standards or criteria for making decisions. However, authority rules and substantive rules interact. For instance, authority rules are justified, in part, by how well particular authorities can be expected to respect and express substantive rules and principles.

Procedural rules. We also defend rules that establish procedures to be followed in certain circumstances. Procedures for determining eligibility for organ transplantation and procedures for reporting grievances to higher authorities are typical examples. We often resort to procedural rules when we run out of substantive rules and when authority rules are incomplete or inconclusive. For example, if substantive or authority rules are inadequate to determine which patients should receive scarce medical resources, we resort to procedural rules such as queuing and lottery.[21] (See pp. 277–78 in Chapter 7.)

Virtues, Emotions, and Other Moral Considerations

This framework of principles and rules does not mention character and virtues, moral ideals, or moral emotions. Yet they are as important as principles and rules for a comprehensive vision of the moral life. These aspects of the moral life receive attention in Chapters 2, 9, and 10.

CONFLICTING MORAL NORMS

Norms as Prima Facie Binding

Principles, rules, obligations, and rights are not wooden standards that disallow compromise. Although "a person of principle" is sometimes regarded as strict and unyielding, we must specify principles so they can function in particular circumstances, and we must often weigh them against other moral norms. It is no objection to moral norms that, in some circumstances, they can be justifiably overridden by other moral norms with which they conflict. All general moral norms are justifiably overridden in some circumstances. For example, we might justifiably not tell the truth to prevent someone from killing another person; and we might justifiably disclose confidential information about a person to protect the rights of another person. Principles, duties, and rights are not absolute merely because they are universal.

W. D. Ross's distinction between *prima facie* and *actual* obligations informs our analysis. A *prima facie* obligation is one that must be fulfilled unless it conflicts, on a particular occasion, with an equal or stronger obligation. This type of obligation is always binding *unless* a competing moral obligation outweighs it in a particular circumstance. Some acts are at once prima facie wrong and prima facie right, because two or more norms conflict in the circumstances. Agents must then determine what they ought to do by finding an actual or overriding (in contrast to prima facie) obligation. That is, they must locate what Ross called "the greatest balance" of right over wrong. Agents can determine their *actual* obligations in such situations by examining the respective weights of the competing prima facie obligations (the relative weights of all competing prima facie norms). What agents ought to do is, in the end, determined by what they ought to do all things considered.[22]

For example, imagine that a psychiatrist has confidential medical information about a patient who also happens to be an employee in the hospital where the psychiatrist practices. The employee is seeking advancement in a stress-filled position, but the psychiatrist has good reason to believe that this advancement would be devastating for both the employee and the hospital. The psychiatrist has several duties in these circumstances, including those of confidentiality, nonmaleficence, beneficence, and respect for autonomy. Should the psychiatrist break confidence in this circumstance to meet these other duties? Could the psychiatrist make "confidential" disclosures to a hospital administrator and not to the personnel office? Addressing such questions through a process of moral deliberation and justification is required to establish an agent's actual duty in the face of conflicting prima facie duties.

No moral theory or professional code of ethics has successfully presented a system of moral rules free of conflicts and exceptions, but this fact should not generate either skepticism or alarm. Ross's distinction between prima facie and actual obligations conforms closely to our experience as moral agents and provides indispensable categories for biomedical ethics. Almost daily we confront situations that force us to choose among conflicting values in our personal lives. Some choices are moral, and many are nonmoral. For example, a person's financial situation might require that he or she choose between buying books and buying a train ticket to see friends. Not having the books will be an

inconvenience and a loss, and not visiting home will leave the friends disap-
pointed. Such a choice is not easy, but we are usually able to think through the
alternatives, deliberate, and reach a conclusion. The moral life presents similar
problems of choice.

Moral Regret and Residual Obligation

An agent who is able to determine which act is the best act to perform under
circumstances of a conflict of obligations may still not discharge all aspects of
moral obligation by performing the selected act. Even the morally best action
under many circumstances of conflict is regrettable and will leave a moral residue, which is also referred to as a "moral trace."[23] Regret and residue can arise
even if the right choice of action is clear and uncontested.

This point is about *continuing obligation,* not merely about *feelings* of regret
and residue. Moral residue results because an overridden prima facie obligation does not simply go away when overridden. Often persons have residual
obligations because the obligations they were unable to discharge create new
obligations. As Ross puts it in the case of breaking a promise, we feel not only
"compunction" (here meaning deep regret and a sting of conscience) but realize
that "it is our duty to make up somehow to the promisee for the breaking of the
promise."[24] We both feel regret and recognize continuing obligation. Although
we cannot keep an obligation that we failed to perform, we can make up for it
in a variety of ways, depending on the circumstance. For example, we may be
able to notify persons in advance that we will not be able to keep a promise; we
may be able to apologize in a manner that heals a relationship; we may be able
to create a change of circumstance so that the conflict does not occur again; or
we may be able to provide adequate compensation.

Regret and a sense of moral residue may exist whether or not residual obligations can be discharged. They are the natural result of the fact that an over-
ruled prima facie obligation does not mean that the obligation winds up counting
for nothing.

Specifying Principles and Rules

The four clusters of principles we present in this book do not constitute a general
ethical theory and provide only a framework of norms with which we can start in
biomedical ethics. Our framework is spare, because prima facie principles do not
contain sufficient content to address the nuances of moral problems. However,
the principles can be specified to provide more specific guidance. The reason
why directives in particular moralities often differ is that abstract starting points
in the common morality can be coherently specified in more than one way to
create practical guidelines and procedures.

Specification is a process of reducing the indeterminate character of abstract norms and generating more specific, action-guiding content.[25] For example, without further specification, "do no harm" is too bare a starting point for thinking through problems such as whether it is permissible to hasten the death of a terminally ill patient. Specification is not a process of producing or defending general norms such as those in the common morality; it assumes that they are available. Specifying the norms with which one starts (whether those in the common morality or norms previously specified to some extent) is accomplished by narrowing the scope of the norms, not by explaining what the general norms mean. The scope is narrowed, as Henry Richardson puts it, by "spelling out where, when, why, how, by what means, to whom, or by whom the action is to be done or avoided."[26] For example, the norm that we are obligated to "respect the autonomy of persons" cannot, unless specified, handle complicated problems of what to disclose or demand in clinical medicine and research involving human subjects. A definition of "respect for autonomy" (as, say, "allowing competent persons to exercise their liberty rights") might clarify one's meaning in using the norm, but would not narrow the general norm or render it more specific.

Specification, then, does not merely analyze meaning; it adds content. For example, as noted previously, one possible specification of "respect the autonomy of persons" is "respect the autonomy of competent patients by following their advance directives when they become incompetent." This specification will work well in some medical contexts, but it will confront limits in others, necessitating additional specification. Progressive specification can continue indefinitely, but to qualify all along the way as a specification some transparent connection must be maintained to the initial general norm that gives moral authority to the resulting string of specifications.

An example of specification arises when psychiatrists conduct forensic evaluations of patients in a legal context. Psychiatrists cannot always obtain an informed consent and risk violating their obligations to respect autonomy. However, obtaining informed consent is a vital rule of medical ethics. A specification aimed at handling this problem is "Respect the autonomy of persons who are the subjects of forensic evaluations, where consent is not legally required, by disclosing to the evaluee the nature and purpose of the evaluation." We do not claim that this formulation is the best specification, but it is roughly the provision recommended in the "Ethical Guidelines for the Practice of Forensic Psychiatry" of the American Academy of Psychiatry and the Law.[27] This specification attempts to guide forensic psychiatrists in discharging their diverse moral obligations.

A more extended example of specification involves the oft-cited rule "Doctors should put their patients' interests first." In some countries patients can receive the best treatment strategy only if their physicians falsify information on insurance forms or at least thinly spread the truth; yet the rule of patient priority does not imply that a physician should act illegally by lying or distorting the description of a patient's problem on an insurance form. Rules against deception, on the one hand, and for patient priority, on the other, are not categorical demands. When they conflict, they need specification.

A survey of practicing physicians' attitudes toward deception illustrates how some physicians reconcile their dual commitment to patients and to nondeception. Dennis H. Novack and several colleagues used a questionnaire to obtain physicians' responses to four difficult ethical problems that potentially could be resolved by deception. In one scenario, a physician recommends an annual screening mammography for a fifty-two-year-old woman who protests that last year her insurance company would not cover the test and that she had to pay herself, although she could not afford it. A secretary suggests that the patient's insurance company would cover the costs of the mammography if the physician stated the reason as "rule out cancer" rather than "screening mammography," although the latter alone was the true reason. Almost 70% of the physicians responding to this survey indicated that they would state that they were attempting to "rule out cancer," and 85% of this group (85% of the 70%) insisted that their act would not involve "deception."[28]

We can interpret these physicians' decisions as crude attempts to specify the rule that "Doctors should put their patients' interests first." Some doctors seem to think that it should be specified as follows: "Doctors should put their patients' interests first by withholding information from or misleading someone who has no *right* to that information, including an insurance company with unjust policies of coverage, who thereby forfeits his or her right to accurate information." In addition, most physicians in the study apparently did not operate with the definition of deception favored by the researchers, which is "to deceive is to make another believe what is not true, to mislead." Some physicians apparently believed that "deception" occurs when one person *unjustifiably* misleads another, and that it was *justifiable* to mislead the insurance company in these circumstances. It appears that these physicians would not agree on how to specify rules against deception or rules assigning priority to patients' interests.

All moral rules are, in principle, subject to specification. They all will need some additional content, because, as Richardson puts it, "the complexity of the moral phenomena always outruns our ability to capture them in general norms."[29] Many already specified rules will need further specification to handle new circumstances of conflict. Progressive specification often must occur to handle the variety of problems that arise, gradually reducing the conflicts that abstract principles themselves cannot resolve.

These conclusions are connected to our earlier discussion of *particular moralities*. Different persons and groups will offer conflicting specifications, potentially creating multiple particular moralities. In any problematic case, competing specifications are likely to be offered by reasonable and fair-minded parties, all of whom are committed to the common morality. Nothing in the model of specification suggests that we can avoid all circumstances of conflicting judgments.

To say that a problem or conflict is resolved or dissolved by specification is to say that norms have been made sufficiently determinate in content that, when cases fall under them, we know what ought to be done. Obviously some *proposed* specifications will not provide the most adequate or justified resolution. When competing specifications emerge, we should seek to discover which is superior. Proposed specifications should be based on deliberative processes of reasoning. The specification best supported by argument would seem the one that ought to prevail. In Chapter 10, we argue that we also need to link specification to a method of justification that allows for a reflective testing of our moral principles and other relevant moral beliefs to make them as coherent as possible. The goal is to adjust specifications, as needed, to render them coherent with the premises of other justified moral commitments. If proposed specifications are shown to have incoherent results, we must continue to readjust the guides further. (See Chapter 10, pp. 381–87.) In this way, we connect specification as a method with a model of justification that will support some specifications and not others.

Finally, some specified norms are virtually absolute and need no further specification. Examples include prohibitions of cruelty that involve the unnecessary infliction of pain and suffering.[30] More interesting are norms that are intentionally formulated with the goal of including all legitimate exceptions. An example is, "Always obtain oral or written informed consent for medical interventions with competent patients, *except* in emergencies, in forensic examinations, in low-risk situations, or when patients have waived their right to adequate information." This norm needs further interpretation, including an analysis of what constitutes an informed consent, an emergency, a waiver, a forensic examination, and a low risk. However, this rule would be absolute if it were correct that all legitimate exceptions had successfully been incorporated in its formulation.

If such rules exist, they are rare. In light of the range of possibilities for contingent conflicts among rules, even the firmest rules are likely to encounter exceptive cases. If professional medical associations, health care institutions, religious groups, and government bureaus had more often taken this lesson to heart, we would have been spared many stubbornly imperious pronouncements in biomedical ethics.

Weighing and Balancing

The process of weighing and balancing. Principles, rules, professional obligations, and rights often need to be balanced. Is balancing different from specification? Each conception seems to address a separate dimension of moral norms.

Balancing is the process of finding reasons to support beliefs about which moral norms should prevail. Balancing is concerned with the relative weights and strengths of different moral norms, whereas specification is concerned primarily with their scope (i.e., range). Accordingly, balancing consists of deliberation and judgment about the relative weights or strengths of norms. At first glance, balancing seems best suited for reaching judgments in particular cases, whereas specification seems especially useful for developing more specific policies from already accepted general norms. But are the two conceptions really different?

The metaphor of larger and smaller weights moving a scale up and down has often been invoked to depict the balancing process, but this metaphor may obscure what happens in balancing. Justified acts of balancing can be supported by good reasons. They need not rest merely on intuition or feeling (although intuitive balancing is one form of balancing). Suppose a physician encounters an emergency case that would require her to extend an already long day, making her unable to keep a promise to take her son to the local library. She then engages in a process of deliberation that leads her to consider how urgently her son needs to get to the library, whether they could go later to the library, whether another physician could handle the emergency case, and so on. If she determines to stay deep into the night with the patient, this obligation will have become overriding because, let us assume, she has found a good and sufficient reason for her action. The reason might be that a life hangs in the balance and she alone may have the knowledge to deal adequately with the circumstances. Canceling her evening with her son, distressing as it may be, could be justified by the significance of her reason for doing what she does.

One way of viewing the process of balancing merges it with specification. David DeGrazia and Henry Richardson have argued that the reasons offered in balancing are simply specifications that incorporate those reasons. In our example, the physician's reasons can be generalized for similar cases: "If a patient's life hangs in the balance and the attending physician alone has the knowledge to deal adequately with the full array of the circumstances, then the physician's conflicting domestic obligations must yield." Even if we do not always state the way we balance considerations in the form of a specification, might not all deliberative judgments conform to this model? If so, then deliberative balancing *is* deliberative specification.

The goal of merging specification and balancing is appealing, but it is too streamlined to handle all situations of balancing. Specification requires that a moral agent extend norms by both narrowing their scope and generalizing to relevantly similar circumstances. Thus, "respect the autonomy of competent patients when they become incompetent by following their advance directives" is a rule suited for all incompetent patients with advance directives. However, it often seems that the responses of caring moral agents, such as physicians and nurses, are specific to the needs of *this* patient or *this* family in *this* circumstance.

Numerous considerations must be weighed and balanced and any generalizations that could be formed might not hold even in related cases. For example, cases in which risk of harm and burden are involved for a patient are often circumstances unlikely to be decided by expressing *by rule* how much risk is allowable or how heavy the burden can be to secure a certain stated benefit. After levels of risk and burden are determined, these considerations must be balanced with the likelihood of the success of a procedure (in this specific case), the uncertainties involved, whether an adequately informed consent can be obtained, whether the family has a role to play, and the like. In this way, balancing allows for a due consideration of all norms bearing on a complex, very particular circumstance.

Consider the following discussion with a young woman who has just been told that she is HIV-infected, as recorded by physician Timothy Quill and nurse Penelope Townsend:[31]

> PATIENT: Please don't tell me that. Oh my God. Oh my children. Oh Lord have mercy. Oh God, why did He do this to me? . . .
> DR. QUILL: First thing we have to do is learn as much as we can about it, because right now you are okay.
> PATIENT: I don't even have a future. Everything I know is that you gonna die anytime. What is there to do? What if I'm a walking time bomb? People will be scared to even touch me or say anything to me.
> DR. QUILL: No, that's not so.
> PATIENT: Yes they will, 'cause I feel that way . . .
> DR. QUILL: There is a future for you . . .
> PATIENT. Okay, alright. I'm so scared. I don't want to die. I don't want to die, Dr. Quill, not yet. I know I got to die, but I don't want to die.
> DR. QUILL: We've got to think about a couple of things.

Quill and Townsend work to calm down and reassure this patient, while engaging sympathetically with the patient's feelings and conveying the presence of knowledgeable medical authorities. Their emotional investment in the patient's feelings is joined with a detached evaluation of the patient. Too much compassion and emotional investment may doom the task at hand; too much detachment will be cold and may destroy the patient's trust. A balance in the sense of a right mixture between engagement and detachment must be found. Quill and Townsend could try to *generalize* from norms of respect and beneficence to a specification regarding how caring physicians and nurses should respond to patients who are desperately upset. However, any such generalization will ring hollow and will not be subtle enough to provide practical guidance for this patient, and certainly not for all desperately upset patients. Each encounter calls for a response not adequately captured by general rules and their specifications. Behavior that in the context of one desperate patient is a caring response will intrude on privacy or irritate the next desperate patient. A physician may, for example, find it appropriate to touch or caress a patient in a circumstance in which such behavior would be entirely inappropriate for another patient. How physicians and nurses balance different moral considerations often involves sympathetic insight, humane responsiveness, and the practical wisdom of evaluating a particular patient's circumstance and needs.[32] Balancing is more complex than the simple case of balancing two principles that are in conflict. Considerations of trust, compassion, objective assessment, caring responsiveness, reassurance, and the like must be balanced. For example, to act compassionately may be to undercut objective assessment. Not all of the norms at work can reasonably be said to be specifications, nor is there a final specification.

In many clinical contexts it may be impossibly complicated to engage in specification. For example, in cases of balancing harms of treatment against the benefits of treatment for incompetent patients, the cases are often so exceptional that it is perilous to generalize a conclusion that would reach out to other cases. These problems are sometimes complicated by disagreements among family members about what constitutes a benefit, poor decisions and indecision by a marginally competent patient, limitations of time and resources, and the like.

We do not suggest that balancing is a matter of on-the-fly, unreflective intuition without reasons. Instead, we propose a model of moral judgment that focuses on how balancing and judgment occur through practical astuteness, discriminating intelligence, and sympathetic responsiveness that are not reducible to the specification of norms. The capacity to balance many moral considerations is connected to what we discuss in Chapter 2 as capacities of moral character. Capacities such as compassion, attentiveness, discernment, caring, and kindness are integral to the way wise moral agents balance diverse, sometimes competing, moral considerations. These capacities tutor us in "what to notice, how to care, what to be sensitive to, how to get beyond one's own biases and narrowness of vision," and the like.[33]

Practicability supplies another reason why the model of specification needs supplementation by the model of balancing. Progressive specification would eventually mushroom into a body of norms so bulky that the normative system would become unwieldy. A scheme of comprehensive specification would constitute a package of potentially hundreds, thousands, or millions of rules, each suited to a narrow range of conduct. In the ideal of specification, every type of action in a circumstance of the contingent conflict of norms would be covered by a rule, but the formulation of rules for every circumstance of contingent conflict would be a body of rules so cumbersome as to become ineffective. The larger the number of rules and the more complex each rule, the less likely it becomes that the system will be achievable, and practicable were it achievable. Moreover, every rule is subject at any time to challenge if a contingent conflict arises or in the face of a newly detected problem of lack of coherence in the rules.

Conditions that constrain balancing. To allay concerns that the model of balancing is too intuitive or too open-ended and lacking in a commitment to firm principles and rigorous reasoning, we here list six conditions that should help reduce intuition, partiality, and arbitrariness. These conditions must be met to justify infringing one prima facie norm to adhere to another. (To the extent these conditions incorporate norms, the norms are prima facie, not absolute.)

1. Good reasons can be offered to act on the overriding norm rather than on the infringed norm.
2. The moral objective justifying the infringement has a realistic prospect of achievement.
3. No morally preferable alternative actions are available.[34]
4. The lowest level of infringement, commensurate with achieving the primary goal of the action, has been selected.
5. Any negative effects of the infringement have been minimized.
6. All affected parties have been treated impartially.

Although some of these conditions are obvious and noncontroversial, some are often not observed in moral deliberation and would lead to different conclusions were they observed. For example, some proposals to use life-extending technologies, despite the objections of patients or their surrogates, violate condition 2 by endorsing actions in which no realistic prospect exists of achieving the goals of a proposed intervention. Typically, this occurs when health professionals regard the intervention as legally required, but in some cases the standard invoked is merely a traditional or prevailing one.

More commonly violated is condition 3. Actions are frequently performed without serious consideration of alternative actions that might be performed. As a result, agents fail to identify a morally preferable alternative. For example, in animal care and use committees a common conflict involves the obligation to approve a good scientific protocol and the obligation to protect animals against unnecessary suffering. A protocol is often approved if it proposes a *standard* form of anesthesia. However, standard forms of anesthesia are not always the best way to protect the animal, and further inquiry would be required to determine the best anesthetic for the particular interventions proposed. In our schema of conditions, it is unjustifiable to approve the protocol or to conduct the experiment without this additional inquiry, which affects conditions 4 and 5 as well as 3.

Finally, consider this example: The principle of respect for autonomy and the principle of beneficence (which requires acts intended to prevent harm to others) sometimes conflict in responding to the HIV/AIDS epidemic. Respect for autonomy sets a prima facie barrier to invasions of privacy and the mandatory testing of people at risk of HIV infection, yet their actions may put others at risk under conditions in which society has a prima facie obligation to act to prevent harm to those at risk. To justify overriding respect for autonomy, one must show that mandatory testing that invades the privacy of certain individuals is necessary to prevent harm to others and has a reasonable prospect of preventing such harm. If it meets these conditions, mandatory testing still must pass the least-infringement test (condition 4), and health workers must seek to reduce negative effects, such as the consequences that individuals fear from testing (condition 5). As we will see in Chapter 8, many proposed forms of mandatory testing and invasions of privacy are not justified because other available alternatives would have a higher probability of success without infringing rights of autonomy.[35]

Accordingly, the preceding six conditions are morally demanding, at least in some circumstances. When conjoined with requirements of coherence that we propose in Chapter 10, these conditions should help us achieve a reasonable measure of protection against purely intuitive, subjective, or partial balancing judgments. We could try to introduce further criteria or safeguards, such as "rights override nonrights" and "liberty principles override nonliberty principles," but these rules are certain to fail in circumstances in which rights claims and liberty interests are relatively minor. Honesty about the process of balancing, as well as the process of specification, compels us to return to our earlier discussion of moral dilemmas and perplexity and to acknowledge that in some circumstances we will not be able to determine which moral norm to follow.

Moral Diversity and Moral Disagreement

Conscientious and reasonable moral agents understandably disagree over moral priorities in circumstances of a contingent conflict of norms. Morally conscientious persons may disagree, for example, about whether disclosure of a life-threatening condition to a fragile patient is appropriate, whether religious values about brain death have a place in secular biomedical ethics, whether teenagers should be permitted to refuse life-sustaining treatments, and hundreds of other issues in biomedical ethics. Such disagreement does not indicate moral ignorance or moral defect. We simply lack a single, entirely reliable way to resolve many disagreements, despite methods of specifying and balancing.

Neither morality nor ethical theory has the resources to provide a single solution to every moral problem. Moral disagreement can emerge because of (1) factual disagreements (e.g., about the level of suffering that an action will cause), (2) disagreement resulting from insufficient information or evidence, (3) disagreements about which norms are applicable or relevant in the circumstances, (4) disagreement about the relative weights or rankings of the relevant norms, (5) disagreements about appropriate forms of specification or balancing, (6) the presence of a genuine moral dilemma, and (7) scope disagreements about who should be protected by a moral norm (e.g., whether embryos, fetuses, and sentient animals are protected; see Chapter 3); or (8) conceptual disagreements about a crucial moral notion (such as whether removal of nutrition and hydration at a family's request constitutes *killing*).

Different parties may emphasize different principles or assign different weights to principles even when they agree on which principles are relevant. Such disagreement may persist even among morally committed persons who conform to all the demands that morality makes on them. If evidence is incomplete and different sets of evidence are available to different parties, one individual or group may be justified in reaching a conclusion that another individual or group is justified in rejecting. Even when both parties have incorrect beliefs, each party may be justified in holding its beliefs. We cannot hold persons to a higher practical standard than to make judgments conscientiously in light of the relevant norms and relevant evidence. (See our account of justification in Chapter 10, where we argue that we cannot know whether a moral disagreement is irresolvable until we have examined competing views using an appropriate method of justification.)

Disagreement in the moral life may discourage persons who deal with practical problems, but the phenomenon of moral disagreement provides no basis for skepticism about morality or about moral thinking. It offers a reason for taking morality seriously and using the best tools we have to carry our moral projects as far as we can. We frequently do obtain near-complete agreement in our moral judgments, and we always have available the thin set of four clusters of universal principles mentioned earlier in this chapter.

When moral disagreements arise, a moral agent can—and often should—defend his or her decision without disparaging or reproaching others who reach different decisions. Recognition of *legitimate* diversity (by contrast to moral violations that warrant criticism and perhaps even punishment) is vital when we evaluate the actions of others. One person's conscientious assessment of his or her obligations may differ from another's, even when they confront the same moral problem. Both evaluations may be solidly grounded in the common morality. Similarly, what one institution or government determines it should do may differ from what another institution or government determines it should do. In such cases, we can assess one position as morally preferable to another only if we can show that the position rests on a more coherent specification or interpretation of the common morality.[36]

CONCLUSION

In this chapter we have explained and initiated a defense of what is sometimes called the *four-principles approach* to biomedical ethics,[37] now increasingly called *principlism*.[38] The four clusters of principles derive from considered judgments in the common morality and professional traditions in health care, particularly medicine and nursing, although we have been critical of certain aspects of medical codes and traditional medical ethics. Our goal in later chapters is to develop, specify, and balance these principles.

NOTES

1. See Albert R. Jonsen, *The Birth of Bioethics* (New York: Oxford University Press, 1998), pp. 3ff; Jonsen, *A Short History of Medical Ethics* (New York: Oxford University Press, 2000); Edmund D. Pellegrino and David C. Thomasma, *The Virtues in Medical Practice* (New York: Oxford University Press, 1993), pp. 184–89.

2. These distinctions should be used with caution. Metaethics frequently takes a turn toward the normative, as our discussion of the justification of moral standards later in this chapter indicates. Likewise, normative ethics relies on metaethics. Just as no sharp distinction should be drawn between practical ethics and general normative ethics, so no clear line should be drawn to distinguish normative ethics and metaethics.

3. Although there is only one universal common morality, there is more than one theory of the common morality. For a diverse set of theories of the common morality, see Alan Donagan, *The Theory of Morality* (Chicago: University of Chicago Press, 1977); Bernard Gert, *Common Morality: Deciding What to Do* (New York: Oxford University Press, 2007); Bernard Gert, Charles M. Culver, and K. Danner Clouser, *Bioethics: A Return to Fundamentals* (New York: Oxford University Press, 1997); W. D. Ross, *The Foundations of Ethics* (Oxford: Oxford University Press, 1939); and the special issue of the *Kennedy Institute of Ethics Journal* 13 (2003), especially the introductory article by Robert Veatch, pp. 189–92.

4. Compare the thesis of Martha Nussbaum that, in an Aristotelian philosophy, certain "non-relative virtues" are objective and universal. "Non-Relative Virtues: An Aristotelian Approach," in Peter French et al., eds., *Ethical Theory, Character, and Virtue* (Notre Dame, IN: University of Notre Dame Press, 1988), pp. 32–53, especially pp. 33–34, 46–50.

5. This charge is mistakenly directed at us by Leigh Turner, "Zones of Consensus and Zones of Conflict: Questioning the 'Common Morality' Presumption in Bioethics," *Kennedy Institute of Ethics Journal* 13 (2003): 193–218; and Turner, "An Anthropological Exploration of Contemporary Bioethics: The Varieties of Common Sense," *Journal of Medical Ethics* 24 (1998): 127–33.

6. At least in all cultures in which there is the requisite core of morally committed persons.

7. See Turner, "Zones of Consensus and Zones of Conflict"; Donald C. Ainslee, "Bioethics and the Problem of Pluralism," *Social Philosophy and Policy* 19 (2002): 1–28; David DeGrazia, "Common Morality, Coherence, and the Principles of Biomedical Ethics," *Kennedy Institute of Ethics Journal* 13 (2003): 219–30.

8. See Richard B. Brandt, "Morality and Its Critics," in his *Morality, Utilitarianism, and Rights* (Cambridge: Cambridge University Press, 1992), chap. 5.

9. Talcott Parsons, *Essays in Sociological Theory,* rev. ed. (Glencoe, IL: The Free Press, 1954), p. 372.

10. The American Medical Association Code of Ethics of 1847 was largely adapted from Thomas Percival's *Medical Ethics; or a Code of Institutes and Precepts, Adapted to the Professional Conduct of Physicians and Surgeons* (Manchester, England: S. Russell, 1803). See Donald E. Konold, *A History of American Medical Ethics 1847–1912* (Madison, WI: State Historical Society of Wisconsin, 1962), chaps. 1–3; and Chester Burns, "Reciprocity in the Development of Anglo-American Medical Ethics," in *Legacies in Medical Ethics,* ed. Burns (New York: Science History Publications, 1977).

11. Cf. the conclusions reached about medicine today in N. D. Berkman, M. K. Wynia, and L. R. Churchill, "Gaps, Conflicts, and Consensus in the Ethics Statements of Professional Associations, Medical Groups, and Health Plans," *Journal of Medical Ethics* 30 (2004): 395–401; Robert D. Orr et al., "Use of the Hippocratic Oath: A Review of Twentieth Century Practice and a Content Analysis of Oaths Administered in Medical Schools in the U.S. and Canada in 1993," *Journal of Clinical Ethics* 8 (1997): 377–88; A. C. Kao and K. P. Parsi, "Content Analyses of Oaths Administered at U.S. Medical Schools in

2000," *Academic Medicine* 79 (2004): 882–87; E. Dickstein, J. Erlen, and J. A. Erlen, "Ethical Principles Contained in Currently Professed Medical Oaths," *Academic Medicine* 66 (1991): 622–24.

12. Jay Katz, ed., *Experimentation with Human Beings* (New York: Russell Sage Foundation, 1972), pp. ix–x.

13. Omnibus Budget Reconciliation Act of 1990. Public Law 101–508 (Nov. 5, 1990), §§ 4206, 4751. See 42 USC, scattered sections.

14. See Will Kymlicka, "Moral Philosophy and Public Policy: The Case of New Reproductive Technologies," in *Philosophical Perspectives on Bioethics,* ed. L. W. Sumner and Joseph Boyle (Toronto: University of Toronto Press, 1996); Dennis Thompson, "Philosophy and Policy," *Philosophy and Public Affairs* 14 (Spring 1985): 205–18; and a symposium on "The Role of Philosophers in the Public Policy Process: A View from the President's Commission," with essays by Alan Weisbard and Dan Brock, in *Ethics* 97 (July 1987): 775–95.

15. *Tarasoff v. Regents of the University of California,* 17 Cal. 3d 425, 551 P.2d 334, 131 Cal. Rptr. 14 (Cal. 1976).

16. See John Lemmon, "Moral Dilemmas," *Philosophical Review* 71 (1962): 139–58; Daniel Statman, "Hard Cases and Moral Dilemmas," *Law and Philosophy* 15 (1996): 117–48; H. E. Mason, "Responsibilities and Principles: Reflections on the Sources of Moral Dilemmas," in *Moral Dilemmas and Moral Theory,* ed. H. E. Mason (New York: Oxford University Press, 1996).

17. William R. Bascom, *African Dilemma Tales* (The Hague, Netherlands: Mouton, 1975), p. 145 (relying on anthropological research by Roland Fletcher).

18. See Christopher W. Gowans, ed., *Moral Dilemmas* (New York: Oxford University Press, 1987); Walter Sinnott-Armstrong, *Moral Dilemmas* (Oxford: Basil Blackwell, 1988); and Edmund N. Santurri, *Perplexity in the Moral Life: Philosophical and Theological Considerations* (Charlottesville, VA: University Press of Virginia, 1987).

19. Some writers in biomedical ethics express reservations about these principles. See numerous essays in *Principles of Health Care Ethics,* ed. Raanan Gillon and Ann Lloyd (London: Wiley, 1994); *Principles of Health Care Ethics,* 2nd ed., ed. Richard E. Ashcroft et al. (Chichester, England: Wiley, 2007); K. Danner Clouser and Bernard Gert, "A Critique of Principlism," *The Journal of Medicine and Philosophy* 15 (April 1990): 219–36; K. Danner Clouser, "Common Morality as an Alternative to Principlism," *Kennedy Institute of Ethics Journal* 5 (1995): 219–36; and Peter Herissone-Kelly, "The Principlist Approach to Bioethics, and Its Stormy Journey Overseas," in *Scratching the Surface of Bioethics,* ed. Matti Hayry and Tuija Takala (Amsterdam: Rodopi, 2003), pp. 65–77.

20. Thomas Percival, *Medical Ethics.* See note 10 earlier.

21. These rules might also be interpreted as grounded in substantive rules of equality. If so interpreted, the procedural rules could be said to have a justification in substantive rules.

22. W. D. Ross, *The Right and the Good* (Oxford: Clarendon, 1930), esp. pp. 19–36, 88; and *The Foundations of Ethics* (Oxford: Clarendon, 1939).

23. See Robert Nozick, "Moral Complications and Moral Structures," *Natural Law Forum* 13 (1968): 1–50; James J. Brummer, "Ross and the Ambiguity of Prima Facie Duty," *History of Philosophy Quarterly* 19 (2002): 401–22; and Thomas E. Hill, Jr., "Moral Dilemmas, Gaps, and Residues: A Kantian Perspective"; Walter Sinnott-Armstrong, "Moral Dilemmas and Rights"; and Terrance C. McConnell, "Moral Residue and Dilemmas"—all in *Moral Dilemmas and Moral Theory,* ed. Mason.

24. Ross, *The Right and the Good,* p. 28.

25. Henry S. Richardson, "Specifying Norms as a Way to Resolve Concrete Ethical Problems," *Philosophy and Public Affairs* 19 (Fall 1990): 279–310; and "Specifying, Balancing, and Interpreting Bioethical Principles," *Journal of Medicine and Philosophy* 25 (2000): 285–307, as in *Belmont Revisited: Ethical Principles for Research with Human Subjects,* ed. James F. Childress, Eric M. Meslin, and Harold T. Shapiro (Washington, D.C.: Georgetown University Press, 2005), pp. 205–27. See also David DeGrazia, "Moving Forward in Bioethical Theory: Theories, Cases, and Specified Principlism," *Journal of Medicine and Philosophy* 17 (1992): 511–39; and DeGrazia and Tom L. Beauchamp, "Philosophical Foundations and Philosophical Methods," in *Methods of Bioethics,* ed. D. Sulmasy and J. Sugarman (Washington, D.C.: Georgetown University Press, 2000), pp. 31–46.

26. Richardson, "Specifying, Balancing, and Interpreting Bioethical Principles," p. 289.

27. As revised October, 1991, p. 2: "The informed consent of the subject of a forensic evaluation is obtained when possible. Where consent is not required, notice is given to the evaluee of the nature of the evaluation. If the evaluee is not competent to give consent, substituted consent is obtained in accordance with the laws of the jurisdiction."

28. Dennis H. Novack et al., "Physicians' Attitudes Toward Using Deception to Resolve Difficult Ethical Problems," *Journal of the American Medical Association* 261 (May 26, 1989): 2980–85. We return to these problems in Chapter 8.

29. Richardson, "Specifying Norms," p. 294. "Always" in this formulation should be understood to mean "in principle always." Specification may, in some cases, reach a final form.

30. Other prohibitions, such as rules against murder, are absolute only because of the meaning of their terms. For example, to say "murder is categorically wrong" is to say "unjustified killing is unjustified."

31. Timothy Quill and Penelope Townsend, "Bad News: Delivery, Dialogue, and Dilemmas," *Archives of Internal Medicine* 151 (March 1991): 463–64.

32. See Alisa Carse, "Impartial Principle and Moral Context: Securing a Place for the Particular in Ethical Theory," *Journal of Medicine and Philosophy* 23 (1998): 153–69. For a defense of balancing as the best method in such situations, see Joseph P. DeMarco and Paul J. Ford, "Balancing in Ethical Deliberations: Superior to Specification and Casuistry," *Journal of Medicine and Philosophy* 31 (2006): 483–97, esp. 491–93.

33. Lawrence Blum, *Moral Perception and Particularity* (New York: Cambridge, 1994), p. 204.

34. This condition is redundant if condition 3 cannot be violated when all of the other conditions are satisfied; but we think it is best to be clear on this point, even if redundant.

35. See James F. Childress, "Mandatory HIV Screening and Testing," in *Practical Reasoning in Bioethics* (Bloomington and Indianapolis, IN: Indiana University Press, 1997), chap. 6.

36. Cf. Sinnott-Armstrong, *Moral Dilemmas,* pp. 216–27; and D. D. Raphael, *Moral Philosophy* (Oxford: Oxford University Press, 1981), pp. 64–65.

37. See essays in Gillon and Lloyd, eds. *Principles of Health Care Ethics.*

38. See B. Gert, C. M. Culver, and K. D. Clouser, *Bioethics: A Return to Fundamentals* (New York: Oxford University Press, 1997), chap. 4; Clouser and Gert, "A Critique of Principlism," pp. 219–36; John H. Evans, "A Sociological Account of the Growth of Principlism," *Hastings Center Report* 30 (Sept.–Oct. 2000): 31–38; Earl Winkler, "Moral Philosophy and Bioethics: Contextualism versus the Paradigm Theory," in *Philosophical Perspectives on Bioethics,* ed. L. W. Sumner and J. Boyle; John D. Arras, "Principles and Particularity: The Roles of Cases in Bioethics," *Indiana Law Journal* 69 (1994): 983–1014; Jeffrey Blustein, "Character-Principlism and the Particularity Objection,"

Metaphilosophy 28 (1997): 135–55; Richard B. Davis, "The Principlism Debate: A Critical Overview," *Journal of Medicine and Philosophy* 20 (1995): 85–105; Ana Smith Iltis, "Bioethics as Methodological Case Resolution: Specification, Specified Principlism, and Casuistry," *Journal of Medicine and Philosophy* 25 (2000): 271–84; and Carson Strong, "Specified Principlism," *Journal of Medicine and Philosophy* 25 (2000): 285–307.

2
Moral Character

In Chapter 1 we concentrated on moral norms in the form of principles, rules, obligations, and rights. In this chapter, we concentrate on *moral virtues, moral character, moral ideals*, and *moral excellence*. These categories complement the analysis in the previous chapter without undermining principles, rules, obligations, and rights. Whereas moral norms principally govern right action, character ethics or virtue ethics emphasizes the agent who performs actions.[1]

What often counts most in the moral life is not adherence to moral rules, but reliable character, good moral sense, and emotional responsiveness. Even specified principles and rules do not convey what occurs when parents lovingly play with and nurture their children or when physicians and nurses exhibit compassion, patience, and responsiveness in encounters with patients and families. Our feelings and concerns for others lead us to actions that cannot be reduced to instances of rule-following, and most people appreciate that morality would be a cold and uninspiring practice without appropriate sympathy, emotional responsiveness, and heartfelt ideals that reach beyond principles and rules.

MORAL VIRTUES

Some philosophers have questioned the place of virtues in moral theory. They see virtues as less central than actions and as difficult to unify in a systematic theory, in part because there are many largely independent virtues to be considered.[2] Although it is clear that principles and virtues are different and taught differently, virtues should not be regarded as less important. To the contrary, the goals and structure of medicine, health care, and research call for a deep appreciation of virtues.[3] We begin an argument to these conclusions by analyzing the concept of virtue and by considering the special status of virtues. We then examine virtues in professional roles, treat care (or caring) as a primary virtue in health care, and explicate five other focal virtues in both health care and research. We close by considering how moral virtues are related to action guides, both through principles corresponding to particular virtues and through examining what a virtuous agent would do.

The Concept of Virtue

A *virtue* is a trait of character that is socially valuable,[4] and a *moral virtue* is a trait of character that is morally valuable. It is not sufficient to qualify as a moral virtue that social groups approve a trait and regard it as moral. Some communities disvalue persons who are virtuous, and some communities admire persons for their vices, such as meanness and churlishness. Moral virtue, then, is more than a trait that is socially approved.

Some define moral virtue as a disposition to act or a habit of acting in accordance with moral principles, obligations, or ideals.[5] For example, they understand the moral virtue of nonmalevolence as the trait a person has of abstaining from causing harm to others when it would be wrong to harm them. However, this definition unjustifiably renders virtues wholly dependent on principles and also fails to capture the importance of moral motives. We care morally about people's motives, and we care especially about their *characteristic* motives; that is, the motivational structures deeply embedded in their character. Persons who are motivated through sympathy and personal affection, for example, meet our moral approval, whereas others who act in the identical way, but from motives of personal ambition, generally do not.

Imagine a person who discharges a moral obligation *because* it is an obligation, but who intensely dislikes being placed in a position in which the interests of others override his or her own interests. This person does not feel friendly toward or cherish others, and he or she respects their wishes only because obligation requires it. This person nonetheless performs morally right actions and has a disposition to perform right actions. But if the motive is improper, a critical moral ingredient is missing; and if a person *characteristically* lacks this motivational structure, a necessary condition of virtuous character is absent. The act may be right and the actor blameless, but neither the person nor the act is *virtuous*. In short, people may be disposed to do what is right, intend to do it, and do it, while simultaneously yearning to avoid doing it. Persons who characteristically perform morally right actions from this motivational structure are not morally virtuous even if they invariably perform the morally right action.

Aristotle drew an important (although underdeveloped) distinction between right action and proper motive, which he also analyzed in terms of the distinction between external performance and internal state. An action can be right without being virtuous, he maintained, but an action can be virtuous only if performed in the right state of mind. Both right action and right motive are present in a virtuous action: "The agent must...be in the right state when he does [the actions]. First, he must know [that he is performing virtuous actions]; second, he must decide on them, and decide on them for themselves; and third, he must also do them from a firm and unchanging state," including the right state of emotion and desire. "The just and temperate person is not the one who [merely] does these actions, but the one who also does them in the way in which just or temperate people do them."[6]

Aristotle is right. In addition to being properly motivated, a virtuous person will experience appropriate feelings, such as sympathy and regret, even when the feelings are not motives and no action results from the feelings. However, not all virtues have a clear link to either motives or feelings. Moral discernment and moral integrity, two virtues treated later in this chapter, are examples. Here psychological properties other than feelings are paramount, as we will see.[7]

The Special Status of the Virtues

Some writers on the subject of moral character maintain that the language of obligation is derivative from what they view as the basic moral language of virtue. They think that a person disposed by character to have good motives and desires provides the model of the moral person and that this model determines our expectations of persons, which are then expressed as obligations.[8] They regard this model as more important than a model of action done from obligation, on grounds that right motives and character tell us more about moral worth than do right actions performed under the goad of obligation.

This position is attractive. We are often more concerned about the character and motives of persons than about the conformity of their acts to rules. When a friend performs an act of "friendship," we expect it not to be motivated entirely from a sense of obligation to us, but because the person has a desire to be friendly, feels friendly, wants to keep friends, and values friendship. The friend who acts only from obligation lacks the virtue of friendliness, and in the absence of this virtue, the relationship lacks the moral quality of friendship.[9]

Some writers in biomedical ethics argue that the attempt in obligation-oriented theories to replace the virtuous judgments of health care professionals with rules, codes, or procedures will not produce better decisions and actions.[10] Rather than relying on institutional rules and government regulations to protect subjects in research, they claim that the most reliable protection is the presence of an "informed, conscientious, compassionate, responsible researcher."[11] From this perspective, character is more important than conformity to rules, and virtues should be inculcated and cultivated over time through educational interactions, role models, and the like.

This conclusion provides a compelling reason for incorporating the virtues into biomedical ethics and into medical and nursing education, but it needs both qualification and elaboration. A morally good person with the right configuration of desires and motives is more likely than others to understand what should be done, more likely to perform attentively the acts required, and even more likely to form and act on moral ideals. A person we trust is one who has an ingrained motivation and desire to perform right actions. Thus, the person we will recommend, admire, praise, and hold up as a moral model is the person disposed by character to be generous, caring, compassionate, sympathetic, fair, and the like.

A person's character frequently informs our assessment of his or her actions. If a virtuous person makes a mistake in judgment, leading to a morally wrong act, he or she would be less blameworthy than a habitual offender who performed the same act. In his chronicle of life under the Nazi SS in the Jewish ghetto in Cracow, Poland, Thomas Keneally describes a physician faced with a grave dilemma: either inject cyanide into four immobile patients or abandon them to the SS, who were at that moment emptying the ghetto and had already demonstrated that they would brutally torture and kill captives and patients. This physician, Keneally reports, "suffered painfully from a set of ethics as intimate to him as the organs of his own body."[12] Here is a person of the highest moral character and virtue, motivated to act rightly and even heroically, yet who at first had no idea what the morally right action was. Ultimately, with uncertainty and reluctance, the physician elected active euthanasia (using forty drops of hydrocyanic acid) without the consent or knowledge of the four doomed patients—an act almost universally denounced by the canons of professional medical ethics. Even if one thinks that the physician's act was wrong and blameworthy—a judgment we reject—no reasonable person would make a judgment of blame or demerit directed at the physician's motives or character. Having already risked death by choosing to remain at his patients' bedside in the hospital rather than take a prepared escape route, this physician is a moral hero who displayed an extraordinary moral character.

We have been arguing that judgments of agents' praiseworthiness and blameworthiness are directly tied to their motives, which are signs of character. Nonetheless, the merit of an action does not reside entirely in motive or character. The action must be gauged to bring about the desired results and must conform to relevant principles and rules. For example, the physician or nurse who is appropriately motivated to help a patient, but who acts incompetently in seeking the desired result, does not act in a praiseworthy or acceptable manner.

VIRTUES IN PROFESSIONAL ROLES

Although persons differ in the character traits they possess, all persons with normal moral capacities can cultivate the traits of importance to morality. In professional life, the traits that warrant encouragement and admiration often derive from role responsibilities. Accordingly, we begin with virtues that are critically important in professional and institutional roles and practices.

Virtues in Roles and Practices

Professional roles are usually tied to institutional expectations and standards of professional practice. Roles internalize conventions, customs, and procedures of teaching, nursing, doctoring, and the like. Professional practice has a tradition that requires professionals to cultivate certain virtues. Standards of virtue incorporate criteria of professional merit, and possession of these virtues disposes a person to act in accordance with the objectives of the practices.[13]

Roles and practices in medicine and nursing reflect social expectations as well as standards and ideals internal to these professions. The traditional virtues in these professions derive primarily from health care relationships.[14] The virtues we highlight here are care—a fundamental virtue for traditional health care relationships—along with five focal virtues: compassion, discernment, trustworthiness, integrity, and conscientiousness, all of which support and promote caring. Elsewhere in this chapter and in later chapters, we discuss other virtues, such as respectfulness, nonmalevolence, benevolence, justice, truthfulness, and faithfulness.

To illustrate the difference between professional standards of moral character and professional standards that define technical skills, we begin with an instructive study of surgical error. Charles L. Bosk's *Forgive and Remember: Managing Medical Failure* presents an ethnographic study of the way two surgical services in "Pacific Hospital" handle medical failure, especially failures by surgical residents.[15] Bosk found that both surgical services distinguish, at least implicitly, between several different forms of error or mistake. The first is *technical*: The professional discharges role responsibilities conscientiously, but his or her technical training or information falls short of what the task requires. Every surgeon will occasionally make this sort of mistake. The second sort of error is *judgmental*: A conscientious professional develops and follows an incorrect strategy. These errors are also to be expected. Attending surgeons forgive momentary technical and judgmental errors but remember them in case a pattern develops indicating that a surgical resident lacks the technical and judgmental skills to be a competent surgeon.

The third sort of error is *normative*: A physician committing this kind of error violates a norm of conduct, particularly by failing to discharge moral obligations conscientiously. Bosk contends that surgeons view technical and judgmental errors as less important than these moral errors, because every conscientious person can be expected to make "honest errors" or "good faith errors." However, moral errors such as failures of conscientiousness are considered profoundly serious when a pattern indicates a defect of character.

As Bosk's study suggests, persons of high moral character acquire a reservoir of goodwill in assessments of the praiseworthiness or blameworthiness of their actions. If a conscientious surgeon and another surgeon who is defective in conscientiousness make the same technical or judgmental errors, the conscientious surgeon will not be subjected to moral blame to the same degree as the other surgeon.

The Virtues in Alternative Professional Models

Professional virtues were historically integrated with professional obligations and ideals in codes of health care ethics. Insisting that the medical profession's "prime objective" is to render service to humanity, an American Medical Association (AMA) code in effect from 1957 to 1980 urged the physician to be "upright" and "pure in character and...diligent and conscientious in caring for the sick." It endorsed the virtues that Hippocrates commended: modesty, sobriety, patience, promptness, and piety. However, in contrast to its first code in 1847, the AMA over the years has deemphasized virtues in codes. The 1980 version for the first time eliminated all trace of the virtues except for the admonition to expose "those physicians deficient in character or competence." That pattern continues.

Thomas Percival, who wrote the most influential treatise on medical ethics in the last two centuries, provides a classic example of an attempt to establish the proper set of virtues in medicine. Starting from the assumption that the patient's best medical interest is the proper goal of medicine, Percival reached conclusions about the good physician's traits of character, which were invariably tied to responsibility for the patient's medical welfare.[16]

Likewise, in traditional nursing, where the nurse was often viewed as the "handmaiden" of the physician, the nurse was counseled to cultivate the passive virtues of obedience and submission. In contemporary models, however, active virtues have become more prominent. For example, when the nurse's role is viewed as one of advocacy for patients, prominent virtues include respectfulness, considerateness, justice, persistence, and courage.[17] Attention to patients' rights and preservation of the nurse's integrity dominate some contemporary models.

The conditions under which virtues may be present in morally unworthy and condemnable actions present some thorny ethical issues. Virtues such as loyalty, courage, kindness, and benevolence at times lead persons to act inappropriately and unacceptably.[18] For instance, the physician who acts kindly and loyally by not reporting the incompetence of a fellow physician acts improperly. Such a failure to report professional misconduct does not, however, suggest that loyalty and kindness are not virtues, only that the virtues need to be accompanied by an understanding of what is right and good, and of what deserves our kindness, generosity, and the like. Virtues warranting special caution include respectfulness, generosity, and patriotism, which may easily be misdirected by obedience, zeal, or excessive devotion.

THE VIRTUE OF CARING

As the language of *health care, medical care*, and *nursing care* suggests, the virtue of care, or caring, is prominent in this context. We treat it here as a fundamental and directional virtue of relationships, practices, and actions in health care. In explicating this virtue, or family of virtues, in health care, we draw on the *ethics of care*, an influential form of virtue ethics.[19] The ethics of care emphasizes traits valued in intimate personal relationships such as sympathy, compassion, fidelity, and love. *Caring,* in particular, refers to care for, emotional commitment to, and deep willingness to act on behalf of persons with whom one has a significant relationship. "Caring for" is also expressed in such actions as "care-giving," "taking care of," and "due care."

The ethics of care emphasizes not only *what* physicians and nurses do—for example, whether they break or maintain confidentiality—but also *how* they perform those actions, which motives underlie them, and whether their actions promote or thwart positive relationships. The nurse's or physician's trustworthiness and quality of care and sensitivity in the face of problems encountered with patients are integral to their professional moral lives.

The Origins of the Ethics of Care

The ethics of care originated primarily in feminist writings. The earliest works emphasized how women display an ethic of care, by contrast to men, who predominantly exhibit an ethic of rights and obligations. Psychologist Carol Gilligan advanced the influential hypothesis that "women speak in a different voice"—a voice that traditional ethical theory drowned out. She discovered "the voice of care" through empirical research involving interviews with girls and women. This voice, she said, stresses empathic association with others, not based on "the primacy and universality of individual rights, but rather on...a very strong sense of being responsible."[20]

Gilligan identified two modes of moral thinking: an ethic of care and an ethic of rights and justice. She did not claim that these two modes of thinking strictly correlate with gender or that all women or all men speak in the same moral voice.[21] Rather, she maintained that men *tend* to embrace an ethic of rights and justice that uses quasi-legal terminology and impartial principles, accompanied by dispassionate balancing and conflict resolution, whereas women *tend* to affirm an ethic of care that centers on responsiveness in an interconnected network of needs, care, and prevention of harm. The core notion in an ethics of care, then, is caring for and taking care of others. [22]

Criticisms of Traditional Theories

Proponents of the care perspective often criticize traditional ethical theories that deemphasize virtues of caring. Two criticisms merit special attention.[23]

Challenging impartiality. According to the care perspective, theories of norms of obligation (as we discuss them in Chapters 1, 9, and 10) can unduly telescope morality by overemphasizing detached fairness. This orientation is suitable for some moral relationships, especially those in which persons interact as equals in a public context of impersonal justice and institutional constraints. But moral detachment may turn out to be a lack of caring responsiveness. In the extreme case, detachment becomes uncaring indifference. Lost in the *detachment* of impartiality is an *attachment* to what we care about most and is closest to us—for example, our loyalty to friends and to groups. In the absence of public and institutional constraints, partiality toward others is morally permissible and is the expected form of interaction. It is also a feature of the human condition that cannot be eliminated. Without exhibiting partiality, we would impair or sever our most important relationships.[24]

Proponents of care ethics do not recommend a general abandonment of principles as long as principles allow room for discretionary and contextual judgment. At the same time, like many other proponents of virtue ethics, defenders of the ethics of care do find principles often irrelevant, unproductive, ineffectual, or unduly constrictive in the moral life. A defender of principles could say that *principles* of care, compassion, and kindness tutor our responses in caring, compassionate, and kind ways. But this effort to rescue principles seems hollow. Moral experience suggests that we often do rely on our emotions, our capacity for sympathy, our sense of friendship, and our sensitivity to determine appropriate moral responses. Although we can produce rough generalizations about how caring physicians and nurses should respond to patients, these generalizations are not subtle enough to provide guidance for all interactions with patients. Each situation calls for a set of responses beyond any generalization, and behavior that is caring in one context may be offensive in another setting. (See our discussion of this sort of behavior in Chapter 3, when treating the place of *sympathy*.)

Relationship and emotion. The ethics of care places special emphasis on mutual interdependence and emotional responsiveness. Many human relationships in health care and research involve persons who are vulnerable, dependent, ill, and frail. Feeling for and being immersed in the other person are vital aspects of the moral relationship.[25] They involve forms of empathy that a rights-based account may ignore because of its focus on protecting persons from wrongdoing by others.

Having a certain emotional attitude and expressing the appropriate emotion in action are morally relevant factors, just as having appropriate motives is morally relevant. A person seems morally deficient who acts according to norms of obligation without appropriately aligned feelings, such as concern and sympathy for a suffering friend. Good health care often involves insight into the needs of patients and considerate attentiveness to their circumstances, which often derives more from emotion than reason.[26]

In the history of human experimentation, those who first recognized that some subjects of research were being brutalized, subjected to misery, or placed at unjustifiable risk were persons who were able to feel sympathy, compassion, disgust, and outrage through insight into the situation of these research subjects. They exhibited perception of and sensitivity to the feelings of subjects, where others lacked comparable perceptions, sensitivities, and responses. This emphasis on the emotional dimension of the moral life does not reduce moral response to emotional response. Caring itself has a cognitive dimension and requires a range of moral skills, because it involves insight into and understanding of another's circumstances, needs, and feelings. (See our discussion of compassion and empathy later in this chapter.)

One proponent of the ethics of care argues that in a defensible ethical theory, action should at times be principle-guided, but not necessarily always governed by or derived from principles.[27] This statement moves in exactly the right direction in the quest for a comprehensive framework. We need not and should not reject principles in favor of the virtues of caring, but if we agree that moral judgment involves more than applying abstract principles, we will have a better grasp on the full range of essential moral skills and ways of coming to moral judgments and actions. An ethic that emphasizes the many virtues of caring can potentially serve health care well because it is close to the processes of decision making and attachment found in clinical contexts, gives insight into basic commitments of caring and caretaking, and liberates health professionals from narrow conceptions of role responsibilities often found in professional codes of ethics.

Five Focal Virtues

We now treat five focal virtues for health professionals: compassion, discernment, trustworthiness, integrity, and conscientiousness. These virtues are important in part for the development and expression of caring, which we have presented as the fundamental orienting virtue. These six virtues provide a moral compass of character for health professionals. Of course, several other virtues are also important, and we treat some of them later.

Compassion

Compassion has been called "the prelude to caring."[28] The virtue of compassion combines an attitude of active regard for another's welfare with an imaginative awareness and emotional response of sympathy, tenderness, and discomfort at another's misfortune or suffering.[29] Compassion presupposes sympathy, has affinities with mercy, and is expressed in acts of beneficence that attempt to alleviate the misfortune or suffering of another person. Unlike the virtue of integrity, which is focused on the self, compassion is focused on others.

Nurses and physicians need to understand the feelings and experiences of patients to respond appropriately to them and their illnesses and injuries. Hence, the importance of empathy, which involves the "imaginative reconstruction of another person's experience," whether that experience is negative or positive.[30] As important as empathy may be for compassion and other virtues, it must not be confused with compassion, and it does not always lead to compassion. Much of the literature on education for and professionalism in medicine and health care now focuses on empathy rather than compassion, making the mistake of viewing empathy alone as sufficient for humanizing medicine and health care.[31]

Compassion generally focuses on others' pain, suffering, disability, and misery—the typical occasions for compassionate responses in health care. Using the language of *sympathy*, eighteenth-century philosopher David Hume pointed to a typical circumstance of compassion in health care and explained how it arises:

> Were I present at any of the more terrible operations of surgery, 'tis certain,
> that even before it begun, the preparation of the instruments, the laying of
> the bandages in order, the heating of the irons, with all the signs of anxiety
> and concern in the patient and assistants, wou'd have a great effect upon
> my mind, and excite the strongest sentiments of pity and terror. No passion
> of another discovers itself immediately to the mind. We are only sensible
> of its causes or effects. From *these* we infer the passion: And consequently
> *these* give rise to our sympathy.[32]

Physicians and nurses who express no compassion in their behavior often fail to provide what patients need most. The physician or nurse lacking altogether in the appropriate display of compassion has a moral weakness. However, compassion also may cloud judgment and preclude rational and effective responses. In one reported case, a long-alienated son wanted to continue indefinitely a futile and painful treatment for his near-comatose father in an intensive-care unit (ICU) to have time to "make his peace" with his father. Although the son understood that his alienated father had no cognitive capacity, the son wanted to work through his sense of regret. Some hospital staff argued that the patient's grim prognosis and pain, combined with the needs of others waiting to receive care in the ICU, justified stopping the treatment, as had been requested by the patient's close cousin and informal guardian. Another group in the unit regarded continued treatment as an appropriate act of compassion toward the son, who they thought should have time to express his farewells and regrets to make himself feel better about his father's death. The first group, by contrast, viewed compassion as misplaced because of the patient's prolonged agony and dying. In effect, those in the first group believed that the second group's compassion prevented clear thinking about primary obligations to this patient.[33]

Many writers in the history of ethical theory, most notably Spinoza and Kant, have suggested a cautious approach to compassion. They have maintained that a passionate, or even a compassionate, engagement with others can blind reason and impartial reflection. Health care professionals understand and appreciate this phenomenon. Constant contact with suffering can overwhelm and even paralyze a compassionate physician or nurse. Impartial judgment can give way to impassioned decisions, and emotional burnout sometimes occurs. To counteract this problem, medical education and nursing education are designed to inculcate detachment alongside compassion. The language of *detached concern* and *compassionate detachment* appropriately appears in health care ethics expressly to identify a complex characteristic of the good physician or good nurse.

Discernment

The virtue of discernment brings sensitive insight, astute judgment, and understanding to action. Discernment involves the ability to make fitting judgments and reach decisions without being unduly influenced by extraneous considerations, fears, personal attachments, and the like.

Some writers closely associate discernment with practical wisdom, or *phronesis*, to use Aristotle's term. A person of practical wisdom knows which ends to choose, knows how to realize them in particular circumstances, and carefully selects from among the range of possible actions, while keeping emotions within proper bounds. In Aristotle's model, the practically wise person understands how to act with the right intensity of feeling, in just the right way, at just the right time, with a proper balance of reason and desire.[34]

More generally, the person of discernment is disposed to understand and perceive what circumstances demand in the way of human responsiveness. For example, a discerning physician will see when a despairing patient needs comfort rather than privacy, and vice versa. If comfort is the right choice, the discerning physician will find the right type and level of consolation to be helpful rather than intrusive. If a rule guides action in a particular case, seeing *how* to follow the rule involves a form of discernment that is independent of seeing *that* the rule applies.

The virtue of discernment thus involves understanding both *that* and *how* principles and rules apply in a variety of circumstances. Acts of respect for autonomy and beneficence will vary in health care contexts, and the ways in which clinicians manifest these principles and virtues in the care of patients will be as different as the ways in which devoted parents care for their children.

Trustworthiness

Virtues, according to Annette Baier, "are personal traits that contribute to a good climate of trust between people, when trust is taken to be acceptance of being, to some degree and in some respects, in another's power."[35] As this assessment suggests, trustworthiness is essential in medical and health care, where patients are vulnerable and must put themselves in the hands of health care profession-als. "Trustworthiness" is sometimes considered a virtual synonym for character or virtue, but this is overstatement. Even though trustworthiness necessarily shares features in common with some other virtues, such as honesty and integrity, here we treat it simply as one of the most important virtues in medicine and health care.

Trust itself is a confident belief in and reliance on the moral character and competence of another person, often but not always a person with whom one has an intimate or established relationship. Trust entails a confidence that another will act with the right motives and in accordance with appropriate moral norms.[36] To be *trustworthy* is to merit confidence in one's character and conduct. Trustworthiness has the practical outcome of promoting the image of the professional and making health care effective. Nothing is more important in health care organizations than the maintenance of a culture of trust.

Traditional ethical theories rarely mention trustworthiness. However, Aristotle took note of one aspect of trust and trustworthiness. He maintained that when relationships are voluntary and among intimates, in contrast to legal relationships among strangers, it is appropriate for the law to forbid lawsuits for harms that occur. Aristotle reasoned that, in intimate relationships, "dealings with one another as good and trustworthy," rather than "bonds of justice," hold persons together. The former bond he regarded as a matter of character.[37]

It is hard to fault Aristotle's ideal. At the same time, a climate of trust is endangered in contemporary health care institutions, as is evidenced by the number of medical malpractice suits and adversarial relations between health care professionals and the public. Overt distrust has been engendered by mechanisms of managed care, because of the incentives some health care organizations create for physicians to limit the amount and kinds of care they provide to patients. Talk has increased of the need for ombudsmen, patient advocates, legally binding "directives" to physicians, and the like. Among the contributing causes of the erosion of a climate of trust are the loss of intimate contact between physicians and patients, the increased use of specialists, and the growth of large, impersonal, and bureaucratic medical institutions.[38]

Integrity

Some writers claim that the primary virtue in health care is integrity.[39] People commonly justify some of their actions or refusals to act on grounds that they would otherwise compromise or sacrifice their integrity. Later in this chapter we discuss such appeals to integrity as they appear in invocations of *conscience*, but at present we confine attention to the virtue of integrity.

The *value of* moral integrity is beyond serious dispute, but what we *mean* by the term is less clear. In its most general sense, *moral integrity* means soundness, reliability, wholeness, and integration of moral character. In a more restricted sense, *moral integrity* means fidelity in adherence to moral norms. Accordingly, the virtue of integrity represents two aspects of a person's character. The first is a coherent integration of aspects of the self: emotions, aspirations, knowledge, and the like, so that each complements and does not frustrate the others. The second is the character trait of being faithful to moral values and standing up in their defense when necessary. A person can lack moral integrity in several respects— for example, through hypocrisy, insincerity, bad faith, and self-deception. These vices represent breaks in the connections among a person's moral convictions, emotions, and actions. Perhaps the most common deficiency is the simple lack of sincerely held, firm moral convictions; but no less important is the failure to act on the moral beliefs that one does hold.

Problems in maintaining integrity sometimes arise not from a lack of moral conviction or even from a conflict of moral norms, but from moral demands that require persons to sacrifice in a way that causes them to abandon their personal goals and projects. Persons can feel violated by having to abandon their personal commitments to pursue moral objectives created by the conduct of others. For example, if a sister who is a nurse is the only person in the family who can properly manage her sister's health, health care, prescription medications, nursing home arrangements, explanations to relatives, and negotiations with physicians, little time may be left for her personal projects and commitments. Such situations can deprive us of the liberty to structure and integrate our lives as we choose. If a person has structured his or her life around personal goals that are ripped away by the needs and agendas of others, a loss of personal integrity occurs.

Sometimes the issues concern so-called *professional* integrity. These issues are largely about lack of integrity and wrongful conduct in the profession. Breaches of professional integrity involve violations of professional standards of conduct, and so are often said to be violations of the rules of professional associations. This vision is too narrow.[40] It is a breach of professional integrity for any physician to prescribe a drug that is not effective, to enter into a sexual relationship with a patient, or to follow a living will that asks for a medically outrageous "treatment"—whether or not professional associations disallow such conduct and whether or not the physician feels bound by the standards of conduct.

In other cases the issue is *personal* rather than professional integrity. An example is found in medical practitioners who, because of their religious commitments to the sanctity of life, find it difficult to participate in decisions not to do everything possible to prolong life. To them, participating in removing ventilators and intravenous fluids from patients, even from patients with a clear advance directive, violates their integrity. Their evaluative commitments may create morally troublesome situations in which they must either compromise their fundamental commitments or withdraw from the care of the patient. Yet compromise seems what a person or an organization of integrity cannot do, because it involves the sacrifice of deep moral commitments.[41]

Modern health care facilities cannot entirely eliminate problems of staff disagreement and the like, but persons with the virtues of patience, humility, and tolerance can ameliorate these problems. Situations that compromise integrity can usually be avoided if participants anticipate the problem before it arises and recognize the limits and fallibility of their own moral views. Participants in a dispute may also have recourse to consultative institutional processes, such as a hospital ethics committee. However, it would be morally impoverished advice to recommend that a person of integrity can and should always negotiate and compromise in an intrainstitutional confrontation. There is something ennobling and admirable about the person or organization that refuses to compromise beyond a certain carefully delineated, deeply considered moral threshold. To compromise below the threshold of integrity is simply to lose it.

Conscientiousness

These points about integrity and compromise lead directly to the virtue of conscientiousness and to accounts of conscience. An individual acts *conscientiously* if he or she is motivated to do what is right because it is right, has tried with due diligence to determine what is right, intends to do what is right, and exerts an appropriate level of effort to do so. *Conscientiousness* is the character trait of acting in this way.

Conscience and conscientiousness. Many people view *conscience* as a mental faculty of, and authority for, moral decision making.[42] Slogans such as, "Let your conscience be your guide" suggest that conscience is the final authority in moral justification. However, this account fails to capture the nature of either conscience or conscientiousness. We can see why by examining the following case, which is derived from Bernard Williams: Having recently completed his Ph.D. in chemistry, George has not been able to find a job. His family has suffered from his failure: They are short of money, his wife has had to take additional work, and their small children have been subjected to considerable strain, uncertainty, and instability. An established chemist can get George a position in a laboratory that pursues research in chemical and biological warfare. Despite his perilous financial and familial circumstances, George feels that he cannot accept this position because of his conscientious opposition to chemical and biological warfare. The older chemist notes that the research will continue no matter what George decides. Furthermore, if George does not take this position, it will be offered to another young man who would probably pursue the research with great vigor. Indeed, the older chemist confides, his concern about this other candidate's nationalistic fervor and uncritical zeal for research in chemical and biological warfare motivated him to recommend George for the job. George's wife is puzzled and hurt by George's reaction. She sees nothing wrong with the research. She is profoundly concerned about their children's problems and the instability of their family.[43] Nonetheless, George forgoes this opportunity both to help his family and to prevent a destructive fanatic from obtaining the position because his conscience stands in the way.

Conscience, as this example suggests, is not a special moral faculty or a self-justifying moral authority. It is a form of self-reflection on, and judgment about, whether one's acts are obligatory or prohibited, right or wrong, good or bad. It is an internal sanction that comes into play through critical reflection. This sanction often appears as a bad conscience—in the form of feelings of remorse, guilt, shame, disunity, or disharmony—as the individual recognizes his or her acts as wrong. A conscience that sanctions in this way does not signify bad moral character. This experience of conscience is most likely to occur in persons of strong moral character and it may even be a necessary condition of morally good character.[44] For example, kidney donors have been known to say, "I had to do it. I couldn't have backed out, not that I had the feeling of being trapped, because the doctors offered to get me out. I just had to do it."[45] Such poignant statements indicate that some ethical standards are sufficiently powerful that violating them would diminish integrity and result in guilt or shame.[46]

When people claim that their actions are conscientious, they sometimes feel compelled by conscience to resist others' apparently authoritative demands. Instructive examples are found in military physicians who believe they must answer first to their consciences and cannot plead "superior's orders" when commanded by a superior officer to commit what they believe to be a moral wrong. In some cases agents even act out of character to perform what they judge to be the morally appropriate action. For example, a normally cooperative and cheerful physician may angrily, but justifiably, protest an insurance company's decision not to cover the costs of a patient's treatment. Such moral indignation and outrage are sometimes appropriate and even admirable.

Conscientious refusals. Conscientious objections by physicians, nurses, pharmacists, and other health care professionals raise issues for public policy, professional organizations, and health care institutions, as well as for patients and others who may be affected by conscience-based refusals to provide some legal service. Examples include a physician's refusal to honor a patient's valid advance directive to withdraw artificial nutrition and hydration under certain circumstances, a nurse's refusal to participate in an abortion or sterilization procedure, and a pharmacist's refusal to fill a woman's prescription for an emergency contraception. On the one hand, there are strong reasons to promote conscientiousness and to respect conscience; on the other hand, some conscientious refusals adversely affect patients' and others' legitimate interests. Public policy, the professions, and institutions should seek to recognize and accommodate conscientious refusals, as long as they can do so without seriously compromising patients' rights and interests.

No single model of appropriate response to conscientious refusal will be satisfactory for all affected parties in all cases.[47] Frequently, institutions such as hospitals and pharmacies can ensure the timely performance of needed or requested services while allowing particular conscientious objectors not to perform those services. But ethical complexities arise when, for example, a pharmacist, on grounds of complicity in moral wrongdoing, refuses to refer or transfer a consumer's prescription or even to inform the consumer of pharmacies that would fill the prescription. According to one study, 14% of U.S. physicians surveyed do not feel obligated to disclose information about morally controversial medical procedures, and 29% do not recognize an obligation to refer patients for such procedures.[48]

At a minimum, health care professionals have an ethical duty to inform prospective employers and prospective patients, clients, or consumers of their conscientious objections to performing any services that could reasonably be expected. They also always have an ethical duty to disclose options for obtaining legal, albeit morally controversial, services and, in many cases, a duty to provide a referral for those services.

MORAL VIRTUES AND ACTION GUIDES

A common criticism of virtue ethics is that it provides little, if any, guidance for actions. Although we are here primarily developing a place for virtue in ethics, we should also consider implications for action by asking, "What would a virtuous moral agent do?"

The Relationship between Moral Virtues and Moral Principles

There is a rough, although imperfect, correspondence between some virtues and moral norms, including principles, rules, and ideals. The following (radically incomplete) list illustrates the correspondence between a few select virtues and norms that are prominent in this book.

Principles	Corresponding Virtues
Respect for autonomy	Respectfulness
Nonmaleficence	Nonmalevolence
Beneficence	Benevolence
Justice	Justice (or fairness)

Rules	Corresponding Virtues
Veracity	Truthfulness
Confidentiality	Confidentiality

| Privacy | Respect for privacy |
| Fidelity | Faithfulness |

Ideals of Action	**Ideals of Virtue**
Exceptional forgiveness	Exceptional forgiveness
Exceptional generosity	Exceptional generosity
Exceptional compassion	Exceptional compassion
Exceptional kindness	Exceptional kindness

We could expand this list to include many additional norms and virtues, but the list would never amount to a comprehensive schema of correspondence. Many virtue standards do not directly correspond to norms in the one-to-one correspondence just indicated. For example, caring, concern, compassion, sympathy, courage, modesty, and patience are virtues that do not correspond well to principles and rules of obligation. Other examples of such virtues are cautiousness, integrity (in the sense of consistently upholding and standing firm in one's values), cheerfulness, unpretentiousness, sincerity, appreciativeness, cooperativeness, and commitment.[49] Some of these, such as courage and integrity, are important for morality as a whole and thus for more than one principle or rule of obligation. Some of the virtues that lack corresponding norms of *obligations* do have corresponding moral *ideals*. Before we turn to moral ideals and moral excellence, we consider how a framework of virtues can provide action guidance, even apart from correspondent, although independent, norms.

What Would a Virtuous Moral Agent Do?

It is often assumed that a virtuous health care professional who embodies a wide range of virtues will both discern what he or she should do and be motivated to do it in particular circumstances. However, this expectation is overly optimistic. In the course of deliberation, a health care professional may find valuable guidance for action not only from norms of obligation and ideals, but also by asking, "What would a virtuous health care professional do in these circumstances?" This question may focus on specific virtues—for example, compassion or courage—or on the agent's character as a whole, including specific virtues. According to Rosalind Hursthouse,

> Virtue ethics provides a specification of "right actions"—as "what a virtuous agent would, characteristically, do in the circumstances"—and such a specification can be regarded as generating a number of moral rules or principles (contrary to the usual claim that virtue ethics does not come up with rules or principles). Each virtue generates an instruction—"Do what is honest", "Do what is charitable", and each vice a prohibition— "Do not...do what is dishonest, uncharitable".[50]

This is an insightful and straightforward way to address the question "What would a virtuous agent do?" However, specification of the "instruction" will not be clear-cut,[51] and it will render virtue ethics very similar to the theory of moral norms that we proposed in Chapter 1. For example, proponents will have to bring these "instructions" (i.e., rules) to bear on dilemmas and conflict situations. Proponents of virtue ethics do not lament that their approach lacks a complete decision procedure for such conflicts. Rather, they rightly note the limitations of principles, rules, and so on, as well as of the virtues, in resolving moral dilemmas; and they stress that, in irresolvable and tragic dilemmas, the virtues help direct agents to appropriate responses, including appropriate attitudes and emotions, such as moral distress.[52] We accept this conclusion. At the same time, this theory does not prove some sort of triumph of virtues over principles and rules of obligation. Rather, it shows their close connections.[53]

MORAL IDEALS

Ordinary moral standards apply to everyone; extraordinary moral standards do not. Standards in the common morality, we argued in Chapter 1, pertain to everyone. These standards form the moral minimum. Extraordinary moral standards come from a morality of aspiration in which individuals and particular communities adopt moral ideals that need not hold for everyone—although many general ideals such as extraordinary generosity are universally admired and endorsed. This level of moral standards does not *require* impartial actions and permits agents to pursue the particular moral objectives they choose. Other persons can praise and admire those who fulfill these ideals, but they cannot blame or criticize persons who do not pursue these ideals. Persons who do not accept these ideals are not bound by them and cannot be criticized for not adopting them.

With the addition of moral ideals, we now have four categories of moral action: (1) actions that are right and obligatory (e.g., truth-telling); (2) actions that are wrong and prohibited (e.g., murder); (3) actions that are optional and morally neutral (neither wrong nor obligatory; e.g., playing chess with a friend); and (4) actions that are optional but morally meritorious and praiseworthy (e.g., sending flowers to a sick friend). We concentrated on the first two in Chapter 1, occasionally mentioning the third. We now focus exclusively on the fourth, using the language of "moral ideals" and "supererogation."

Supererogatory Acts

Supererogation is a category of moral ideals pertaining principally to ideals of *action*, but it has important links to *virtues* and to Aristotelian ideas of *moral excellence*.[54] The etymological root of *supererogation* means paying or performing beyond what is owed or, more generally, doing more than is required. Supererogation has four defining conditions (which collectively specify category 4 listed immediately above on p. 47). First, supererogatory acts are optional; they are neither required nor forbidden by common-morality standards. Second, supererogatory acts exceed what the common morality demands, but at least some moral ideals are shared by all who accept the common morality. Third, supererogatory acts are intentionally undertaken to promote the welfare of others. Fourth, supererogatory acts are morally good and praiseworthy in themselves, not merely undertaken from good intentions.

Despite the first condition, individuals who hold moral ideals do not always *consider* the quality of their actions (or their characters) to be morally optional. Many heroes and saints describe their actions in the language of *ought*, *duty*, and *necessity*: "I had to do it." "I had no choice." "It was my duty." The point of this language is to express a personal sense of obligation. The agent accepts, as a pledge or assignment of personal responsibility, a personal norm that lays down what ought to be done, despite the fact that it is not obligatory in the common morality or in a code of professional ethics. At the end of Albert Camus's *The Plague,* Dr. Rieux decides to make a record of those who fought the pestilence. It is to be a record, he says, of "what *had to be done*...despite their personal afflictions, by all who, while unable to be saints but refusing to bow down to pestilences, strive their utmost to be healers."[55] Such healers accept exceptional risks and thereby exceed the obligations of both the common morality and their professional tradition.

Many supererogatory acts would be morally required were it not for some abnormal adversity or risk in the face of which the individual elects not to invoke an exemption introduced by the presence of the adversity or risk.[56] If persons have the strength of character that enables them to resist extreme adversity or assume additional risk to fulfill their own conception of their obligations, then it makes sense to accept their view that they are under a self-imposed obligation. The hero who says, "I was only doing my duty," is, from his or her perspective, speaking correctly, as one who accepts a standard of moral excellence. Such a person does not make a mistake in regarding the action as personally required, and can view failure as grounds for guilt, although no one else is free to so evaluate the act.

Not all supererogatory acts are *exceptionally* arduous, costly, or risky. Examples of less demanding forms of supererogation include generous gift-giving, volunteering for public service, forgiving another's costly error, and exceptional kindness. Many everyday actions exceed obligation without reaching the highest level of supererogation. For example, a nurse may put in extra hours of work during the day and return to the hospital at night to visit patients without becoming a saint or hero. Many of these acts spring from virtues of character.

Often we are uncertain whether an action exceeds obligation because the boundaries of obligation and supererogation are ill defined. There may be no clear norm of action, only a virtue of character. For example, what is a nurse's role obligation to desperate, terminally ill patients who cling to the nurse for comfort in their few remaining days? If the obligation is that of spending forty hours a week in conscientiously fulfilling a job description, then the nurse exceeds that obligation by a few off-duty visits to patients. If the obligation is simply to help patients overcome burdens and meet a series of challenges, then a nurse who does this while displaying exceptional patience, fortitude, and friendliness exceeds the demands of obligation. There are also cases of health care professionals living up to what would ordinarily be a role obligation (e.g., standard care of a patient), while making a large sacrifice or taking an exceptional risk.

The Continuum from Obligation to Supererogation

Our analysis thus far may suggest that we should classify an action as either obligatory or as beyond obligation. However, some actions do not fit neatly into these categories because they fall between the two. The common morality and ethical theory are not precise enough to determine whether these actions are morally required or morally elective. This problem is compounded in professional ethics, because professional roles engender obligations that do not bind persons who do not occupy the relevant professional roles. From this perspective, the two "levels" of the obligatory and the supererogatory lack sharp boundaries both in the common morality and in professional ethics.

We need to distinguish between actions that are strictly obligatory, actions that are borderline, and still other actions that are not obligatory. More precisely, there is a continuum running from strict obligation (the core principles and rules in the common morality) through weaker obligations (the periphery of ordinary expectations in the common morality) and on to the domain of the morally nonrequired and the exceptionally virtuous. The nonrequired starts with lower level supererogation, such as walking a visitor lost in a hospital's corridors to a doctor's office. Here an absence of charitableness or generosity constitutes a defect in the moral life, although not a failure of obligation. The continuum ends with higher level supererogation, such as heroic acts of self-sacrifice. A continuum exists on each level and across their boundaries. The following diagram represents the continuum.

Obligation		Beyond Obligation (Supererogation)	
Strict obligation [1]	Weak obligation [2]	Ideals beyond the obligatory [3]	Saintly and heroic ideals [4]

This continuum moves from the strictest obligation to the most arduous and elective moral ideal. The horizontal line represents a continuum with rough rather than sharply defined breaks; the middle vertical line divides the two general categories, but does not represent a sharp break. The horizontal line expresses a continuum across the four lower categories.

Joel Feinberg argued that supererogatory acts are "located on an altogether different scale than obligations."[57] The preceding diagram suggests that this comment is correct in one respect, but misleading in another. The right half of the diagram is not scaled by obligation, whereas the left half is. In this respect, Feinberg's comment is correct. However, the full horizontal line is connected by a single scale of moral value in which the right is continuous with the left. For example, obligatory acts of beneficence and supererogatory acts of beneficence are on the same scale because they are morally of the same kind. The domain of supererogatory ideals is continuous with the domain of norms of obligation by *exceeding* those obligations in accordance with the several defining conditions of supererogation listed previously.

The Place of Ideals in Biomedical Ethics

Many beneficent actions by health care professionals straddle the territory marked in the preceding diagram between Obligation and Beyond Obligation (in particular, between (2) and (3)). Matters become more complicated by distinguishing between professional obligations and obligations incumbent on everyone. Many moral *obligations* established by roles in health care are moral *ideals* from the perspective of the common morality. These obligations in medicine and nursing are profession-relative, and some are role obligations even when not formally stated in professional codes. For example, the expectation that physicians and nurses will encourage and cheer patients is a profession-imposed obligation, but not one usually incorporated in a professional code of ethics.

Some customs in the medical community are not well established as obligations, such as the belief that physicians and nurses have an obligation to efface self-interest and take risks in attending to patients. A relevant issue is the nature of "obligations" when caring for patients with severe acute respiratory syndrome (SARS) and other serious transmissible diseases. Proposed policies have been controversial, and professional codes and medical association pronouncements have varied.[58] These issues cannot be resolved without considering the level of risk that professionals are expected to assume and setting a threshold beyond which the level of risk is so high as to be optional rather than obligatory. This problem should help us appreciate why some medical associations urged their members to exhibit the virtue of courage and treat these patients, while other associations advised their members that treatment is optional.[59] Still others insisted that both virtue and obligation converge to the conclusion that health

care professionals should set aside self-interest and that the health care professions should take actions to ensure appropriate care.[60]

It is doubtful that health care professionals fail to discharge moral *obligations* when they fall short of the highest possible standards in the profession
(the so-called gold standard). Confusion arises because of the indeterminate
boundaries of what is required in the common morality, what is required in
professional communities, and what is a matter of moral character beyond the
requirements of such moral norms.

MORAL EXCELLENCE

Aristotelian ethical theory has rightly insisted that moral excellence is intimately
connected to moral character. We now draw on this Aristotelian tradition and on
our prior analysis of moral ideals and supererogation for an account of moral
excellence.

The Place of Moral Excellence

We begin with four reasons that motivate us to attend to this subject. First, we
hope to overcome an undue imbalance in contemporary ethical theory, which
too often focuses narrowly on the moral minimum of obligations while largely
ignoring supererogation and moral ideals.[61] This concentration on minimal obligations dilutes the moral life, including our expectations for ourselves, our close
associates, and health professionals. If we expect only the moral minimum, we
may lose an ennobling sense of excellence.

Second, we aspire to overcome a suppressed skepticism in contemporary
ethical theory concerning high ideals in the moral life. This skepticism is evident in some influential philosophical works, including those written by Susan
Wolf, Philippa Foot, Bernard Williams, and Thomas Nagel. They note that high
moral ideals must compete with other goals and responsibilities in life, and
consequently that these ideals can demand too much morally or cause persons
to neglect other matters worthy of attention, including personal projects, family
relationships, friendships, and experiences that broaden outlooks.

We do not wholly reject this view, but these writings too unqualifiedly suggest that high moral ideals are only one of life's major considerations and that
moral excellence is no more valuable or worthwhile than hobbies, recreational
activities, and other so-called agent-relative projects. Lost is the Aristotelian
goal of aspiring to an admirable life. As a result, the model of a moral person is
uninspiring and devoid of moral challenge for reflective persons. As John Stuart
Mill once noted, "The contented man, or the contented family, who have no
ambition to make any one else happier, to promote the good of their country or
their neighborhood, or to improve themselves in moral excellence, excite in us
neither admiration nor approval."[62]

Our third reason concerns what we call in Chapter 9 the criterion of *comprehensiveness* in an ethical theory. Recognizing the value of moral excellence will allow us to incorporate a broad range of moral virtues and forms of supererogation beyond the obligations and virtues that comprise ordinary morality. We can include virtues such as tactfulness, courage, patience, hospitality, and what Aristotle called "greatness of soul" without maintaining that these virtues are conditions of morality that everyone is somehow required to meet or that there are *principles* of patience, hospitality, courage, and the like. These features of the moral life merit inclusion in a comprehensive account.

Fourth, and finally, a model of moral excellence merits pursuit because it indicates that which is worthy of aspiration. Morally exemplary lives provide ideals that help guide and inspire us to higher goals and morally better lives. These models exemplify high moral achievement. They illustrate why excellence and the pursuit of moral ideals are important in the moral life, alongside moral norms and moral virtues.

Aristotelian Ideals of Moral Character

Aristotle maintained that we acquire virtues much as we do skills such as carpentry, playing a musical instrument, and cooking. Obligations play a less central role in his account. Consider, for example, a person who undertakes to expose scientific fraud in an academic institution. It is easy to frame this objective as a matter of obligation, especially if the institution has a policy on fraud; but suppose this person's reports to superiors are ignored and eventually her job is in jeopardy and her family receives threats. At some point, she has fulfilled her obligations and is not morally required to pursue the matter further. However, her continued pursuit is praiseworthy. Her efforts to bring about institutional reform could even take on heroic dimensions. Aristotelian theory frames this situation in terms of the person's level of commitment, the perseverance and endurance shown, the resourcefulness and discernment in marshalling evidence, and the courage, as well as the decency and diplomacy, displayed in confronting superiors.

An analogy to educational goals illustrates why setting goals beyond the moral minimum is important. Most of us are trained to aspire to an ideal of education. We are taught to prepare ourselves as best we can. No educational aspirations are too high unless they exceed our abilities and thus cannot be attained. If we stop at a level below our educational potential, we will consider our achievement a matter of disappointment and regret even if we obtain a degree. As we fulfill our aspirations, we sometimes expand our goals beyond what we had originally planned. We think of getting another degree, learning another language, or reading widely beyond our specialized training. We do not say, however, that we have an *obligation* to achieve as high a level of education as we can achieve.

The Aristotelian model suggests that moral character and moral achievement similarly are functions of self-cultivation and aspiration. Goals of moral excellence can and should enlarge as moral development advances. Each individual should aspire to a level as elevated as his or her ability permits. Just as persons vary in the quality of their performances in athletics and medical practice, so too in the moral life some persons are more capable than others and deserve more acknowledgment, praise, and admiration. Some persons are sufficiently advanced morally that what they can achieve is elevated above what those who are less morally developed can expect to achieve.

Wherever a person is on the continuum of moral development, there will be a goal of excellence that exceeds what he or she has already achieved. This analysis explains why ideals are so centrally important in Aristotelian ethics and in the account that we are now recommending. This account is not for persons who merely want to know what social obligations require. For example, the investigator who uses human subjects in research might ask (as is typical in protocol review), "What am I obligated to do to protect human subjects?" The presumption is that once this question has been addressed (using a checklist of obligations), the researcher can proceed with the research. By contrast, in the Aristotelian model, this approach is only the starting point. The most important question is, "How could I conduct this research to maximally protect and minimally inconvenience subjects, commensurate with achieving the objectives of the research?" Evading this question indicates that one is morally less serious than one could be.

The Aristotelian model does not expect perfection, only that persons strive toward perfection. The model might seem impractical, but a fairer assessment is that moral ideals are practical instruments. As *our* ideals, they motivate us and set out a path that we can climb in stages, with a renewable sense of progress and achievement.

Exceptional Moral Excellence: Saints, Heroes, and Others

Extraordinary persons function as models of excellence whose examples we aspire to follow. Among the many models, the moral hero and the moral saint are the most celebrated, and deservedly so.

The term *saint* has a long history in religious, especially Christian, traditions, but it also has a secular use, just as *hero* does. Other-directedness, altruism, and benevolence are prominent features of the moral saint.[63] Saints do their duty and realize moral ideals where most people would fail to do so. Saintliness requires regular fulfillment of duty and realization of ideals over time; it demands consistency and constancy. We likely cannot make a final judgment about a person's moral saintliness until the record is complete. By contrast, a person may become a moral hero through one exceptional action, such as accepting extraordinary risk while discharging duty or realizing ideals. The hero resists fear and the desire for self-preservation in undertaking risky actions that most people would avoid, but the hero also may lack the constancy over a lifetime that distinguishes the saint.

Many persons who serve as moral models or as persons from whom we draw moral inspiration are not so advanced morally that they qualify as saints or heroes. We learn about good moral character from persons with a limited repertoire of exceptional virtues, such as conscientious health professionals. Consider, for example, John Berger's biography of the English physician John Sassall, who chose to practice medicine in a poverty-ridden, culturally deprived country village in a remote region of northern England. Under the influence of works by Joseph Conrad, Sassall chose this village from an "ideal of service" that reached beyond "the average petty life of self-seeking advancement." Sassall was aware that he would have almost no social life and that the villagers had few resources with which to pay him, to develop their community, and to attract better medicine, but he focused on their needs rather than his own. Progressively, Sassall grew morally as he interacted with members of the community. He developed a deep understanding of, and profound respect for, the villagers and learned how to attend to them as whole human beings. He became a person of exceptional caring, devotion, discernment, conscientiousness, and patience when taking care of the villagers. His moral character grew and deepened year after year in caring for them. They, in turn, trusted him under the most adverse and personally difficult circumstances.[64]

From exemplary lives like that of John Sassall and from our previous analysis, we can extract four criteria of moral excellence.[65] First, Sassall is faithful to a *worthy moral ideal* that he keeps constantly before him in making judgments and performing actions. The ideal is deeply devoted service to a poor and needy community. Second, he has a *motivational structure* that conforms closely to our earlier description of the motivational patterns of virtuous persons, which include being prepared to forgo benefits to oneself in the service of a moral ideal. Third, he has an *exceptional moral character*; that is, he possesses moral virtues that dispose him to perform supererogatory actions to an exceptional extent.[66] Fourth, he is a *person of integrity*—both of moral integrity and of a deep personal integrity—and thus is not overwhelmed by distracting conflicts, self-interest, or personal projects, in making judgments and performing actions.

These four conditions are sufficient conditions of moral *excellence*. They are also relevant, but not sufficient, conditions of moral *saintliness* and moral *heroism*. John Sassall, exceptional as he is, is neither a saint nor a hero. To achieve this elevated status, he would have to satisfy additional conditions. Sassall is not a person who faces deep adversity (although he faces modest adversity), extremely difficult tasks, or a high level of risk, and these are typically the sorts of conditions that contribute to making a person a saint or a hero.

Examples of prominent moral saints include St. Francis, Mother Teresa, and Albert Schweitzer. Examples of prominent moral heroes include soldiers, political prisoners, and ambassadors who take substantial risks to save endangered persons by such acts as falling on hand grenades and resisting political tyrants. Scientists and physicians who experiment on themselves to generate knowledge that may benefit others are sometimes heroes. There are many examples: Daniel Carrion injected blood into his arm from a patient with verruga peruana (an unusual disease marked by many vascular eruptions of the skin and mucous membranes as well as fever and severe rheumatic pains), only to discover that it had given him a fatal disease (Oroya fever). Werner Forssman performed the first heart catheterization on himself, walking to the radiological room with the catheter sticking into his heart.[67] A French researcher, Dr. Daniel Zagury, injected himself with an experimental AIDS vaccine, maintaining that his act was "the only ethical line of conduct."[68]

A person can qualify as a moral hero or a moral saint only if he or she meets some combination of the previously listed four conditions of moral excellence. While it is not clear that a person must satisfy all four conditions to qualify as a moral hero, a person must satisfy all four to qualify as a moral saint. This appraisal does not imply that moral saints are more valued or more admirable than moral heroes. We are simply proposing conditions of moral excellence that are more stringent for moral saints than for moral heroes. We will not consider whether these conditions point to another and still higher form of moral excellence: the combination of saint and hero in one person. There have been such extraordinary persons, and we could make a case that some of these extraordinary figures are more excellent than others. But at this level of moral exemplariness, such fine distinctions serve no purpose.

Finally, physician David Hilfiker's *Not All of Us Are Saints* offers an instructive model of very exceptional but not quite saintly or heroic conduct in medicine—in his case resulting from his efforts to practice "poverty medicine" in Washington, D.C.[69] His decision to leave a rural medical practice in the Midwest to provide medical care to the very poor, including the homeless, reflected both an ambition and a felt obligation. Many health problems he encountered stemmed from an unjust social system, in which his patients had limited access to health care and to other basic social goods that contribute to health. He experienced severe frustration as he encountered major social and institutional barriers to providing poverty medicine, while his patients were often difficult and uncooperative. His frustrations generated stress, depression, and hopelessness, along with vacillating feelings and attitudes, including anger, pain, impatience, and guilt. His wellspring of compassion exhausted by his sense of endless needs and personal limitations, he one day failed to respond as he felt he should have: "Like those whom on another day I would criticize harshly, I harden myself to the plight of a homeless man and leave him to the inconsistent mercies of the city police and ambulance system. Numbness and cynicism, I suspect, are more often the products of frustrated compassion than of evil intentions."

Hilfiker realized that he is "anything but a saint." He considered the label "saint" to be inappropriate for people, like himself, who have a safety net to protect them. Blaming himself for "selfishness," he redoubled his efforts, but he recognized "the gap between who I am and who I would like to be," and he considered that gap "too great to overcome." He abandoned "in frustration the attempt to be Mother Teresa," observing that "there are few Mother Teresas, few Dorothy Days who can give everything to the poor with a radiant joy." Hilfiker did think that many of the people with whom he worked counted as heroes, in the sense that they "struggle against all odds and survive; people who have been given less than nothing, yet find ways to give."

These observations about ordinary persons who act in extraordinary ways pertain to what has been called moral heroism in living organ and tissue donation—a topic to which we now turn.

Living Organ Donation and Tissue Donation

Health care professionals frequently function as moral gatekeepers to determine who may undertake living donation of organs and tissues for transplantation. Blood donation raises few questions, but in cases of bone marrow donation and the donation of kidneys or portions of livers or lungs, health care professionals have to consider whether, when, and from whom to invite, accept, and effectuate acts of donation. Living organ donation raises complex ethical issues because the transplant team subjects a healthy person to a variably risky surgical procedure, with no medical benefit to him or her. It is therefore appropriate for transplant teams to probe the donor's understanding, voluntariness, and motives.

Transplant teams have generally been suspicious of living, genetically unrelated donors—not only of strangers and mere acquaintances but often even of spouses and friends who are emotionally bonded. This suspicion has several sources, including concerns about donors' motives and worries about their competence to decide and the voluntariness of their decisions. However, in contrast to professionals' attitudes,[70] a majority of the public in the United States accepts the premise that the gift of a kidney to a stranger is reasonable and proper and that the transplant team should accept it.[71] The offer to donate a kidney by a friend, acquaintance, or stranger typically does not involve such high risks that questions should automatically emerge about the donor's competence, voluntariness, and motivations.[72]

Transplant teams can and should decline some heroic offers of organs for moral reasons—even when the donors are competent, their decisions informed and voluntary, and their moral excellence beyond question. For instance, transplant teams have good grounds to decline a mother's offer to donate her heart to

save her dying child, because the donation would involve others in directly causing her death. A troublesome case arose when an imprisoned, 38-year-old father
who had already lost one of his kidneys wanted to donate his remaining kidney
to his 16-year-old daughter whose body had already rejected one kidney transplant.[73] The family insisted that medical professionals and ethics committees
had no right to evaluate, let alone reject, the father's act of donation. However,
questions arose about the voluntariness of the father's offer (in part because he
was in prison), about the risks to him (many patients without kidneys do not
thrive on dialysis), about the probable success of the transplant (because of his
daughter's problems with her first transplant), and about the costs to the prison
system (approximately $40,000 to $50,000 a year for dialysis for the father if he
donated the remaining kidney).

Society and health care professionals should start with the presumption that
living organ donation is praiseworthy but optional. Transplant teams need to subject
their criteria for selecting and accepting living donors to public scrutiny to ensure
that the teams do not inappropriately use their own values about sacrifice, risk, and
the like as the basis for their judgments. Whether or not they rise to the level of
heroes, many organ donors have clearly risen to a level of moral excellence.

CONCLUSION

In this chapter we have moved to a moral territory distinct from the principles,
rules, obligations, and rights treated in Chapter 1. However, we have tried to
render the two domains entirely consistent and not to give priority to one over
the other. Often we have emphasized that standards of virtue and character are
closely connected to the moral norms discussed in Chapter 1. Virtues, ideals, and
aspirations of moral excellence both support and enrich the morality of obligations, rights, and actions that are grounded in a framework of principles and
rules. There is no reason to consider one domain inferior to or merely derivative
from the other. There is reason to think, however, that there are domains of the
moral life other than those of moral norms and moral character. In Chapter 3 we
turn to the chief domain not yet addressed: criteria of moral status.

NOTES

1. For relevant literature, see Stephen Darwall, ed., *Virtue Ethics* (Oxford: Blackwell Publishing,
2003); Roger Crisp and Michael Slote, eds., *Virtue Ethics* (Oxford: Oxford University Press,
1997); Roger Crisp, ed., *How Should One Live? Essays on the Virtues* (Oxford: Oxford University
Press, Clarendon, 1996); Daniel Statman, ed., *Virtue Ethics: A Critical Reader* (Washington, D.C.:
Georgetown University Press, 1997). Many discussions of virtue theory are indebted to Aristotle;
for a range of treatments, see Nancy Sherman, *The Fabric of Character: Aristotle's Theory of Virtue*
(Oxford: Clarendon, 1989); Alasdair MacIntyre, *After Virtue: A Study in Moral Theory*, 3rd ed. (Notre
Dame, IN: University of Notre Dame Press, 2007) and *Dependent Rational Animals: Why Human*

Beings Need the Virtues (Chicago: Open Court, 1999); Timothy Chappell, ed., *Values and Virtues: Aristotelianism in Contemporary Ethics* (Oxford: Clarendon, 2006). For departures from Aristotelian perspectives, while still drawing on Aristotle, see, for example, Christine Swanton, *Virtue Ethics: A Pluralistic View* (Oxford: Oxford University Press, 2003). See also Robert Merrihew Adams, *A Theory of Virtue: Excellence in Being for the Good* (Oxford: Clarendon, 2006).

2. For descriptions of positive character traits, see Christopher Peterson and Martin E. P. Seligman, eds., *Character Strengths and Virtues: A Handbook and Classification* (Washington, D.C.: American Psychological Association; and New York: Oxford University Press, 2004). The chapters identify twenty-four specific character strengths under six broad virtues. Categorization has centuries of tradition behind it in ethical theory. In normative ethical and religious traditions, there are significant variations in lists of virtues (and vices). However, much is also held common in all of these traditions—enough to speak of a common morality of the virtues, as we do.

3. Compare, favorably, the analysis of the virtues presented by Edmund D. Pellegrino and David C. Thomasma, *The Virtues in Medical Practice* (New York: Oxford University Press, 1993).

4. This is not the broadest possible sense of "virtue," inasmuch as machines, tools, horses, and the like are often said to have virtues. Some writers more tightly restrict the meaning of virtue than we do. For example, Aristotle required that virtue involve habituation rather than a natural character trait [*Nicomachean Ethics*, trans. Terence Irwin (Indianapolis, IN: Hackett Publishing, 1985), 1103ª18–19]. Thomas Aquinas (relying on a formulation by Peter Lombard) additionally held that virtue is a good quality of mind by which we live rightly and therefore cannot be put to bad use. See *Treatise on the Virtues* (from *Summa Theologiae*, I–II), Question 55, Arts. 3–4.

5. This definition is the primary use reported in the *Oxford English Dictionary* (*OED*). It is defended by Alan Gewirth, "Rights and Virtues," *Review of Metaphysics* 38 (1985): 751, and R. B. Brandt, "The Structure of Virtue," in *Midwest Studies in Philosophy* 13 (1988): 76. Edmund Pincoffs presents a definition of virtue in terms of desirable dispositional qualities of persons, in *Quandaries and Virtues: Against Reductivism in Ethics* (Lawrence, KS: University Press of Kansas, 1986), pp. 9, 73–100; see also MacIntyre, *After Virtue*, chaps. 10–18, on various definitions; and Raanan Gillon, "Ethics Needs Principles," *Journal of Medical Ethics* 29 (2003): 307–12, especially p. 309.

6. *Nicomachean Ethics,* 1105ª17–33, 1106ᵇ21–23; cf. 1144ª14–20 (trans. Irwin).

7. Robert Adams distinguishes "motivational virtues" (such as benevolence) from "structural virtues" (such as courage and self-control). The latter are structural features of the agent's organization and management of his or her motives. Adams, *A Theory of Virtue*, pp. 33–34, passim.

8. See Philippa Foot, *Virtues and Vices* (Oxford: Basil Blackwell, 1978); Gregory Trianosky, "Supererogation, Wrongdoing, and Vice," *Journal of Philosophy* 83 (1986): 26–40; Jorge L. Garcia, "The Primacy of the Virtuous," *Philosophia* 20 (1990): 69–91; and criticisms of such a view in Lynn A. Jansen, "The Virtues in Their Place: Virtue Ethics in Medicine," *Theoretical Medicine* 21 (2000): 261–76.

9. See Diane Jeske, "Friendship, Virtue, and Impartiality," *Philosophy and Phenomenological Research* 57 (1997): 51–72; and Michael Stocker, "The Schizophrenia of Modern Ethical Theories," *Journal of Philosophy* 73 (1976): 453–66.

10. Cf. Gregory Pence, *Ethical Options in Medicine* (Oradell, NJ: Medical Economics, 1980), p. 177.

11. Henry K. Beecher, "Ethics and Clinical Research," *New England Journal of Medicine* 274 (1966): 1354–60.

12. Thomas Keneally, *Schindler's List* (New York: Penguin Books, 1983), pp. 176–80.

13. This analysis is influenced by Alasdair MacIntyre, *After Virtue*, esp. chap. 14; and Dorothy Emmet, *Rules, Roles, and Relations* (New York: St. Martin's, 1966). See also Justin Oakley and Dean Cocking, *Virtue Ethics and Professional Roles* (Cambridge: Cambridge University Press, 2001).

14. A similar thesis is defended in dissimilar ways in Edmund D. Pellegrino, "Toward a Virtue-Based Normative Ethics for the Health Professions," *Kennedy Institute of Ethics Journal* 5 (1995): 253–77. See also John Cottingham, "Medicine, Virtues and Consequences," in *Human Lives: Critical Essays on Consequentialist Bioethics*, ed. David S. Oderberg (New York: Macmillan, 1997).

15. Charles L. Bosk, *Forgive and Remember: Managing Medical Failure* (Chicago: University of Chicago Press, 1979). Bosk also recognizes a fourth type of error: "quasi-normative errors," based on the attending's special protocols.

16. Thomas Percival, *Medical Ethics; or a Code of Institutes and Precepts, Adapted to the Professional Conduct of Physicians and Surgeons* (Manchester, England: S. Russell, 1803), pp. 165–66. This book formed the substantive basis of the first AMA code.

17. For models of nursing, see Dan W. Brock, "The Nurse–Patient Relation: Some Rights and Duties," in *Nursing: Images and Ideals,* ed. Stuart F. Spicker and Sally Gadow (New York: Spring, 1980), pp. 102–24; Gerald Winslow, "From Loyalty to Advocacy: A New Metaphor for Nursing," *Hastings Center Report* 14 (June 1984): 32–40; and Helga Kuhse, *Caring: Nurses, Women and Ethics* (Oxford: Blackwell, 1997), esp. chap. 3. See also the virtue-based approach to nursing ethics in Alan F. Armstrong, *Nursing Ethics: A Virtue-Based Approach* (Houndmills, England: Palgrave Macmillan, 2007).

18. We thus reject claims about the unity of the virtues to the effect that if one virtue is present all are present.

19. Contrast Virginia Held's argument for a sharp distinction between the ethics of care and virtue ethics on the grounds that the former focuses on relationships and the latter on individuals' dispositions: *The Ethics of Care: Personal, Political, and Global* (New York: Oxford University Press, 2006). We reject this treatment (in part) because both types of ethical framework are more varied and overlapping than her analysis allows.

20. Carol Gilligan, *In a Different Voice* (Cambridge, MA: Harvard University Press, 1982), esp. p. 21. See also her "Mapping the Moral Domain: New Images of Self in Relationship," *Cross Currents* 39 (Spring 1989): 50–63.

21. Gilligan and many others deny that the two distinct voices correlate strictly with gender. See Gilligan and Susan Pollak, "The Vulnerable and Invulnerable Physician," in *Mapping the Moral Domain*, ed. C. Gilligan, J. Ward, and J. Taylor (Cambridge, MA: Harvard University Press, 1988), pp. 245–62.

22. See Gilligan and G. Wiggins, "The Origins of Morality in Early Childhood Relationships," in *The Emergence of Morality in Young Children*, ed. J. Kagan and S. Lamm (Chicago: University of Chicago Press, 1988). See also Margaret Olivia Little, "Care: From Theory to Orientation and Back," *Journal of Medicine and Philosophy* 23 (1998): 190–209.

23. Our formulation of these criticisms is influenced by Alisa L. Carse, "The 'Voice of Care': Implications for Bioethical Education," *The Journal of Medicine and Philosophy* 16 (1991): 5–28, esp. 8–17. For analysis and assessment of such criticisms, see Kuhse, *Caring*.

24. Alisa L. Carse, "Impartial Principle and Moral Context: Securing a Place for the Particular in Ethical Theory," *Journal of Medicine and Philosophy* 23 (1998): 153–69.

25. See Nel Noddings, *Caring: A Feminine Approach to Ethics and Moral Education* (Berkeley, CA: University of California Press, 1984), and the evaluation of her work in Raja Halwani, "Care Ethics and Virtue Ethics," *Hypatia* 18 (2003), esp. pp. 162ff.

26. See Nancy Sherman, *The Fabric of Character* (Oxford: Oxford University Press, 1989), pp. 13–55; and Martha Nussbaum, *Love's Knowledge* (Oxford: Oxford University Press, 1990). On "attention" in medical care, see Margaret E. Mohrmann, *Attending Children: A Doctor's Education* (Washington, D.C.: Georgetown University Press, 2005).

27. Carse, "The 'Voice of Care,'" p. 17.

28. Pellegrino, "Toward a Virtue-Based Normative Ethics," p. 269.

29. See Lawrence Blum, "Compassion," in *Explaining Emotions,* ed. Amélie Oksenberg Rorty (Berkeley, CA: University of California Press, 1980); and David Hume, *A Dissertation on the Passions,* Sect. 3, §§ 4–5 (London, 1772 ed.), pp. 208–09.

30. Martha Nussbaum, *Upheavals of Thought: The Intelligence of Emotions* (Cambridge: Cambridge University Press, 2001), p. 302. Part II of this book is devoted to compassion, which Nussbaum carefully distinguishes from empathy, sympathy, and the like.

31. See Jodi Halpern, *From Detached Concern to Empathy: Humanizing Medical Practice* (New York: Oxford University Press, 2001).

32. David Hume, *A Treatise of Human Nature,* ed. David Fate Norton and Mary Norton (Oxford: Clarendon, 2007), 3.3.1.7.

33. Baruch Brody, "Case No. 25. 'Who Is the Patient, Anyway': The Difficulties of Compassion," in *Life and Death Decision Making* (New York: Oxford University Press, 1988), pp. 185–88.

34. Aristotle, *Nicomachean Ethics,* trans. Irwin, 1106^b15–29, 1141^a15–1144^b17.

35. Annette Baier, "Trust, Suffering, and the Aesculapian Virtues," in *Working Virtue: Virtue Ethics and Contemporary Moral Problems,* ed. Rebecca L. Walker and Philip J. Ivanhoe (Oxford: Clarendon, 2007), p. 137.

36. See Annette Baier's "Trust and Antitrust" and two later essays on trust in her *Moral Prejudices* (Cambridge, MA: Harvard University Press, 1994); Nancy N. Potter, *How Can I Be Trusted: A Virtue Theory of Trustworthiness* (Lanham, MD: Rowman & Littlefield, 2002); Philip Pettit, "The Cunning of Trust," *Philosophy and Public Affairs* 24 (1995): 202–25; and Pellegrino and Thomasma in *The Virtues in Medical Practice,* chap. 5.

37. Aristotle, *Eudemian Ethics,* 1242^b23–1243^a13, in *The Complete Works of Aristotle,* ed. Jonathan Barnes (Princeton, NJ: Princeton University Press, 1984).

38. For a discussion of the erosion of trust in medicine, see David Mechanic, "Public Trust and Initiatives for New Health Care Partnerships," *Milbank Quarterly* 76 (1998): 281–302; Pellegrino and Thomasma in *The Virtues in Medical Practice,* pp. 71–77; and Mark A. Hall, "The Ethics and Empirics of Trust," in W. B. Bondeson and J. W. Jones, ed., *The Ethics of Managed Care: Professional Integrity and Patient Rights* (Dordrecht, Netherlands: Kluwer, 2002), pp. 109–26. Broader explorations of trustworthiness, trust, and distrust appear in Russell Hardin's *Trust and Trustworthiness,* The Russell Sage Foundation Series on Trust, Vol. 4 (New York: Russell Sage Foundation Publications, 2004). Onora O'Neill offers proposals to restore trust in medical and other contexts where mistrust results largely from such factors as bureaucratic structures of accountability, excessive transparency, and public culture. See her *A Question of Trust* (Cambridge: Cambridge University Press, 2002) and *Autonomy and Trust in Bioethics* (Cambridge: Cambridge University Press, 2003).

39. Brody, *Life and Death Decision Making,* p. 35.

40. See Michael Wreen, "Medical Futility and Physician Discretion," *Journal of Medical Ethics* 30 (2004): 275–78.

41. For useful discussions of this question in nursing, see Martin Benjamin and Joy Curtis, *Ethics in Nursing,* 3rd ed. (New York: Oxford University Press, 1992), pp. 105–08; and Betty J. Winslow and Gerald Winslow, "Integrity and Compromise in Nursing Ethics," *Journal of Medicine and Philosophy* 16 (1991): 307–23. For a broader discussion, see also Benjamin, *Splitting the Difference: Compromise and Integrity in Ethics and Politics* (Lawrence, KS: The University Press of Kansas, 1990).

42. For a historically grounded critique of such conceptions and a defense of conscience as a virtue, see Douglas C. Langston, *Conscience and Other Virtues: From Bonaventure to MacIntyre* (University Park, PA: The Pennsylvania State University Press, 2001).

43. Williams, "A Critique of Utilitarianism," in J. J. C. Smart and Williams, *Utilitarianism: For and Against* (Cambridge: Cambridge University Press, 1973), pp. 97–98.

44. We here draw from two sources: Hannah Arendt, *Crises of the Republic* (New York: Harcourt, Brace, Jovanovich, 1972), p. 62; and John Stuart Mill, *Utilitarianism*, chap. 3, pp. 228–29, and *On Liberty*, chap. 3, p. 263, in *Collected Works of John Stuart Mill*, vols. 10, 18 (Toronto, Canada: University of Toronto Press, 1969, 1977).

45. Carl H. Fellner, "Organ Donation: For Whose Sake?," *Annals of Internal Medicine* 79 (October 1973): 591.

46. See Larry May, "On Conscience," *American Philosophical Quarterly* 20 (1983): 57–67. See also C. D. Broad, "Conscience and Conscientious Action," in *Moral Concepts*, ed. Joel Feinberg (Oxford: Oxford University Press, 1970), pp. 74–79, and Childress, "Appeals to Conscience," *Ethics* 89 (1979): 315–35.

47. For several models, see Rebecca Dresser, "Professionals, Conformity, and Conscience," *Hastings Center Report* 35 (November–December 2005): 9–10. See also Mark R. Wicclair, "Conscientious Objection in Medicine," *Bioethics* 14 (July 2000): 2005–27; Alta R. Charo, "The Celestial Fire of Conscience—Refusing to Deliver Medical Care," *New England Journal of Medicine* 352 (2005): 2471–73; Elizabeth Fenton and Loren Lomasky, "Dispensing with Liberty: Conscientious Refusal and the 'Morning-After Pill'," *Journal of Medicine and Philosophy* 30 (2005): 579–92; Julian Savulescu, "Conscientious Objection in Medicine," *British Medical Journal* 332 (2006): 294–97.

48. Farr A. Curlin et al., "Religion, Conscience, and Controversial Clinical Practices," *New England Journal of Medicine* 356 (February 8, 2007): 593–600.

49. For another analysis of "the link between virtues, principles, and duties," see Edmund Pellegrino and David Thomasma, *The Virtues in Medical Practice* (New York: Oxford University Press, 1993), chap. 2.

50. Rosalind Hursthouse, *On Virtue Ethics* (Oxford: Oxford University Press, 2001), p. 17.

51. See Robert Louden, "On Some Vices of Virtue Ethics," *American Philosophical Quarterly* 21 (1984): 229; reprinted in *Virtue Ethics*, ed. Crisp and Slote, pp. 201–16. See also Justin Oakley's discussion of these points in "A Virtue Ethics Approach," in *A Companion to Bioethics*, ed. H. Kuhse and P. Singer (Oxford: Blackwell, 1998), pp. 86–97.

52. See Hursthouse, *On Virtue Ethics*; "Normative Virtue Ethics," in *How Should One Live?: Essays on the Virtues*, ed. Crisp, pp. 16–36; Hursthouse, "Applying Virtue Ethics," in *Virtues and Reasons*, ed. Hursthouse, Gavin Lawrence, and Warren Quinn (New York: Oxford University Press, 1995); and "Virtue Ethics," *The Stanford Encyclopedia of Philosophy*, Fall 2003, http://plato.stanford.edu/archives/fall2003/entries/ethics-virtue/.

53. For a well-argued view that treats the morality of acts as derivative from virtue notions, see Michael Slote, *Morals from Motives* (New York: Oxford University Press, 2001).

54. Our analysis is indebted to David Heyd, *Supererogation: Its Status in Ethical Theory* (Cambridge: Cambridge University Press, 1982); Heyd, "Tact: Sense, Sensitivity, and Virtue," *Inquiry* 38 (1995): 217–31; and Heyd, "Obligation and Supererogation," *Encyclopedia of Bioethics*, 3rd ed. (New York: Thomson Gale, 2004), vol. 4, pp. 1915–20. We are also indebted to J. O. Urmson, "Saints and Heroes," in *Essays in Moral Philosophy*, ed. A. I. Melden (Seattle, WA: University of Washington Press, 1958), pp. 198–216; John Rawls, *A Theory of Justice* (Cambridge, MA: Harvard University Press, 1971; rev. ed. 1999), pp. 116–17, 438–39, 479–85 (1999: 100–01, 385–86, 420–25); Joel Feinberg, "Supererogation

and Rules," *Ethics* 71 (1961); Roderick M. Chisholm, "Supererogation and Offense: A Conceptual Scheme for Ethics," *Ratio* 5 (June 1963): 1–14; and Gregory Mellema, *Beyond the Call of Duty: Supererogation, Obligation, and Offence* (Albany, NY: State University of New York Press, 1991).

55. Albert Camus, *The Plague*, trans. Stuart Gilbert (New York: Knopf, 1988), p. 278.

56. The formulation in this sentence relies in part on Rawls, *A Theory of Justice*, p. 117 (1999: 100).

57. Feinberg, "Supererogation and Rules," 397.

58. See Dena Hsin-Chen and Darryl Macer, "Heroes of SARS: Professional Roles and Ethics of Health Care Workers," *Journal of Infection* 49 (2004): 210–15; Bernard Lo, "Obligations to Care for Persons with Human Immunodeficiency Virus," *Issues in Law & Medicine* 4 (1988): 367–81; Doran Smolkin, "HIV Infection, Risk Taking, and the Duty to Treat," *Journal of Medicine and Philosophy* 22 (1997): 55–74; John Arras, "The Fragile Web of Responsibility: AIDS and the Duty to Treat," *Hastings Center Report* 18 (April–May 1988): S10–S20.

59. See American Medical Association, Council on Ethical and Judicial Affairs, "Ethical Issues Involved in the Growing AIDS Crisis," *Journal of the American Medical Association* 259 (March 4, 1988): 1360–61.

60. Health and Public Policy Committee, American College of Physicians and Infectious Diseases Society of America, "The Acquired Immunodeficiency Syndrome (AIDS) and Infection with the Human Immunodeficiency Virus (HIV)," *Annals of Internal Medicine* 108 (1988): 460–61; and Edmund Pellegrino, "Character, Virtue, and Self-Interest in the Ethics of the Professions," *Journal of Contemporary Health Law and Policy* 5 (1989): 53–73, esp. 70–71.

61. Urmson recognized this problem in "Saints and Heroes," pp. 206, 214. Such imbalance is found in forms of utilitarianism that make strong demands. However, see the attempt to revise consequentialism and bring it in line with common moral intuitions in Douglas W. Portman, "Position-Relative Consequentialism, Agent-Centered Options, and Supererogation," *Ethics* 113 (2003): 303–32.

62. John Stuart Mill, *Considerations on Representative Government*, in *The Collected Works of John Stuart Mill*, vol. 19 (Toronto: University of Toronto Press, 1977), chap. 3, p. 409.

63. Edith Wyschogrod defines a "saintly life" as "one in which compassion for the other, irrespective of cost to the saint, is the primary trait." Wyschogrod, *Saints and Postmodernism: Revisioning Moral Philosophy* (Chicago: University of Chicago Press, 1990), pp. xiii, xxii, et passim.

64. John Berger (and Jean Mohr, photographer), *A Fortunate Man: The Story of a Country Doctor* (London: Allen Lane, the Penguin Press, 1967), esp. pp. 48, 74, 82ff, 93ff, 123–25, 135. Lawrence Blum pointed us to this book and influenced our perspective on it.

65. Our conditions of moral excellence are indebted to Lawrence Blum, "Moral Exemplars," *Midwest Studies in Philosophy* 13 (1988): 204. See also Blum's "Community and Virtue," in *How Should One Live?: Essays on the Virtues*, ed. Crisp.

66. Our second and third conditions are influenced by the characterization of a saint in Susan Wolf's "Moral Saints," *Journal of Philosophy* 79 (1983): 419–39. For a pertinent critique of Wolf's interpretation, see Robert Merrihew Adams, "Saints," *The Journal of Philosophy* 81 (1984), reprinted in Adams, *The Virtue of Faith and Other Essays in Philosophical Theology* (New York: Oxford University Press, 1987), pp. 164–73.

67. Jay Katz, ed., *Experimentation with Human Beings* (New York: Russell Sage Foundation, 1972), pp. 136–40.

68. Philip J. Hilts, "French Doctor Testing AIDS Vaccine on Self," *Washington Post*, March 10, 1987, p. A7; and see Lawrence K. Altman, *Who Goes First?: The Story of Self-Experimentation in Medicine*, 2nd ed. (Berkeley, CA: University of California Press, 1998).

69. David Hilfiker, *Not All of Us Are Saints: A Doctor's Journey with the Poor* (New York: Hill & Wang, 1994). The summaries and quotations that follow come from this book.

70. For the attitudes of nephrologists, transplant nephrologists, and transplant surgeons, see Carol L. Beasley, Alan R. Hull, and J. Thomas Rosenthal, "Living Kidney Donation: A Survey of Professional Attitudes and Practices," *American Journal of Kidney Diseases* 30 (October 1997): 549–57.

71. See Aaron Spital and Max Spital, "Living Kidney Donation: Attitudes Outside the Transplant Center," *Archives of Internal Medicine* 148 (May 1988): 1077–80; and Carl H. Fellner and Shalom H. Schwartz, "Altruism in Disrepute," *New England Journal of Medicine* 284 (March 18, 1971): 582–85.

72. From 1996 to 2005, as living kidney donation overall doubled, the annual percentage of genetically unrelated kidney donors (excluding spouses) rose from 5.9% to 22%. *2006 Annual Report of the U.S. Organ Procurement and Transplantation Network and the Scientific Registry of Transplant Recipients: Transplant Data 1996–2005* (Rockville, MD: Health Resources and Services Administration, Healthcare Systems Bureau, Division of Transplantation, 2006). For an examination of the ethical issues in living organ donation, see James F. Childress and Cathryn T. Liverman, ed., *Organ Donation: Opportunities for Action* (Washington, D.C.: The National Academies Press, 2006), chap. 9.

73. Evelyn Nieves, "Girl Awaits Father's 2nd Kidney, and Decision by Medical Ethicists," *New York Times,* December 5, 1999, pp. A1, A11.

3
Moral Status

The previous two chapters concentrated on moral agents and their obligations, virtues, and relationships. We said little about to whom these obligations are owed, why we owe obligations to some individuals and not to others, and which beings have rights and which do not. We now inquire into these issues of moral status, also referred to as moral standing and moral considerability. A major objective is to determine the scope of the moral community.

THE PROBLEM OF MORAL STATUS

The problem of moral status begins with questions about which individuals and groups are protected by moral norms. For example, what are we to say about human eggs? Embryos? Fetuses? Newborn infants? Anencephalic babies? The mentally disabled? Those who cannot distinguish right from wrong? The seriously demented? Those incurring a permanent loss of consciousness? The brain dead? The corpse? Nonhuman animals used in medical research? Chimeric animals created in research? Do the members of each of these classes deserve moral protections or have moral rights? If so, do they deserve the same complement of protections and rights afforded to autonomous humans? If not, what elevates the autonomous human above members of the groups just listed?

Throughout much of human history, certain groups of human beings (e.g., racial groupings, tribes, or enemies in war) and effectively all nonhuman animals have been treated as less than persons. They have often been treated as not being able to act morally, and, therefore, as either having no moral status or as having a lower moral status. Those without moral status have been regarded as having no moral rights (e.g., historically, slaves in many, and almost certainly most, societies). Those with a lower moral status have fewer or weaker rights (e.g., historically, women in many, and probably most, societies).[1] Thus, having either a full or a partial moral status determines whether an individual or group has a full or a partial set of moral rights. A common, but controversial, presumption in medicine and biomedical ethics is that some groups have no moral rights (e.g., animals used in biomedical research) and that other groups have fewer or weaker rights (e.g., humans who have been judged incompetent have diminished, if any, rights to decide for themselves).

Surrogate decision making is an issue about who qualifies for which moral protections that cuts across many problems of biomedical ethics. (We treat this issue in Chapters 4 and 5.) When a person becomes incompetent and needs a surrogate decision maker, the person judged incompetent does not lose all moral protections and forms of moral respect. Many obligations to these individuals continue, and some may increase. Nonetheless, the recognition of a surrogate as the rightful decision maker entails that the incompetent individual has lost some rights of decision making. A "decision" that such an individual might reach (e.g., to leave a nursing home or mental institution) does not have the same moral authority that it had prior to the determination of incompetency. Generally, we think that our obligations to that person have shifted and that certain ones have even ceased. For example, those related to obtaining first-party informed consent will likely have ceased. The criterion of mental incompetence is one among many in assessing moral status and in determining our precise obligations to persons.

Similar questions arise about what we owe to small children when we involve them in pediatric research that holds out no promise of direct benefit for the subjects (only future benefit for others). Often we think that we owe vulnerable parties more, rather than fewer, protections. Yet children involved in research that is not intended to benefit them are sometimes treated as if they have a diminished moral status and even as utilitarian means to the advancement of research goals.

Consider next the fascinating cases of pregnant women who are brain dead but whose biological capacities are artificially maintained for several weeks to enable the fetus they are carrying to be born.[2] Ordinarily, we would not think of dead people as having a moral status affording them a right to be kept biologically functioning. Indeed, some might argue that maintaining a brain-dead pregnant woman's body against her formerly stated wishes implies that she has been categorized as having a *lower* moral status than other corpses because her body is subjected to extreme measures—sometimes for months—to benefit the fetus, the woman's partner, or next of kin in the family.[3] However, the central ethical question is whether anyone, principally a fetus, has rights stronger than those of a brain-dead pregnant woman who filed an advance directive expressing a wish to have her body cease cardio-respiratory functions at the point of death. Beliefs about the moral status of the fetus clearly are powerful motivating considerations in some cases, but we need to assess carefully whether the fetus is the only individual with moral status and rights at the point of the pregnant woman's brain death. Discussion is ongoing about whether a brain-dead woman has any rights and whether maintaining her body to sustain the pregnancy violates those rights.[4] Even if we recognize the fetus as having moral status, there will still be questions about when in fetal development the fetus acquires this status and whether that status is strong enough to engender a right to be kept alive in the way these fetuses are being maintained.

Finally, we need to consider our views of and practices toward the many nonhuman animals that we use in biomedical research. At times we appear to treat them fundamentally as our utilitarian means to the ends of science, facilitated by the decisions of some person or group said to be their "stewards." The implication seems to be that laboratory animals are not morally protected against invasive, painful, and harmful forms of experimentation, and, indeed, that they lack moral status. However, an outright denial of moral status is implausible in light of the fact that virtually every nation and major scientific association has guidelines to alleviate, diminish, or otherwise limit what can be done to animals in biomedical research. It is today generally accepted that experimental animals have some form of moral status, but it is less clear what warrants this judgment and whether our obligations to these animals also imply that they have rights.

At the root of these and related questions is a rich body of theoretical issues and practical problems about moral status.

Theories of Moral Status

To have moral status is to deserve the protection afforded by moral norms, including the principles, rules, obligations, and rights discussed in Chapter 1. Such protections are afforded only to entities that can be morally wronged by actions. Here is a simple example: We wrong a person by intentionally infecting his or her computer with a virus, but we do not wrong the computer itself even if we damage it irreparably and render it nonfunctional. It is possible to have duties with regard to some entities, such as someone's computer, without having duties to those entities.[5] By contrast, if we deliberately infect a person's dog with a harmful virus, then it seems that we have not only wronged the dog's owner, we have also wronged the dog. Why are persons and dogs different than computers or, for that matter, rocks?

The mainstream approach has been to ask whether a being is *the kind of entity* to which moral principles or other moral categories can and should be applied and, if so, based on which *properties* of the being. Some say that there is one and only one property that confers moral status. For example, some say that this property is human dignity—an unclear notion that moral theory has done little to clarify. Others say that another property, or perhaps several properties, are needed to acquire moral status—for example, sentience, rationality, or moral agency.

We argue in this chapter that the properties identified in prominent theories of moral status will not, by themselves, resolve the main issues about moral status, but that *collectively* these theories can be used to provide us with a general, although untidy, framework for handling problems of moral status. We begin by looking at each of the five theories and assessing why each one is attractive, yet deeply problematic if taken as the only acceptable theory. We argue that each theory presents a plausible perspective on moral status that merits attention, but that no theory by itself is adequate. We identify the conditions presented in each theory that are relevant criteria of moral status, even though we find each theory problematic in some crucial respect. We conclude that each theory fails to account adequately for the ways we do, and should, approach issues of moral status. Nonetheless, progress can be made in understanding both the problems of moral status and why, despite their deficiencies, all five theories merit serious attention.

We doubt that it is possible to resolve definitively all controversies about moral status, and we make no pretense to do so here. However, we do try to show why disagreement persists, and sometimes rages, over the moral status of some individuals, and we suggest plausible ways to reduce the conflict.

A Theory Based on Human Properties

The first theory might be called the traditional account of moral status. It holds that distinctively human properties, those of *Homo sapiens,* confer moral status. All humans have full moral status and only humans have that status. Distinctively human properties demarcate that which has *moral value* and delineate which beings constitute the *moral community.* In this theory, an individual has moral status if and only if that individual is conceived by human parents—or, alternatively, if and only if it is an organism with a human genetic code. To be a living member of the species *Homo sapiens* is a necessary and sufficient condition of moral respect. The following is a concise statement of such a position by two members of the President's Council on Bioethics:

> Fertilization produces a new and complete, though immature, human organism. The same is true of successful cloning. Cloned embryos therefore ought to be treated as having the same moral status as other human embryos. A human embryo is a whole living member of the species Homo sapiens in the earliest stage.... Human embryos possess the epigenetic primordial for self-directed growth into adulthood.... We were then, as we are now distinct and complete.... To deny that embryonic human beings deserve full respect, one must suppose that not every whole living human being is deserving of full respect. To do that, one must hold that those human beings who deserve full respect deserve it not in virtue of the kind of entity they are, but, rather, in virtue of some acquired characteristic that some human beings...have and others do not, and which some human beings have in greater degree than others.... [Even embryos] are quite unlike cats and dogs.... As humans they are members of a natural

kind—the human species.... Since human beings are intrinsically valuable and deserving of full moral respect in virtue of what they are, it follows that they are intrinsically valuable from the point at which they come into beings.[6]

Many find such a theory attractive because it unequivocally covers all human beings and demands that no human be excluded on the basis of a property such as being a fetus, having brain damage, or having a congenital anomaly. We expect a moral theory to cover everyone, without making arbitrary or rigged exceptions. This theory meets that standard. The moral status of human infants, mentally disabled humans, and those with a permanent loss of consciousness (in a persistent vegetative state) is not in doubt or subject to challenge in this theory. This theory is also attractive because it fits well, intuitively, with the moral belief that all humans have "human rights" precisely because they are human, whether or not the rights are legally recognized in a political state.[7] This theory thus reflects the commonsense proposition that all human beings are persons and that the moral obligation of "respect for persons" is a basic moral norm. One way to interpret a "principle of respect for persons" is as a principle of moral status that determines to whom moral principles apply, namely, all human beings.

Despite its attractive features, this theory is problematic as a general theory of moral status. If we were to train nonhuman apes to converse with us and engage in moral relationships with us (as some believe has already occurred), it would be baseless and prejudicial to say that they have a lesser status merely because of a *biological* difference in species. If we were to encounter a being with properties such as intelligence, memory, and moral capacity, we would frame our moral obligations toward that being not only or even primarily by asking whether it is or is not biologically human. We would look to see if such a being has capacities of reasoning and planning, has a conception of itself as a subject of action, is able to act autonomously, is able to engage in speech, or makes moral judgments. If it does have such properties, its moral status (at some level) is assured, whereas if it had no such properties, its moral status would be more in question, depending on the precise properties it had. Accordingly, human biological properties are not necessary conditions, or the only sufficient conditions, of moral status.

The criterion of "human properties" using species criteria is also not as clear as adherents to this first theory often seem to think. Consider the example of a monkey-human chimera created for the purposes of stem-cell research. This research, which has the objective of alleviating or curing neurological diseases and injuries, is conducted by inserting a substantial human cell contribution into a developing monkey's brain. Investigators implant human neural stem cells into a fetal bonnet monkey's brain to see what the cells do and where they are located.[8] Thus far, no such chimeric being has been allowed to progress past early fetal stages, but such a chimera might be born. There are cells in this chimera

that are distinctly human and cells that are distinctly monkey. The monkey's
brain is developing under the influence of the human cells. Should it be born, it
could possibly think and behave in humanlike ways (no one knows as yet). In
theory, the larger the proportion of engrafted human cells relative to host cells,
the higher the likelihood of humanlike features or responses. Such a chimera
would possess a substantial human biological contribution, and could even have
capacities for speech and moral behavior, especially if the great apes were the
selected species. There also are transgenic animals (animals that possess and
express genes from a different species). An example is the much discussed
Harvard oncomouse, which has only mouse cells but also has bits of human
DNA and develops human skin cancers.[9]

There has been little opposition, other than a few concerns about human
safety, to most mixtures of human and animal tissues and cells in the context of
medical care (e.g., transplantation of animal parts or insertion of animal-derived
genes or cells) and biomedical research (e.g., several kinds of insertion of human
stem cells into animals). Matters become more complicated, from an ethical
standpoint, when animal–human *hybrids* are created. The President's Council
on Bioethics in the United States found "especially acute" the ethical concerns
raised by the possibility of mixing human and nonhuman gametes or blastom-
eres to create a hybrid. It opposed creating animal–human hybrid embryos by
ex vivo fertilization of a human using animal sperm or by an animal egg using
human sperm. One reason for this caution is the difficulty society would face
in judging the humanity and the moral status of such an "ambiguous hybrid
entity."[10] These and other possible developments challenge the belief that there
are fixed species boundaries determinative of moral status.[11]

The first theory of moral status also confronts another problem: It is correct to say that the commonsense concept of *person* is, in ordinary language,
functionally identical to the concept of *human being,* but there is no warrant for
the stronger assertion that *only* properties distinctive of the human species count
toward personhood or that species membership determines moral status. Even
if certain properties strongly correlated with membership in the human species
qualify humans for moral status more readily than the members of other species, these properties are only contingently connected to being human. These
properties could be possessed by members of nonhuman species or by entities
outside the sphere of natural species, such as God, chimeras, robots, and genetically manipulated species (and biological humans could, in principle, lack these
properties).[12]

"Person" is itself too vague a category to resolve these problems of moral
status.[13] Some people maintain that what it means to be a person is simply to have
some human biological properties; others maintain that personhood is delineated
not biologically, but in terms of certain cognitive capacities, moral capacities, or
both. What counts as a person seems to expand or contract as theorists construct

their theories so that precisely the entities for which they advocate will be judged to be persons. In one theory, human embryos are declared persons and the great apes are not, whereas in another theory the great apes are persons and human embryos are not. The concept of "personhood" is so inherently contestable that we avoid it in this book insofar as possible. This is one reason, among others, why we shy away from the language of "respect for persons." Our goal is to be as precise as possible about what is and must be respected. Use of the vague language of "person" tends to undercut this goal.

This first theory of moral status might seem salvageable if we include not merely human biological properties but also distinctively human psychological properties; that is, properties exhibiting distinctively human mental functions of awareness, emotion, cognition, motivation, intention, volition, and action. This broader scope, however, will not rescue this theory. If nonhuman animals are not morally protected—in a context of biomedical research, say—because they lack certain psychological characteristics such as self-determination, moral motivation, language use, and moral emotions, then consistency requires us to say that humans who also lack these characteristics lack moral protections for the same reason. For any human psychological property we select, some human beings will lack this characteristic (or lack it to the relevant degree); and frequently some nonhuman animal will possess this characteristic. Primates, for example, often possess humanlike properties that many humans lack, such as intelligence, the capacity to feel pain, and the ability to enter into meaningful social relationships. We have to ask, then, what would make it appropriate to use primate subjects, but not human subjects, in research. It begs the question to say that we should use animal subjects because of the benefits of human health that will accrue to us from their use. In some cases, these same benefits could be obtained by doing research on humans, such as brain-dead corpses or humans with permanent loss of consciousness.

This first theory, then, is not by itself an adequate account of moral status. Undoubtedly, mature human agents supply the initial model of the properties that qualify an individual for moral status, but a theory erected entirely on *species* properties is not a theory premised on mature human *agency*. A shift to psychological properties might incorporate a theory of agency (see the third theory in this chapter), but a theory of this sort would inevitably exclude many humans and invite inclusion of many nonhumans. If the argument thus far is correct, human species properties do not constitute *necessary* conditions of moral status. This conclusion rejects various traditional views still relied on today in the biomedical sciences. Tradition itself is no justification, just as traditions of slavery never constituted a justification of slavery. Stating a preference for tradition is no better than asserting a brute preference in favor of one's own species or culture.

Nonetheless, it would be morally perilous to give up altogether the idea that properties of humanity form a basis of moral status. This position is entrenched in morality and provides the basis of the claim that all humans have human rights. Accordingly, the proposition that some set of human properties is *a sufficient* condition of moral status, although not a necessary condition, is an acceptable position.[14] We leave it an open question precisely which set of properties counts, and we acknowledge that argument is needed to show that some species properties count whereas others do not. It could turn out that this first theory will ultimately be absorbed by a more precise theory that is not developed in terms of *species* properties. It also could turn out that the properties we regard as the critical, distinctively human properties are not distinctively human at all.

However these questions are ultimately answered, the acceptance of a criterion of human properties does not rule out the possibility that properties other than distinctively human ones also constitute sufficient conditions of moral status. We therefore need to consider the other four theories.

A Theory Based on Cognitive Properties

A second theory of moral status moves beyond biological criteria and species membership to a specific set of cognitive psychological properties. "Cognition" here refers to processes of awareness such as perception, memory, understanding, and thinking. This theory does not assume that only humans have such properties, although the starting model for these properties is again the competent human adult. The theory is that individuals have moral status because they are able to reflect on their lives through their cognitive capacities and are self-determined by their beliefs in ways that incompetent humans and nonhuman animals are not.

Properties found in theories of this second type include: (1) self-consciousness (consciousness of oneself as existing over time, with a past and future); (2) freedom to act and capacity to engage in purposeful actions; (3) ability to give and to appreciate reasons for acting; (4) capacity to communicate with other persons using a language; and (5) rationality and higher order volition.[15] The goal of these theories is to identify a set of psychological properties possessed by all and only persons, under the assumption that persons and only persons have moral status. One is a person if and only if one possesses the cognitive properties that distinguish higher level beings from lower level beings. Anything having the higher level properties has moral status. We here set aside disputes internal to these theories about precisely which cognitive properties are jointly necessary and sufficient for personhood, and therefore for moral status. To investigate the problems with this theory, it does not matter whether only one or more than one of these criteria must be satisfied to qualify for moral status.

The model of an autonomous human being—the usual starting place for theories of moral status—is itself conceived in terms of such cognitive properties as self-awareness, processing information, choosing, and authorizing. The theory of such properties as the basis of moral status holds that if a nonhuman animal, a human fetus, or a brain-damaged human is in all relevant respects like a cognitively capable human being, then it has a similar (and presumably identical) moral status. A corollary is that if one is *not* in the relevant respects like a cognitively competent human being, one's moral status is correspondingly reduced or vacated.

This second theory is subject to several different interpretations and to different mixtures of the five above-mentioned criteria. Increasing the number or level of the required cognitive abilities will reduce the number of individuals who satisfy its conditions, and therefore fewer individuals will qualify for moral status, or at least for elevated moral status. For example, if all five of the previously mentioned criteria must be satisfied, many humans would be excluded from moral status. Likewise, reducing the quality or level of required cognitive skill would increase the number of individuals who qualify for protection under the theory. If, say, only understanding and intentional action were required, many children and nonhuman animals would qualify.

A worrisome feature of this theory is that infants, the senile elderly, persons with a severe mental disability, and others we generally view as having a secure moral status lack the cognitive capacities required to attain moral status. Most nonhuman animals also lack such cognitive capacities. The level of cognitive abilities demanded also varies from theory to theory. In explicating a Kantian position, Christine Korsgaard writes that "Human beings are distinguished from animals by the fact that practical reason rather than instinct is the determinant of our actions."[16] If this is so, many biological humans are animals (and not "human beings" in her sense), because they also lack practical rationality.

An objection to this theory, often directed against theories predicated primarily on human dignity and autonomy, is generally referred to as "the argument from marginal cases": This argument sets out to show that every major cognitive criterion of moral status (intelligence, agency, self-consciousness, etc.) excludes some nonautonomous humans, including young children and humans with serious brain damage. These "marginal" cases of cognitive human capacities can be at the same level of cognitive and other capacities as some animals, and hence to exclude these animals is also to exclude comparably situated humans. If animals can be treated as mere means to human ends, then comparable "marginal" cases of human capacity can also be treated as mere means to human ends.[17] This claim is obviously dangerous for all humans who are weak, vulnerable, and incapacitated.

This theory therefore does not function, as does the first theory, to ensure that vulnerable human beings will be morally protected. The more vulnerable the individual, by virtue of cognitive deficiency, the weaker the moral protection afforded. The fact that individuals who are members of the human species will typically exhibit higher levels of cognitive capacities than members of other species does not alleviate this problem. In this theory, a nonhuman animal in principle can overtake a human in moral status once the human loses a measure of mental abilities after a cataclysmic event or a decline of capacity. For example, once the primate in training in a language laboratory exceeds a deteriorating Alzheimer's patient on the relevant scale of cognitive capacities, the primate attains a higher moral status.[18]

Many writers in biomedical ethics assume that nonhuman animals lack the relevant cognitive abilities, including self-consciousness, autonomy, or rationality, and that they are therefore not elevated in status by this theory. However, this premise is more assumed than demonstrated. It ignores evidence of types and degrees of intelligence and awareness of nonhuman animals, not to mention that comparative studies of the brain show many relevant similarities between the human species and some other species. In some behavioral studies, language-trained apes appear to make self-references, and many animals learn from the past and then use their knowledge to forge intentional plans of action for hunting, stocking reserve foods, and constructing dwellings.[19] These animals are aware of their bodies and their interests, and they distinguish those bodies and interests from the bodies and interests of others. In play and social life, they understand assigned functions and either follow designated roles or decide for themselves what roles to play.[20] Moreover, many animals seem to understand and intend in ways that some incapacitated humans cannot. These are all *cognitively* significant properties, and therefore, in this second theory, they are *morally* significant properties that award a more elevated moral status to nonhuman animals with the properties than to humans who lack them. This conclusion should not be taken as a problem for a consistent defender of the second theory. It is a problem only for those who assume a priori that only *humans* have the requisite cognitive capacities.

A problem that defenders of this second theory need to address is how to establish the importance and relevance of the connection asserted between cognitive properties and moral protections. Why do *cognitive* properties of individuals determine anything at all about their *moral* status? This is not to say that a theory of moral status cannot be based on nonmoral properties. It can. But a theory of moral status needs to make a connection between its nonmoral properties and moral status, which will supply the basis of the claim that the lack of a certain property entails a lack of moral status. Defenders need to explain why the absence of this property makes a critical moral difference and precisely what that difference is. If a fetus or a very senile individual lacks cognitive properties, it does not follow that moral protections and moral status are lacking—at least it does not follow without supporting argument.

To conclude this section, this second theory, like the first, fails to establish that cognitive capacity is a *necessary condition* of moral status. However, cognitive capacity is arguably a *sufficient condition* of moral status. Cognitive capacities such as reasoned choice occupy a central place in what we respect in an individual when we invoke moral principles such as "respect for autonomy." The main problem with this second theory is not that it invokes these properties, but rather that it considers *only* cognitive properties and neglects other potentially relevant properties, most notably properties on the basis of which individuals can suffer and enjoy well-being. We will see in Chapters 5 and 6—and in examining the fourth theory of moral status later in this chapter—that these non-cognitive properties ground the principles of nonmaleficence and beneficence in important ways. This problem takes us to the remaining three theories.

A Theory Based on Moral Agency

In the third theory, moral status derives from the capacity to act as a moral agent. The category of a *moral agent* is subject to different interpretations, but it is safe to assume that an individual is a moral agent if two conditions are satisfied: (1) the individual is capable of making moral judgments about the rightness and wrongness of actions, and (2) the individual has motives that can be judged morally. These are moral-capacity criteria, not conditions of morally correct action or character. An individual could make immoral judgments or have immoral motives and still be a moral agent.[21]

There are several theories of this general type, some with more stringent conditions of moral agency than the two just listed. Historically, the most influential theory of moral agency is that of Immanuel Kant, who seems to have intended his theory primarily as an account of moral worth, autonomy, and dignity, although many of its conclusions suggest that he is stating conditions of moral status. In Kant's theory, moral autonomy of the will is central. It occurs if and only if one knowingly governs oneself in accordance with universally valid moral principles. Moral autonomy gives an individual "an intrinsic worth, i.e., dignity," and "hence autonomy is the ground of the dignity of human nature and of every rational creature." One has dignity "only insofar as" one is an autonomous agent.[22]

Whether or not Kant intended his theory as one of moral status, he and others have suggested that capacity for moral agency gives an individual a moral respect and dignity not possessed by individuals incapable of moral agency—human or nonhuman. This account of moral status has one clearly attractive feature: Being a moral agent is indisputably a *sufficient* condition of moral status. Moral agents are paradigmatic bearers of moral status. They know that we can condemn their motives and actions, blame them for irresponsible actions, and punish them for immoral behavior.

Accordingly, this third theory again supplies a *sufficient* condition of moral status, but, like the first two, it fails to identify a *necessary* condition of moral status. If being a moral agent (or being morally autonomous) were a necessary condition of moral status, then many humans to whom we extend moral protections would be stripped of their moral status, as would all nonhuman animals. Many psychopaths, patients with severe brain damage, and patients with advanced dementia would be considered to have no moral status in this theory. Yet individuals in these classes deserve to have their interests attended to by many parties, including institutions of medical care. Obviously the reason for such protections is not a capacity of moral agency, because they have none.

The theory of moral agency as a necessary condition of moral status is, in the final analysis, strongly counterintuitive. A morally appropriate response to vulnerable parties such as young children, the severely retarded, and senile patients is that they deserve *special* protection, not that they merit no protection. Whether these individuals are moral agents is not the primary consideration. They have moral status, and it is not grounded in moral agency.

In sum, the third theory yields a sufficient condition of moral status but not a necessary one. Being a moral agent is not the only way to acquire moral status. We will now see that a fourth theory lends support to this conclusion.

A Theory Based on Sentience

Humans as well as nonhuman animals have properties that are neither *cognitive* nor *moral* properties, and yet count toward moral status. These properties include a range of emotional and affective responses, the single most important being *sentience*—that is, consciousness in the form of feeling, especially the capacity to feel pain and pleasure (as distinguished from consciousness as perception or thought). Proponents of the fourth theory claim that having the capacity of sentience is a sufficient condition of moral status. Some defenders also claim that this capacity is both *necessary and sufficient* for moral status—a more difficult claim to support.[23]

The central line of argument in the fourth theory is the following: Pain is an evil, pleasure a good. To cause pain to any entity is to harm it. Many beings can experience pain and suffering.[24] To harm these individuals is to *wrong* them, even if harming them is justified in certain circumstances.

This simple argument, which is further pursued in Chapter 5, is directly pertinent to the issue of moral status. The properties of experiencing pain and suffering are almost certainly sufficient to confer some measure of moral status. One of the main objectives of morality is to minimize pain and suffering and to prevent or limit indifference and antagonism toward those who are experiencing pain and suffering. If anything is fundamental to morality, it is that actions that cause pain and suffering to others are prohibited unless one has a morally good and sufficient reason for performing those actions. We need look no further than ourselves to find this point convincing: Pain is an evil to you, and the intentional infliction of pain is a moral-bearing action, from your perspective. Even if you were not cognitively capable, morally capable, or biologically human, pain and suffering would be real to you. What matters, in circumstances of pain, is not your species membership or intellectual or moral capacities, but your pain. From this perspective, all entities that can experience pain and suffering have moral status and can be morally wronged when others cause them pain and suffering.

This theory has broad scope. It reaches to vulnerable humans as well as to animals used in research. Most vertebrate animals are sentient (mammals, birds, reptiles, amphibians, and fish), and some invertebrate animals may be sentient or at least capable of subjective experience. We study animals in biomedical research because of their similarities with humans, and here a moral problem arises: The reason to use animals in research is that they are so similar to humans, and the reason not to use animals in research is that they are so similar to us in their experience of pain and suffering. Most notably in the case of primates, their lives are damaged and their suffering is often like human suffering because they resemble us physically, cognitively, and emotionally. To the extent that pain and suffering are real to us, they are real to nonhuman animals. The more we have learned about these animals (our knowledge still being rather rudimentary), the more important problems of pain and suffering have become.

This view underlies Jeremy Bentham's famous statement: "The question is not, Can they *reason?* nor, Can they *talk?* but, Can they *suffer?*"[25] Moral claims on behalf of any individual, human or nonhuman, need have nothing to do with intelligence, capacity for moral judgment, self-consciousness, rationality, personality, or any other such fact about the individual. Sentience, then, seems clearly to be a *sufficient* condition of moral status.

Exactly *who* or *what* is covered by this conclusion, and *when,* is disputed in literature on human fetal research and abortion. If sentience confers moral status, then a human fetus has moral status no later than the point of sentience. Growth to sentience in the sense of a biological process is gradual over time, but the acquisition of sentience, or the first glimmer of sentience, is not itself a gradual process. That point is, in this theory, the point at which moral status is obtained. Some writers argue that development of a functioning central nervous system and brain is the proper point of moral status for the human fetus, because it is the biological condition of sentience.[26] This approach does not protect human blastocysts or embryos and has proved to be an uncertain basis on which to build arguments allowing or disallowing abortion, because there is disagreement about when the brain has developed sufficiently for sentience. However, in this theory a fetus does have moral status at some point after several weeks of development, and thus abortions at that point would be (prima facie) impermissible. This point is prior to the stage of development at which some legal abortions now occur.[27] We are not, in making these observations, presenting objections to sentience theory or to any version of it. We are simply noting that these problems must be handled by a viable theory.

The theory that sentience is a sufficient condition of moral status makes more modest claims than the theory that sentience is a necessary and sufficient condition, and therefore the only criterion of moral status. The latter theory is embraced by several philosophers who hold that properties and capacities other than sentience, such as human biological life and cognitive and moral capacities, are not correct bases of moral status.[28] Nonsentient beings, such as computers, robots, and plants (and also nonsentient animals), lack the stuff of moral status precisely because they have no capacity for pain; and all other beings deserve moral consideration because and only because they are sentient.

Several problems arise for this account of the fourth theory. First, problems confront the claim that any individual lacking the capacity for sentience lacks moral status. On the human side, this theory disallows moral status for early-stage fetuses as well as for all who have irreversibly lost the capacity for sentience, such as patients with severe brain damage. It also has the potential to exclude all nonsentient, nonhuman beings, most notably the lower animals, from any degree of moral status. To see this outcome as a problem, we need not hold that these classes of beings actually do have moral status. It is arguable that they do not. For example, it can be argued that presentient fetuses are morally equivalent to human tissue, that absence of significant brain activity denies moral status to patients in a persistent vegetative state, and the like. Of course, a defense of the fourth theory requires that argument along these lines be successful. It is not satisfactory merely to assert that absence of sentience is sufficient for absence of moral status. Proponents of the sentience theory might seek to defend it in several ways, and some defenses will add another criterion of moral status to that of sentience. This maneuver would give up the claim that sentience is a necessary and sufficient condition of moral status, thereby abandoning the theory itself.

A second problem with some versions of the fourth theory is their *impracticability* (where "practicability" is understood as capability of being effected or put into practice). We could not hope to implement this theory in our conduct with regard to all species whose members are capable of sentience—and certainly we could not do so without grave danger to human beings. Virtually no one believes, or defends the view, that we cannot have public health policies that vigorously control for pests and pestilence by extermination. Here the most plausible argument by a sentience theorist who holds the view that sentience is necessary for moral status is that the theory only grants *some level* of moral status. However, this is a dangerous retreat if the level of moral status is then fixed by features other than sentience itself. For example, if features such as higher cognitive capacities or moral agency are required to attain a higher level of moral status, this supplementation abandons a pure sentience theory.

If the interests of all living beings in avoiding pain and suffering count *equally* in this fourth theory (a thesis not discussed earlier), then the suffering of a human being would count for no more than the suffering of any other creature and practicability would loom as a massive problem. It is implausible to argue that all sentient beings can be treated with the same moral consideration or given an equal level of moral protection against pain and suffering.

We might try to rescue the theory that sentience is both necessary and sufficient for moral status by recognizing (1) that not all sentient creatures have the same level of sentience, and (2) that, even among creatures with the same level of sentience, sentience may not have the same significance because of its interaction with other properties they possess. Some writers believe that there is a gradation of richness or quality of life, depending on complexity of consciousness, social relationships, ability to derive pleasure, creativity, and the like. A continuum of moral status scaled from the autonomous adult human down through the lowest levels of sentience can in this way be layered into the sentience theory. Through this or some similar maneuver, it can be argued that merely because many sentient animals have moral status, it does not follow that humans should be treated no differently than other animals. There may be many good reasons for differential treatment.

In one version of this theory, recognition of a continuum of moral status need not assign different value to different species. We might, as Martha Nussbaum argues, hold that species with more "complex forms of life" are vulnerable to greater and different types of harm and suffering: "The type and degree of harm a creature can suffer varies with its form of life."[29] In a second, quite different, version of such a theory, Raymond Frey argues that a human life with the capacity for richness of consciousness has a higher moral status and value than even a very rich animal life such as that of a dog or a bonobo. This judgment has nothing to do with species membership, but with "the fact that [rich, conscious] human life is more valuable than animal life" by virtue of experiences such as real autonomy.[30]

However, such theories have risks. They hold that, even among sentient beings, the degree of moral status and the level of moral protection can vary according to conditions such as the quality, richness, or complexity of life. A life therefore can lose its value by degrees as conditions of welfare and richness diminish. As loss of capacity occurs, humans and nonhumans will alike have a decreased moral status. In this way, the most vulnerable beings can become the most vulnerable to abuse and exploitation. No theory is morally acceptable that yields this conclusion.

In light of the several problems surrounding the theory of sentience as a necessary condition of moral status, we conclude that this fourth theory—like the first three theories—is best interpreted as providing a sufficient, but not a necessary, condition of some level of moral status. Our analysis leads to the conclusion that this theory needs supplementation by the other theories. Sentience theory could be used to determine what has moral status, whereas the other theories could be called on to determine the degree of moral status. Sentience, in this interpretation, is advanced only as a sufficient condition of *some level* of moral status. Nothing in this theory indicates the precise level of status or the proper scope of moral protections, and the other theories are called on to help resolve this profoundly difficult and complex moral problem.

A Theory Based on Relationships

A fifth and final theory is based on relational properties. This theory holds that relationships between parties account for moral status, primarily relationships that establish roles and obligations. An example is the patient–physician relationship, which is a relationship of medical need and care. Once this relationship is initiated, the patient gains a right to care that other persons who are not the physician's patient lack. The patient does not have this status independent of the established relationship, and the physician does not have the same obligations to those outside such a relationship. This relationship may deepen and gain new dimensions of status as the parties come to know and trust one another. Trusting and caring relationships in which both parties understand and agree are paradigm cases of rights and obligations established and maintained through relationships. Other examples are found in relationships that do *not* involve a formal understanding between the parties, such as our bonds with persons with whom we work closely, our affectionate relations with our pets, and our intimate friendships. These relationships bring value to our lives, and moral obligations often arise from them.

This fifth theory potentially brings many individuals into the moral community that are not moral actors in that community. Babies and companion animals are examples. This theory tries to capture the conditions under which certain relationships, especially those involving social interaction and reciprocity, are stronger and more influential than relationships with strangers and others outside an interpersonal connection. It also tries to account for our degrees of sensitivity to and sympathy for the interests and capacities of other individuals. In the case of both humans and nonhumans, some individuals are in closer contact with us than others; some engage our affections more easily than others; and some become close to us because the relationship occurs over a long period of time. This is apparent with family, friends, and companion animals, but it is not limited to these groups.

One version of this theory of moral status depicts relationships as developing over time and in diverse ways.[31] Moral status does not come through a decisive event that can, independently of communal relationships, be determined at a particular time. Moral status is accorded to classes of beings (human fetuses, Alzheimer's patients, experimental animals, etc.) by virtue of a history in which the human moral community has assessed the importance of its relationship to these classes as well as the burdens of offering moral protections to entities in these classes.

Some proponents of relationship theory argue that the human fetus and the newborn are examples of those who gradually come, through social relationships, to have a significant moral status. Conversely, the less the fetus is part of a nexus of social relationships, the weaker is the fetus's claim to moral status:

> The social role in question develops over time, beginning prior to birth.... A matrix of social interactions between fetus and others is usually present well before parturition. Factors contributing to this social role include the psychological attachment of parents to the fetus, as well as advances in obstetric technology that permit monitoring of the health status of the fetus.... The less the degree to which the fetus can be said to be part of a social matrix, the weaker the argument for regarding her/him as having the same moral status as persons. Near the borderline of viability,... the fetus might be regarded as part of a social network to a lesser degree than at term. If so, the degree of weight that should be given to the fetus's interests varies, being stronger at term but relatively weaker when viability is questionable.[32]

Despite its attractions, this fifth theory faces problems. It leaves a nagging worry that social bonds and attitudes alone determine moral status. Critical rights such as the right to life have no force independent of a community's conferral or rejection of those rights. The theory suggests that if those reasonably expected to value the life of a newborn, the life of someone in a persistent vegetative state, or the life of a research animal do not in fact value these lives, there is no social nexus of value, and thus the life itself has no value or moral status.

It is not clear how determinative this theory is or can be made to be. Once fetuses, for example, are detected in utero by stethoscope or sonogram, they become in significant respects part of a social matrix. They therefore seem to gain some measure of moral status at that point, according to this theory. If fetuses late in pregnancy have a significant moral status, it will be hard to show why fetuses earlier in pregnancy do not have the same form and level of moral status.

This fifth theory also neglects or omits insights in the previous four theories. Those theories recognize moral status on the basis of qualities (cognition, sentience, etc.) that can be acknowledged independently of an established relationship. For example, in the fourth theory, the property of sentience is status conferring. When we wrongfully harm a human research subject or an animal research subject—by inflicting unjustifiable pain, say—it is not correct to say that the harming is wrong because we have an established laboratory or clinical relationship with the individual. We behave wrongly because we cause gratuitous and unnecessary pain, and this would be so whether or not an established relationship exists with the individual. The reason that we should not be cruel to either humans or animals is because they suffer from our cruelty, which is independent of a moral community or relationship.

Finally, and perhaps most important, this fifth theory runs together several different problems about moral status. The problem of moral status is fundamentally about which beings have moral status. This fifth theory does not seem to address this problem. Rather, it addresses related problems having to do with (1) how one gains or loses a specific moral right or obligation, such as the doctor and patient in the earlier example; and (2) the different degrees of moral status, such as moral agents having a higher degree of status than individuals lacking such agency. Many relationships do not themselves determine that an individual has moral status; rather, they determine the nature of the status had by those with moral status.

Accordingly, this fifth theory should not be accepted as supplying a sufficient condition of moral status, and clearly it does not supply a necessary condition.[33] Many kinds of loving and caring relationships, with many kinds of beings, do not confer moral status on those beings. No matter how much we love a favorite plant or institution, neither the plant nor the institution gains status by virtue of this relationship. Nor does the lack of a relationship necessarily indicate a lack of moral status; an individual still may gain status under criteria drawn from one of the four previous theories (humanity, cognition, moral agency, and sentience). This seems the best way to maximally preserve claims of moral status for those individuals who no longer have significant interpersonal relationships. They will not be stripped of moral status merely because certain relationships have been lost.

This fifth theory is unlike the other four theories in that it does not supply a sufficient condition of moral status. This theory's contribution is to show that certain relationships account for how one gains or loses a specific moral right or obligation, and therefore the theory helps account for different degrees of moral status.

FROM THEORIES TO PRACTICAL GUIDELINES

Each of the five theories that we have examined has elements that are worthy of acceptance. However, each theory risks making the mistake of isolating a single property or type of property—biological species, cognitive capacity, moral agency, sentience, or communal relationships—as the sole criterion of moral status. Each theory proposes using its preferred basis for both including certain individuals and excluding those lacking the preferred property. Each theory falls into implausibility when it loses sight of the merit in competing criteria.

It is worrisome that those who defend these theories often seem to select their preferred criteria to match and support their pretheoretical moral position about who deserves moral status and moral protections. This preference

could derive from religious commitment, political orientation, food preferences, or moral intuition. From ancient Hellenic times to the present, we have
witnessed pretheoretical moral positions, and motives are at work when groups
of people (e.g., slaves and women) have been refused a certain social standing
on grounds that they lack some property and therefore do not have full moral
status. Over time, views about the moral acceptability of these presumed criteria
have changed, and therefore beliefs about the moral status of members of these
groups have changed, even though none of their relevant properties has changed.
For example, women and many minority groups who had been denied significant moral status—or at least *equal* moral status—had an increased moral status
socially conferred on them. The worry today is that many groups—especially
vulnerable groups—may still be in a discriminatory social situation: They fail to
satisfy reigning criteria of moral status precisely because these criteria have been
tailored specifically to deny them partial or full moral status.

The evident remedy, and the one we recommend, is to accept the criteria
advanced in each of the first four theories as an acceptable general criterion of
moral status and the fifth theory as adding another relevant dimension to these
theories. Unfortunately, more work than we can undertake here would be needed
to develop the precise nature and limits of these criteria and to determine whether
they are hierarchically ranked. The primary norms in each theory—which we
hereafter refer to as *criteria* of moral status (rather than as *theories* or *conditions*
of moral status)—work well for some problems and circumstances in which
decisions must be made, but not as well for other problems and circumstances.

On Appropriating the Five Theories

Ideally, we will be able to appropriate the best from each of the five theories
and meld these elements together into a multicriterial, coherent account of moral
status.[34] This strategy will help accommodate the diversity of opinion that surrounds issues of moral status, will help us balance the interests of different parties to public controversies such as the interests of scientists in new knowledge
and the interests of research subjects, and will help avoid intractable clashes of
rights, such as conflicts between the rights of scientists to academic freedom and
the rights of human embryos. We hereafter assume that, in principle, the ideal
of a coherent, multicriterial account of moral status can be satisfied. However,
a unified and comprehensive account of moral status will always be a massive
project in the making, and we make no claim to have achieved it here.

Several problems confront this project, four of which we address in this section. First, interpretation and analysis are required of some central concepts. For
instance, the concept of "human life" has long been problematic in the literature
of biomedical ethics, as we hinted in treating the five theories of moral status.
"Human life" carries at least two very different meanings. On one hand, it can

mean *biological human life,* the biological characteristics that set the human species apart from nonhuman species, as in the first theory presented previously. On
the other hand, "human life" can mean *life that is distinctively human*; that is, a
life characterized more by psychological than biological properties or abilities.
This meaning is closer to the second and third theories. For example, the abilities
to use symbols, to imagine, to love, and to perform higher intellectual skills are
among the most distinctive human properties, but not all biologically human
individuals possess these capacities.

A simple example illustrates the gap and the tension between these two
senses of "human life": Some infants with extreme disabilities die shortly after
birth. They are born of human parents and they are biologically human, but they
never exhibit the distinctively human psychological traits mentioned in the second and third theories and in many cases lack the potential to do so. For these
individuals it is not possible to make their human lives, in the biological sense,
human lives in the psychological sense. In discussions of moral status that use
the language of "human life," we need to specify which properties are excluded
and which included in the use of the term.

Second, the problem of potentiality is prominent in theories of moral status.
Human embryos and fetuses are often the centerpiece of discussion because they
are developing individuals with the potential for, without yet having acquired,
cognitive properties, moral agency, and social relationships. If unimpaired and
uninterrupted in development, they have the potential to satisfy every condition
of moral status set out in all five theories. Some writers argue that it is as wrong
to harm or kill beings with the potential for these properties as it is to harm or
kill beings that actually possess them. More generally, the idea is that it is morally wrong to intentionally cause a being with the potential to develop status-
conferring properties to lose or to fail to realize that potential.

Moral responsibilities to the fetus in utero have long been discussed in biomedical ethics, and more recently discussion has focused on moral responsibilities to the embryo created by in vitro fertilization and located in the Petri dish or
freezer. Three general positions have emerged regarding the moral status of the
developing fetus in utero and of the embryo in the Petri dish or freezer: (1) mere
tissue, (2) potential human life (with some, perhaps intermediate, moral status),
and (3) full human life (with full moral status). The first position has many defenders, especially, it appears, among scientists, whereas the third position prominently
appears in certain forms of religious thought. For instance, the official Roman
Catholic position holds that human life (in the normative sense) begins at conception, and it treats this potentiality as morally equivalent to actuality or fulfillment.
The second position (potential human life) seems to be the dominant view in most
Protestant and Jewish traditions, as well as in secular thought. It often includes
a moral presumption against abortion and embryo destruction, while holding
that both can be justified under some conditions. In one such view, early-stage

embryos have an "intermediate moral status" and thus deserve "special respect," but this special respect is compatible with using the embryos for biomedical research if a reasonable prospect exists that such research will save human lives. Although perhaps done with a "heavy heart,"[35] the research is justified if necessary to achieve promising and consequential biomedical goals.

Problems of potentiality are nuanced and compelling, and they need more analysis than we can provide here. We note, however, that whatever degree of moral status is possessed by a being with the potential for status-conferring properties, the individual's rights still may be justifiably overridden by the rights of others under some circumstances. This contingent conflict of rights now propels us to consider degrees of moral status (and, in the next section, to consider conflicts among different parties, where each party has moral status).

Degrees of moral status is the third of the four problems mentioned previously. Not all individuals who have moral status have it categorically, without qualification, or fully. They have it by degrees. For example, consider *rights*, which are one manifestation of moral status. Not all humans who have rights have the full complement of rights. Competent, adult humans generally have a broader array of rights, especially rights of self-determination and liberty, than other individuals. Some of the five theories we have addressed can be expressed in terms of other ways of stating degrees of moral status. For example, in the fourth theory, based on sentience, moral status is arguably proportional to degree of sentience and perhaps to the quality and richness of sentient life. Similarly, the fifth theory, based on relationships, is expressible in terms of degrees of relationship. Relationships vary in importance and come in different degrees of closeness.

However, implementing the idea of degrees of moral status carries major problems of misunderstanding and possible abuse. A comprehensive theory must deal with the fact that not all criteria of moral status are clearly amenable to analysis in terms of degrees, including criteria in the first theory (based on properties of humanity) and the third theory (based on moral agency). It could be philosophically difficult to express these criteria in terms of degrees, and, in some cases, morally dangerous to do so.

A difficult case involves the potential to become a sentient, cognitively aware, moral agent. In some theories this potential is not expressible by degrees; full potential is there from the start of an individual's existence, and therefore the fetus has full moral status in all critical respects. In other theories this potential merely *enhances* moral status. These theories hold that human fetuses, and possibly infants, have a lower degree of moral status precisely because they are merely potential persons. In one version of these theories, the moral standing of zygotes, embryos, fetuses, and newborns increases gradually during gestation.[36] This theory can also be expressed in terms of a limited set of rights—for instance, pregnant women have a higher moral status than their fetuses, at least at some stages of fetal development. The theory can also be developed to make potentiality itself a matter of degree (degree of potential). For example, serious brain defects in a fetus or infant can affect not only potential for cognitive and moral awareness, but the potential for the relationships a human fetus and infant can form with others.

A practically oriented theory of moral status will need to determine with some precision what an individual's or a group's status is, not merely that the individual or group has some form of status. Because "status" refers to a grade or rank of moral importance, the precise grade or rank will need to be specified. A comprehensive theory will explain whether and, if so, how the grade or rank will change as the properties that contribute to status are progressively gained or lost. However, we ought not to be optimistic that such a theory can be developed to cover all problems of moral status, and a coherent theory is unlikely to be the only coherent one. A plausible, philosophically defensible, practical theory of moral status is the most we can expect.

Fourth and finally, the criteria advanced in the five theories themselves come into moral conflict in some circumstances. How can we ease or resolve these conflicts? We treat this problem in the next section. Related questions concern whether these five criteria can be shown to be coherent. We treat some problems of coherence in Chapter 10.

The Connection between Moral Norms and Moral Status

At the beginning of this chapter we distinguished questions of moral status from the question of moral norms addressed in Chapter 1. Moral norms are principles and rules that state obligations and, correlatively, rights. We reaffirm the distinction between problems of moral status and problems of moral norms, but we now qualify it in this important respect: *Criteria of moral status are moral norms in the generic sense of "moral norm."* A norm is a (prima facie) standard that has the authority to judge or direct human belief, reasoning, or behavior. A norm guides, commands, requires, or commends. Failure to follow a norm warrants censure, criticism, disapproval, or some related form of negative appraisal. Criteria of moral status satisfy this description. Although they are not the same type of norm as "principles" and "rules," they are normative.

Criteria of moral status also should be understood in light of the discussions in Chapter 1 of *moral conflict, moral dilemmas, prima facie* norms, and the *specification* of norms. These criteria can and often do come into conflict. For example, the criterion of sentience (drawn from theory 4) and the criterion of human species membership (drawn from theory 1) conflict in the attempt to determine the moral status of the early-stage human fetus. The sentience criterion suggests that the fetus gains status only at the point of sentience; the criterion of human properties (in theory 1) suggests that moral status accrues at biological inception. (Also, to complicate the picture, on one interpretation of the criterion of relational properties, in theory 5, moral status is gained only when certain relationships are formed after birth, but some relationships could be formed in utero—for instance, after ultrasound visualization.) We can address such conflicts by using the account of specification delineated in Chapter 1. Deliberating about and reaching conclusions about specific cases will require becoming more specific about moral status than the five theories discussed thus far allow in the abstract. However, in becoming more specific, we will encounter difficult and even unresolvable moral dilemmas of the sort discussed in Chapter 1.

As we have seen, having moral status does not entail having an absolute claim or right. Satisfying criteria of moral status affords moral protection, but the rights established may be overridden by competing moral considerations in some circumstances. Suppose, for example, that a human fetus (at some designated stage of development) has a level of moral status that includes a right not to be harmed by a research intervention or by an abortion. There still may be cases of justified intervention and abortion. A pregnant woman may legitimately abort the fetus in "self-defense" if she will die unless she terminates the pregnancy. Moral conflict is here reasonably interpreted as a conflict of rights: The unborn possess some rights, including a right to life, and pregnant women also possess some rights, including a right to life. Those who possess rights have a (prima facie) moral claim to be treated in accordance with their rights. It is not possible to avoid all conflicts among rights, and, in exactly the same way, all conflicts among parties with moral status.

Guidelines Governing Moral Status: Putting Specification to Work

The account of specification put forward in Chapter 1 helps us address contingent conflicts between criteria of moral status. We specify norms by narrowing their scope. In this section we adapt the model of specification to create "guidelines" governing moral status. Others might call them rules rather than guidelines, but we reserve the term *rules* for specifications of principles. Tersely expressed, *rules* specify principles, whereas *guidelines* specify criteria of moral status. Our proposals attempt to extract content from the criteria in each of the five theories to show how that content can be shaped into progressively more practical guidelines.

We will state these guidelines in terms of a "*level* of moral status." The idea of a level is interpreted in light of our earlier discussion of degrees of moral status (pp. 81, 84–85). We will assume that there is a continuum of moral status, running from a limited range of moral protections (usually marking out basic rights) to the full complement of moral protections. For example, infants, the mentally handicapped, and many persons who are legally incompetent have some level of moral status, but they do not have the same level of moral status as autonomous persons. Those who lack substantial autonomy simply do not have the same decision-making rights as those who are substantially autonomous.

We turn now to some illustrative specifications that qualify as guidelines of moral status. We are not here *recommending* these guidelines. We are only attempting to clarify their nature and their basis. Presumably reasons can be provided for the selection of one specification over another, although we cannot here present reasoned defenses of the specifications we discuss.

Consider first a circumstance in which the criterion "All living human beings have some level of moral status" comes into conflict with the criterion "All sentient beings have some level of moral status." Here are two possible specifications that engage the criteria put forward in theories 1 (the criterion of human life) and 4 (the criterion of sentience):

Guideline 1. All human beings who are sentient or have the biological potential for sentience have (some level of) moral status; all human beings who are not sentient and have no biological potential for sentience have no moral status.

This specification allows for a further specification to particular groups such as anencephalic individuals (those without a cerebrum and cerebellum) and individuals who have sufficient brain damage that they are not sentient and have no potential for sentience. This guideline says that such groups have no moral status. By contrast, the guideline assigns (some level of) moral status to all healthy human embryos and fetuses because they are either sentient or have the potential to be sentient. Thus, this guideline cannot be used to support human embryonic stem-cell research or abortions. Indeed, it stands opposed to these practices.

A different, and obviously *competitive,* guideline achieved through specification is this:

Guideline 2. All human beings who are sentient have (some level of) moral status; all human beings who are not sentient, including those with a mere potential for sentience, have no moral status.

This second guideline has clear implications for whether embryos and early-stage fetuses have moral status, and therefore implications for moral debates about human embryonic stem-cell research and early-stage abortions. This guideline states that although life prior to sentience is morally unprotected, the fetus is protected against abortion and research interventions once it becomes sentient.[37] Clarifying the exact implications of this second guideline would require further specification(s). In the case of abortion, even when a fetus is sentient its continued existence could threaten the life or health of the pregnant woman. On one line of further specification, sentient fetuses possess the same rights possessed by all human beings, and an abortion is as objectionable as any killing of an innocent person. On a different line of further specification, sentient fetuses would have a diminished set of rights if their presence threatens the life of a pregnant woman. In the abstract form presented above, guideline 2 should be viewed as only a first step in grappling with problems governing several classes of individuals, and therefore a first step in a line of specification.

Here is a third guideline reached by specification that makes an appeal both to theory 4 (sentience) and to theory 2 (cognitive capacity):

> Guideline 3. All sentient beings have some level of moral status; the level of moral status is elevated in accordance with the level of sentience and the level of cognitive complexity.

According to this guideline, the more highly sentient the individual and the richer the mental life of the individual, the higher the level of moral status. This guideline is a first step toward working out the common intuition that great apes deserve stronger protections than pigs, which deserve more protection than rats, and so forth. However, there is no guarantee that this guideline will support any intuition of species preference; for example, pigs could turn out to have a richer mental life than dogs.

Consider now a fourth guideline, this one a specification of the criterion of moral agency (theory 3) in conflict with the criterion of human-species properties (theory 1):

> Guideline 4. All human beings capable of moral agency have equal basic rights; all sentient human beings not capable of moral agency have a diminished set of rights.

This guideline elevates the status of moral agents and gives a lesser status to all other sentient creatures, including all other members of the human species. A defense of this guideline would need an account of equal basic rights and of which rights are not held by those incapable of moral agency (a subject treated in Chapter 4).

Consider, finally, an example of a possible guideline that engages the demands of the fifth theory (of status through relationships) and the fourth theory (of sentience). This specification tailors the two criteria to the circumstance of laboratory animals. The following formulation assumes the moral proposition that the "communal" relationship between persons in charge of a laboratory and the animals in it is morally significant:

> Guideline 5. All sentient laboratory animals have a level of moral status that affords them some level of protections against being caused pain or suffering; as the likelihood or the magnitude of potential pain or suffering increases, the level of special protections must be increased.

This guideline is the first step in making precise the idea that laboratory animals who benefit human communities gain a stronger moral status than would be acquired merely by sentience alone. This guideline is, in the context of laboratory animals, meant to express what historically has often been referred to as stewardship: careful and responsible management of the situation of another entrusted to one's care.

These five guidelines are still so abstract and indeterminate that they may seem of doubtful practicability. If their abstractness cannot be further reduced, this would be unfortunate because practicability is an important criterion of an ethical theory. (See earlier, pp. 22, 77–78, and, later, Chapter 9, pp. 337.) We recognize, of course, that these guidelines need further development and defense and that they will be difficult to bring to bear on the world of biomedical experimentation and all areas of medical practice that present difficult cases. There will be ample room for disagreement at each stage of specification.

Nonetheless, these and other guidelines can be progressively specified to the point of practicability, just as moral principles can (as we argued in Chapter 1). To become a practical instrument, the account of moral status that we have presented in this chapter would have to be developed in richer detail and tested for implications and counterexamples. Still, the criteria in our account of moral status are not so abstract as to leave us without practical guidance. Acceptance of these criteria would powerfully refocus and restructure some of our moral obligations to and relationships with many individuals, human and nonhuman. This is a matter of great importance. Practices of slavery as well as abuses of human research subjects have thrived historically in part as a result of defective criteria of moral status. In our lifetimes, some children who were institutionalized as mentally infirm, some elderly patients in chronic disease hospitals, and some racial groups were treated in the United States as if they had little or no moral status by some of the finest centers of biomedical research in the world and by funders of that research as well.[38] It is easy to forget how recognition of moral status can generate interest in and support vital moral protections.[39]

VULNERABLE POPULATIONS

Much of the concern about moral status in biomedical ethics has derived from concern about so-called vulnerable populations. Vulnerable persons in biomedical contexts are incapable of protecting their own interests because of sickness, debilitation, mental illness, immaturity, cognitive impairment, and the like. They are often unprotected by relevant rights, exposed to potentially harmful circumstances, lacking in decision-making capacity, and socioeconomically impoverished. Those who are easily susceptible to intimidation, manipulation, coercion, or exploitation are commonly classified among the vulnerable. Accordingly, even populations such as homeless families, political refugees,

and illegal aliens—whose members have often been human research subjects—
can be grouped as *vulnerable*. However, this term should be used with caution,
because it can function to stereotype and overly protect.

Historically, many populations were manipulated or coerced into "service"
as research subjects, and they became paradigm instances in biomedical ethics
of vulnerable populations. Fetuses, children, the mentally incapacitated, those
housed in impersonal institutions, and laboratory animals, among others, have
been and continue to be vulnerable populations in research settings. This history
reminds us that those who are socially devalued are subject to abuse and exploitation in a variety of contexts. The paradigm case is, of course, the Nazi program
of extermination in the name of euthanasia and service to medical research.[40]

Guidelines for Vulnerable Populations

In controversies that have arisen over research uses of vulnerable populations,
one of three positions might be taken on the justification of any particular
research practice:

1. Do not allow the practice (a policy of full prohibition).
2. Allow the practice without regard to conditions (a policy of full
   permissibility).
3. Allow the practice only under certain conditions (a policy of partial
   permissibility).

Public opinion is deeply divided over which of these three is the most appropriate
policy to govern various uses of fetuses in research—in utero and after deliberate abortions. Many prefer the first, many the second, and many the third. Split
opinions are less typical of debates about experimentation with animals, experimentation with children, and experimentation with incompetent individuals. Few
today defend either full prohibition or full permissibility on research with these
groups, but many would support a prohibition on the use of certain classes of
these individuals, such as the great apes or seriously ill children. To reject the first
two guidelines is to accept the third, which in turn requires that we establish the
precise set of moral protections afforded (in accord with the level of moral status)
and determine the conditions that allow us to proceed or not to proceed.[41]

Problems of moral coherence hang over these issues. Near universal agreement exists that humans who lack certain capacities should not be used in
biomedical research that is risky and does not offer them a prospect of direct
benefit. Protections for these vulnerable populations should be high because of
their vulnerability. Nonhuman animals are usually not treated equivalently. Their
limited cognitive and moral capacities become the substantive justification *for*
rather than *against* their use in biomedical research when human subjects cannot
ethically be used. How we can justify causing harm and premature death to these

animals, but not to humans with similarly limited capacities, is an unresolved issue of coherence in biomedical ethics.[42]

Practices of abortion, particularly where fetuses are capable of sentience, raise directly related issues of coherence. The struggle over abortion primarily concerns two questions: (1) What is the moral status of the fetus (at various developmental points)? (2) What should we do when the rights generated by this status conflict with the rights of women to control their futures? Near universal agreement exists that a very late-term fetus is not relevantly different from a newborn. Another month earlier in development will also show little difference in morally relevant differences, and coherence threatens any point on the continuum at which a decision is made about moral status. As with animal subjects, the status of human fetuses tends to be downgraded because of their lack of sentient, cognitive, and moral capacities, which becomes the substantive justification for abortion. Questions about whether we can justify such downgrading and whether we can justify causing premature death to the fetus remain some of the most difficult questions in biomedical ethics.

There are human benefits of a system in which the lives of fetuses and research animals can be terminated. The range of impressive, truly indispensable, benefits produced by animal research, in particular, raises questions about whether such research should be restricted, and, if so, in which ways. However, research that involves, but is not intended to benefit, vulnerable humans raises the same questions as research involving animals. All research involves some level of risk or harm, and it often has a compelling justification because of its potential benefits. The moral challenge is to make our answers to these questions coherent, allowing different levels of risk of harm for different classes of individuals only when a criterion of moral status permits unequal treatment.

Sympathy and Impartiality

Problems of moral status and vulnerable populations can be profitably discussed in terms of our capacity to sympathize with the predicament of others. In previous sections of this chapter we have connected our reflections on moral status to the discussion of *moral norms* in Chapter 1. Now we connect these reflections to our account of *moral character* in Chapter 2, by focusing briefly on moral sympathy, a trait similar to compassion and usually involving empathy, both of which we discussed in Chapter 2.

The capacity for sympathy enables us to enter into, although imperfectly, the thoughts and feelings of another being. Through sympathy, we form a concern for the welfare of others. Such sympathizing does not necessarily imply generosity or favorable responsiveness. A convicted criminal who is put to death may engage our sympathy without engaging our generosity, mercy, leniency, or assistance. Research investigators, veterinarians, and animal trainers may have a rich and sympathetic understanding of the humans or the nonhuman animals they encounter, without necessarily exhibiting generosity or mercy toward them.

David Hume discerningly argued that most human beings have only a *limited* sympathy with the plight of others, but also have some level of capacity to overcome these limits through calm, reflective judgments:

> [T]he generosity of men is very limited, and...seldom extends beyond their friends and family, or, at most, beyond their native country.... [T]ho' [our] sympathy [for others] be much fainter than our concern for ourselves, and a sympathy with persons remote from us much fainter than that with persons near and contiguous; yet we neglect all these differences in our calm judgments concerning the characters of men.[43]

Hume notes that bias and partiality enter into many relationships and judgments. Our sympathy for others, he judges, is almost always fainter than our concern for ourselves. After we attend to ourselves, our sympathy reaches out most naturally to our intimates, such as the members of our family. From there sympathy typically moves to some wider, but still relatively small, group of acquaintances, such as those with whom we have the most frequent contact or in whose lives we have most heavily invested. Our sympathy with those truly remote from us (strangers or persons in other nations, say) is usually diminished, by comparison to sympathy with those close to us. The "distance or contiguity," as Hume puts it, between others and us makes a critical motivational difference in how we regard and think about our obligations to them. Both *dissimilarity to* and *distance from* other persons function to limit our sympathy. People in nursing homes are often both dissimilar to and distant from other persons, as are people with diseases such as Lesch-Nyhan, human embryos, and animals used in research, among others. Hence, it is harder for us to view these individuals as having a significant moral status that places demands on us. Even though we know that many in vulnerable populations suffer, our sympathy and moral responsiveness do not come easily. Not surprisingly, many among the "moral saints" we discussed in Chapter 2 are persons who exhibit an *expanded* sympathy with the plight of those who suffer—a form of sympathy beyond the level most of us achieve or even hold as a moral ideal.

Severely limited sympathy, together with severely limited generosity, help explain such social phenomena as child abuse, animal abuse, and the neglect of enfeebled elderly persons in nursing homes. It is regrettable, of course, that enlarged affections are not commonplace in human interactions, but this fact is predictable given what we know about human nature.

One way Hume proposes to address limited sympathy for those different from us is the deliberate exercise of impartiality through "calm judgments": "It is necessary for us, in our calm judgments and discourse...to neglect all these differences, and render our sentiments more public and social."[44] He asks us to make as strong an effort as we can to realize a more extensive sympathy. His proposal is in line with our discussion in Chapter 2 of "moral excellence." A morally excellent person will work both to enlarge his or her affections for those who suffer and to reach calm and unbiased judgments. Hume characterizes his ideal as a "common" or "general" point of view in moral judgment—an impartial viewpoint. This perspective, which some philosophers call "the moral point of view," controls for the distortions and biases created by our closeness to some individuals, and also opens us up to a more extensive sympathy.[45]

This attitude could help address the problems encountered in this chapter. At the same time, it would be unreasonable to insist on a moral point of view with such a deep sympathy and extensive impartiality that, for example, it is applied equally across time (to ancient civilizations), cultures (to those culturally very dissimilar to us), geography (to those very far from us), and species (to those with few, if any, humanlike qualities). Extensive sympathy therefore should be viewed as a regulative but arduous ideal of character and conduct. The arduously ideal nature of extensive sympathy is one reason why issues of moral status are intractable and problems of coherence are so difficult.

CONCLUSION

In this chapter we have used the language of "theories," "criteria," and "guidelines" of moral status, rather than the language of "principles," "virtues," and "character" that dominated Chapters 1 and 2. It is best to distinguish these forms of discourse and the territories of morality they cover, even though all are normative. We have not argued that the common morality—as discussed in Chapters 1 and 2—gives us an adequate and workable framework of criteria of moral status. We return to this problem near the end of Chapter 10, where we discuss both the common morality and the possibility of "moral change" in conceptions of moral status.

NOTES

1. This history and its relevance for biomedical ethics—with special attention to slavery—are presented in Ronald A. Lindsay, "Slaves, Embryos, and Nonhuman Animals: Moral Status and the Limitations of Common Morality Theory," *Kennedy Institute of Ethics Journal* 15 (December 2005): 323–46. On the history of problems about moral status for nonhuman animals, see Andrew N. Rowan, *Of Mice, Models, and Men: A Critical Evaluation of Animal Research* (Albany, NY: State University of New York Press, 1984), especially chaps. 3–4.

2. D. J. Powner and I. M. Bernstein, "Extended Somatic Support for Pregnant Women after Brain Death," *Critical Care Medicine* 31 (2003): 1241–49; David R. Field et al., "Maternal Brain Death During Pregnancy," *Journal of the American Medical Association* 260 (August 12, 1988): 816–22; Xavier Bosch, "Pregnancy of Brain-Dead Mother to Continue," *Lancet* 354 (December 18–25, 1999): 2145; "Brain-Dead Va. Woman Dies," *Boston Globe*, August 4, 2005, p. A4.

3. See Hilde Lindemann Nelson, "The Architect and the Bee: Some Reflections on Postmortem Pregnancy," *Bioethics* 8 (1994): 247–67; D. Sperling, "From the Dead to the Unborn: Is There an Ethical Duty to Save Life?" *Medicine and Law Journal* 23 (2004): 567–86; and Christoph Anstotz, "Should a Brain-Dead Pregnant Woman Carry Her Child to Full Term?: The Case of the 'Erlanager Baby,'" *Bioethics* 7 (1993): 340–50.

4. Sarah Elliston, "Life after Death? Legal and Ethical Considerations of Maintaining Pregnancy in Brain Dead Women," in *Intersections: Women on Law, Medicine and Technology,* ed. Kerry Petersen (Aldershot, England: Ashgate, 1997), pp. 145–65; and Jay E. Kantor and Iffath Abbasi Hoskins, "Brain Death in Pregnant Women," *Journal of Clinical Ethics* 4 (Winter 1993): 308–14.

5. On this distinction, see Mary Midgley, "Duties Concerning Islands," in *Environmental Ethics,* ed. Robert Elliott (Oxford: Oxford University Press, 1995).

6. Robert P. George and Alfonso Gomez-Lobo, "The Moral Status of the Human Embryo," *Perspectives in Biology and Medicine* 48 (2005): 201–05.

7. Cf. the Preamble and Articles in the *United Nations Universal Declaration of Human Rights.* http://www.un.org/Overview/rights.html (accessed May 19, 2007).

8. On September 7, 2001, V. Ourednik et al. published an article entitled "Segregation of Human Neural Stem Cells in the Developing Primate Forebrain," *Science* 293 (2001): 1820–24. This is the first report of the implanting of human neural stem cells into the brain of a primate, creating a monkey–human chimera. The copy of the human cells was taken from the brain of a fifteen-week-old fetal cadaver. One motive prompting this research is that it is considered unethical to graft, for experimental purposes, human neural cells into human beings.

9. "Chimeric" usually refers to the cellular level, whereas "transgenic" concerns the genetic level. We here follow the reports and argument in Mark K. Greene et al., "Moral Issues of Human–Non-human Primate Neural Grafting," *Science* 309 (July 15, 2005): 385–86. Cf. Jason Robert and Francoise Baylis, "Crossing Species Boundaries," *American Journal of Bioethics* 3 (2003): 1–13 (and commentaries following); Henry T. Greely, "Defining Chimeras…and Chimeric Concerns," *American Journal of Bioethics* 3 (2003): 17–20; and Robert Streiffer, "At the Edge of Humanity: Human Stem Cells, Chimeras, and Moral Status," *Kennedy Institute of Ethics Journal* 15 (2005): 347–70.

10. Although some argue for permitting the creation of animal–human hybrids for research purposes, as long as they are destroyed within a specified period of time, the President's Council recommended a federal ban on their creation. See The President's Council on Bioethics, *Reproduction & Responsibility: The Regulation of New Biotechnologies* (Washington, DC: The President's Council on Bioethics, 2004); also available at www.bioethics.gov (accessed August 21, 2007). See also Scottish Council on Human Bioethics, *Embryonic, Fetal and Post-natal Animal–Human Mixtures: An Ethical Discussion* (Edinburgh, U.K.: Scottish Council on Human Bioethics, 2006); http://www.schb.org.uk/ (accessed August 12, 2006). The Scottish body worried that pluripotent stem cells might participate in the tissue of the germline and in the brain and recommended a ban on the incorporation of human pluripotent stem cells into a nonhuman blastocyst (and its early embryonic stage) or postblastocyst and a similar ban on the incorporation of nonhuman pluripotent stem cells into a human blastocyst (and its early embryonic stage) or postblastocyst.

11. National Research Council, National Academy of Science, Committee on Guidelines for Human Embryonic Stem Cell Research, *Guidelines for Human Embryonic Stem Cell Research* (Washington, DC: National Academies Press, 2005); Amendments 2007 available online. Some human–nonhuman grafting has, technically, already taken place through xenografting, using, for example, fetal pig cells. See J. S. Fink et al., "Porcine Xenografts in Parkinson's Disease and Huntington's Disease Patients: Preliminary Results," *Cell Transplant* 9 (2000): 273–78.

12. The language of "person" has a long history in theology, especially in Christian theological efforts to explicate the three individualities of the Trinity. On the potential of chimeras, see Greene et al.,

"Moral Issues of Human–Nonhuman Primate Neural Grafting." On the relevance of robots and physical-mental systems that imitate human traits, see John Pollock, *How to Build a Person* (Cambridge, MA: MIT Press, 1989) and Ausunio Marras, "Pollock on How to Build a Person," *Dialogue* 32 (1993): 595–605.

13. See further Tom L. Beauchamp, "The Failure of Theories of Personhood," *Kennedy Institute of Ethics Journal* 9 (1999): 309–24. For early and influential analysis of this problem, see Jane English, "Abortion and the Concept of a Person," *Canadian Journal of Philosophy* 5 (1975): 233–43; and Roland Puccetti, *Persons* (London: Methuen, 1970).

14. At least one adherent of the first theory reaches precisely this conclusion. See Patrick Lee, "Personhood, the Moral Standing of the Unborn, and Abortion," *Linacre Quarterly* (May 1990): 80–89, esp. 87.

15. See a variety of accounts in Michael Tooley, *Abortion and Infanticide* (Oxford: Clarendon, 1983); Harry G. Frankfurt, *Necessity, Volition, and Love* (Cambridge: Cambridge University Press, 1999), chaps. 9, 11; Mary Anne Warren, *Moral Status* (Oxford: Oxford University Press, 1997), chap. 1; H. Tristram Engelhardt, Jr., *The Foundations of Bioethics,* 2nd ed. (New York: Oxford University Press, 1996), chaps. 4, 6; and Lynne Rudder Baker, *Persons and Bodies* (Cambridge: Cambridge University Press, 2000), chaps. 4, 6.

16. Korsgaard, "Kant's Formula of Humanity," in *Creating the Kingdom of Ends* (Cambridge: Cambridge University Press, 1996), pp. 110–11. See also her considerable elaboration of the position in her Tanner Lecture, "Fellow Creatures: Kantian Ethics and Our Duties to Animals," http://www.tannerlectures.utah.edu/lectures/volume25/korsgaard_2005.pdf (accessed August 27, 2007). Korsgaard has a very difficult time with the basis of moral status for humans who seem to lack all rationality, and consequently with what is later here called the argument from marginal cases.

17. See Tom Regan, *The Case for Animal Rights* (Berkeley, CA: University of California Press, 1983; updated ed. 2004), pp. 178, 182–84.

18. Exactly how this conclusion should be developed is morally disputable. It would clearly be wrong to treat a late-stage Alzheimer patient in the way in which biomedical researchers often treat experimental animals, but it can be argued for the same reasons that we should treat primate research subjects as well as we treat late-stage Alzheimer patients. Similarly, to return to the argument in the previous paragraph, if it is outlandish to assert that "marginal" cases of human capacity can be treated as mere means to human ends, then it is arguably the case that the way researchers often use animals as mere means is morally outlandish.

19. See Donald R. Griffin, *Animal Minds: Beyond Cognition to Consciousness,* 2nd ed. (Chicago: University of Chicago Press, 2001); and Rosemary Rodd, *Ethics, Biology, and Animals* (Oxford: Clarendon, 1990), esp. chaps. 3–4, 10.

20. Cf. Gordon G. Gallup, "Self-Recognition in Primates," *American Psychologist* 32 (1977): 329–38; David DeGrazia, *Taking Animals Seriously: Mental Life and Moral Status* (New York: Cambridge University Press, 1996), esp. p. 302.

21. These criteria also would require, in a deeper analysis than we can provide here, explication in terms of some of the cognitive conditions discussed previously. For example, the capacity to make moral judgments requires a certain level of the capacity for understanding.

22. Kant, *Grounding for the Metaphysics of Morals,* trans. James W. Ellington, in Kant, *Ethical Philosophy* (Indianapolis, IN: Hackett, 1983), pp. 38–41, 43–44 (Preussische Akademie, pp. 432, 435–36, 439–40).

23. See two opposed theories on the latter issue in L. Wayne Sumner, *Abortion and Moral Theory* (Princeton, NJ: Princeton University Press, 1981) and Bonnie Steinbock, *Life Before Birth: The Moral and Legal Status of Embryos and Fetuses* (New York: Oxford University Press, 1992).

24. Although we use both terms—pain and suffering—and although they are sometimes used interchangeably, a distinction is often drawn between them on the grounds that suffering requires more cognitive abilities than the mere experience of pain.

25. Bentham, *An Introduction to The Principles of Morals and Legislation,* ed. J. H. Burns and H. L. A. Hart; with a new introduction by F. Rosen; and an interpretive essay by Hart (Oxford: Clarendon, 1996).

26. Baruch Brody, *Abortion and the Sanctity of Life* (Cambridge, MA: MIT Press, 1975). Brain birth is said to be analogous to brain death at critical transition points.

27. This point is made in Stephen Griffith, "Fetal Death, Fetal Pain, and the Moral Standing of a Fetus," *Public Affairs Quarterly* 9 (1995): 117.

28. Peter Singer, *Animal Liberation,* 2nd ed. (London: Pimlico, 1995), p. 8; Sumner, *Abortion and Moral Theory.*

29. Nussbaum, *Frontiers of Justice: Disability, Nationality, Species Membership* (Cambridge, MA: Harvard University Press, 2006), p. 361. Nussbaum argues that species membership is not "morally and politically irrelevant" in that, properly understood, it can give us "the appropriate benchmark for judging whether a given creature has decent opportunities for flourishing." Hence, efforts should be undertaken to bring a child with mental retardation up to a certain level of function, for instance, in the use of language, whereas such efforts are not required for a chimpanzee who has a comparable level of mental function, but for whom language use is a not essential. *Frontiers of Justice,* pp. 357–66.

30. In this theory, life is valuable and has moral status only under certain conditions of quality of life. Life, therefore, can lose its value and moral status by degrees as conditions of welfare and richness of experience decrease. Because nonhuman animals and seriously ill humans lead lives that are less rich in such elements than in healthy humans, these lives are, by degrees, reduced in quality, value, and moral status. This theory acknowledges that "animals are indisputably harmed" in some biomedical research, but insists that there is "an especially compelling case that such uses benefit humans." Frey, "Moral Standing, the Value of Lives, and Speciesism," *Between the Species* 4 (Summer 1988): 191–201; "Animals," in *The Oxford Handbook of Practical Ethics* (New York: Oxford University Press, 2003), esp. pp. 163, 178; and "Autonomy and the Value of Animal Life," *Monist* 70 (January 1987): 50–63.

31. See Ronald Green, "Stem Cell Research:…Determining Moral Status," *American Journal of Bioethics* 2 (Winter 2002): 20–30.

32. Carson Strong and Garland Anderson, "The Moral Status of the Near-Term Fetus," *Journal of Medical Ethics* 15 (1989): 25–26.

33. See the argument in Nancy Jecker, "The Moral Status of Patients Who Are Not Strict Persons," *The Journal of Clinical Ethics* 1 (1990): 35–38.

34. This strategy is proposed in Warren, *Moral Status.*

35. Quoted notions are in the voice of some members of the President's Council on Bioethics who support human cloning-for-biomedical-research. See The President's Council on Bioethics, *Human Cloning and Human Dignity* (New York: Public Affairs, 2002), pp. 153–58.

36. See Carson Strong, "The Moral Status of Preembryos, Embryos, Fetuses, and Infants," *The Journal of Medicine and Philosophy* 22 (1997): 457–78.

37. Cf. the similar conclusion, with an argued defense, in Mary Anne Warren, "Moral Status," in *A Companion to Applied Ethics,* ed. R. G. Frey and Christopher Wellman (Oxford: Blackwell, 2003), p. 163.

38. Classic cases in the United States are the Tuskegee syphilis experiment, the use of mentally retarded children at the Willowbrook State School, and the injection of cancer cells into debilitated patients at the Jewish Chronic Disease Hospital in Brooklyn. For the first, see James H. Jones, *Bad Blood: The Tuskegee Syphilis Experiment*, rev. ed. (New York: Free Press, 1993); for the others, see Jay Katz, *Experimentation with Human Beings: The Authority of the Investigator, Subject, Professions, and State in the Human Experimentation Process* (New York: Russell Sage Foundation, 1972).

39. Parallel debates in environmental ethics focus on the moral status or considerability of nature beyond human and nonhuman animals; for example, whether individual trees, plants, species, and ecosystems have moral status. See Kenneth Goodpaster, "On Being Morally Considerable," *Journal of Philosophy* 75 (1978): 308–25; Paul Taylor, *Respect for Nature: A Theory of Environmental Ethics* (Princeton, NJ: Princeton University Press, 1986); Thomas Birch, "Moral Considerability and Universal Consideration," *Environmental Ethics* 15 (1993): 313–32; Holmes Rolston, III, "Duties to Endangered Species," *BioScience* 35 (1985): 718–26; and Lawrence E. Johnson, *A Morally Deep World: An Essay on Moral Significance and Environmental Ethics* (Cambridge: Cambridge University Press, 1993).

40. See Patricia Backlar, "Human Subjects Research Ethics: Research on Vulnerable Populations," in *Encyclopedia of Ethical, Legal, and Policy Issues in Biotechnology*, ed. T. H. Murray and M. J. Mehlman, vol. 2 (New York: Wiley, 2001); Kenneth Kipnis, "Vulnerability in Research Subjects: A Bioethical Taxonomy," in *Ethical and Policy Issues in Research Involving Human Participants*, National Bioethics Advisory Commission (NBAC), vol. 2 (Bethesda, MD: NBAC, 2001), pp. G-1– G-13; and Mary C. Ruof, "Vulnerability, Vulnerable Populations, and Policy," Scope Note 44, *Kennedy Institute of Ethics Journal* 14 (2004): 411–25.

41. Basic to all discussions of vulnerable research populations is U.S. federal research policy, 45 CFR 46, available online.

42. See David Thomas, "Laboratory Animals and the Art of Empathy," *Journal of Medical Ethics* 31 (2005): 197–202, and a response ("Pain, Vivisection, and the Value of Life") by Raymond Frey on pp. 202–04, both © 2005 BMJ Publishing Group Ltd & Institute of Medical Ethics, available at www. jmedethics.com (accessed February 22, 2007).

43. Hume, *A Treatise of Human Nature*, ed. David Fate Norton and Mary J. Norton (Oxford: Oxford University Press, 2000, 2006), 3.3.3.2 [SBN 602–3]. (Two different editions exist: One is in the Clarendon Hume (2006), the other is a student edition in Oxford Philosophical Texts (2000).)

44. Hume, *An Enquiry Concerning the Principles of Morals*, ed. Tom L. Beauchamp (Oxford: Oxford University Press, 1998), 5.42. (Two different editions exist: One is in the Clarendon Hume, the other is a student edition in Oxford Philosophical Texts.)

45. Even though we are here concentrating on the role impartiality can play in expanding our sympathy, it can also help to correct misdirected and exaggerated sympathy that borders on sentimentality. For a critique of a kind of sentimentality that stands opposed to potentially effective measures to obtain transplantable organs from brain-dead individuals, see Joel Feinberg, "The Mistreatment of Dead Bodies," *Hastings Center Report* 15 (February 1985): 31–37.

PART II

MORAL PRINCIPLES

4
Respect for Autonomy

Respect for the autonomous choices of persons runs as deep in common morality as any principle, but little agreement exists about its nature, scope, or strength. We use the concept of autonomy in this chapter to examine individuals' decision making in health care and research, as patients and as subjects, now often called "participants."[1]

Although we begin our discussion of principles of biomedical ethics with respect for autonomy, our order of presentation does not imply that this principle has moral priority over other principles. We do not hold, as some critics suggest, that the principle of respect for autonomy overrides all other moral considerations. Furthermore, we attempt to show that, in a properly structured theory, respect for autonomy is not excessively individualistic (thereby neglecting the social nature of individuals and the impact of individual choices and actions on others), not excessively focused on reason (thereby neglecting the emotions), and not unduly legalistic (thereby highlighting legal rights and downplaying social practices and responsibilities).

THE NATURE OF AUTONOMY

The word *autonomy,* derived from the Greek *autos* ("self") and *nomos* ("rule," "governance," or "law"), originally referred to the self-rule or self-governance of independent city-states. Autonomy has since been extended to individuals, but the precise meaning of the term is disputed. Personal autonomy encompasses, at a minimum, self-rule that is free from both controlling interference by others and from certain limitations such as an inadequate understanding that prevents meaningful choice. The autonomous individual acts freely in accordance with a self-chosen plan, analogous to the way an independent government manages its territories and establishes its policies. A person of diminished autonomy, by contrast, is in some respect controlled by others or incapable of deliberating or acting on the basis of his or her desires and plans. For example, cognitively challenged individuals and prisoners often have diminished autonomy. Mental incapacitation limits the autonomy of a severely retarded person, whereas coercive institutionalization constrains the autonomy of prisoners.

Virtually all theories of autonomy view two conditions as essential for autonomy: _liberty_ (independence from controlling influences) and _agency_ (capacity for intentional action). However, disagreement exists over the meaning of these two conditions and over whether additional conditions are required.[2]

Theories of Autonomy

Some theories of autonomy feature the abilities, skills, or traits of the _autonomous person,_ which include capacities of self-governance such as understanding, reasoning, deliberating, managing, and independent choosing.[3] However, our focus in this chapter on decision making leads us to concentrate on _autonomous choice_ rather than on general capacities for governance and self-management. Even autonomous persons who have self-governing capacities and are generally good managers of their health sometimes fail to govern themselves in particular choices because of temporary constraints caused by illness, depression, ignorance, coercion, or other conditions that restrict their options. An autonomous person who signs a consent form for a procedure without reading or understanding the form can act autonomously, but fails to do so. Of course we could redescribe the act as one of placing trust in one's physician, which could be an autonomous act of authorizing the physician to proceed; but it is not an autonomous authorization of the procedure because it is not informed regarding the procedure. Similarly, some persons who are generally incapable of autonomous decision making can at times make autonomous choices. For example, some patients in mental institutions who cannot care for themselves and have been declared legally incompetent may still make some autonomous choices, such as stating preferences for meals, refusing medications, and making telephone calls to acquaintances.

Some writers maintain that autonomy involves having the capacity to reflectively control and identify with one's basic (first-order) desires or preferences through higher level (second-order) desires or preferences.[4] For example, an alcoholic may have a desire to drink, but also a higher order desire to stop drinking. An autonomous person, in this account, has the capacity to reflectively accept, identify with, or repudiate a lower order desire independent of others' manipulations of that desire. Such acceptance or repudiation of first-order desires at the higher level (i.e., the capacity to change one's preference structure) constitutes autonomy.

This theory is problematic. An overriding second-order desire that is simply _stronger_ does not make the act autonomous. Potent first-order desires from a condition such as alcohol addiction are antithetical to autonomy and can cause second-order desires. If second-order desires (decisions, volitions, etc.) are generated by prior desires or commitments, then the process of identifying with one desire rather than another does not distinguish autonomy from nonautonomy. The second-order desires would not significantly differ from first-order desires.

This theory needs more than a convincing account of second-order preferences: It needs a way for ordinary persons to qualify as deserving respect for their autonomy even when they have not reflected on their preferences at a higher level. Few choosers and few choices would be autonomous if held to the standards of higher order reflection in this theory, which presents an aspirational ideal of autonomy. An appropriate test of the adequacy of any theory of autonomy is whether it coheres with the moral requirement that we respect the ways in which we govern our lives, such as the ways we take care of our health and take care of our children, as well as our everyday choices, such as opening bank accounts, purchasing goods in stores, and authorizing repair of an automobile. A theory of autonomy should be kept consistent with pretheoretical assumptions implicit in the principle of respect for autonomy (as analyzed later on pp. 103–05). No theory of autonomy is acceptable if it presents an ideal beyond the reach of normal agents and choosers.

Instead of depicting an ideal of this sort, our analysis of autonomy focuses on nonideal conditions that fit with the moral requirements of "respect for autonomy." We analyze autonomous action in terms of normal choosers who act (1) intentionally, (2) with understanding (see pp. 119–20, 127ff later), and (3) without controlling influences that determine their action (see pp. 132ff later). The first of these three conditions of autonomy is not a matter of degree: Acts are either intentional or nonintentional. However, acts can satisfy both the conditions of understanding and absence of controlling influences to a greater or lesser extent. Actions therefore can be autonomous by degrees, as a function of satisfying these two conditions to different degrees. For both conditions, a broad continuum exists on which autonomy stretches from being fully present to being wholly absent. Many children and many elderly patients, for example, exhibit various degrees of understanding and independence found on this continuum and thus varying degrees of autonomous action.

For an action to qualify as autonomous in our account, it needs only a substantial degree of understanding and freedom from constraint, not a full understanding or a complete absence of influence. To restrict adequate decision making by patients and research subjects to the ideal of fully or completely autonomous decision making strips their acts of any meaningful place in the practical world, where people's actions are rarely, if ever, fully autonomous. A person's appreciation of information and independence from controlling influences in the context of health care need not exceed, for example, a person's information and independence in making a financial investment, hiring a new

employee, buying a new house, or deciding to attend a university. Such consequential decisions must be *substantially* autonomous, but being *fully* autonomous is a mythical ideal.

The line between what is substantial and what is insubstantial may appear
arbitrary. However, thresholds marking substantially autonomous decisions can
be carefully fixed in light of specific objectives such as meaningful decision
making. Patients and research subjects can achieve substantial autonomy in their
decisions, just as substantially autonomous choice occurs in other areas of life
such as buying a car. The appropriate criteria for substantial autonomy are best
addressed in a particular context.

Autonomy, Authority, and Community

Some theorists argue that autonomous action is incompatible with the authority
of governments, religious organizations, and other communities that prescribe
behavior. They maintain that autonomous persons must act on their own reasons
and can never submit to an authority or choose to be ruled by others without
losing their autonomy.[5] We believe, however, that no fundamental inconsistency
exists between autonomy and authority if individuals exercise their autonomy
in choosing to accept an institution, tradition, or community that they view as a
legitimate source of direction.

Choosing to follow medical authority is a prime example. Other examples are
a Jehovah's Witness who accepts the authority of that tradition and who refuses a
recommended blood transfusion, and a Roman Catholic who accepts the authority of the church and chooses against an abortion. That persons share moral principles with authoritative institutions does not prevent these principles from being
autonomously accepted, even when these principles derive from cultural tradition
and institutional authority. If a Jehovah's Witness who insists on adhering to the
doctrines of his faith in refusing a blood transfusion is deemed nonautonomous,
and therefore unworthy of respect, many of our choices based on our confidence
in institutional authority will be deemed unworthy of respect. In our judgment, a
theory of autonomy that takes this course is morally unacceptable.

We encounter many problems of autonomy in medical contexts because of
the patient's dependent condition and the medical professional's authoritative
position. On some occasions authority and autonomy are incompatible, but not
because the two *concepts* are incompatible. Conflict arises because authority has
not been properly delegated or accepted. In these circumstances, the patient's
autonomy is sometimes compromised because the physician has assumed an
unwarranted degree of authority, as in certain paternalistic actions.

Some critics of the prominent role played by autonomy in biomedical ethics
question the model of an independent, rational will that is inattentive to emotions, communal life, reciprocity, and the development of persons over time.

They charge that such an account of autonomy focuses too narrowly on the self as independent and rationally controlling. For instance, some feminist critics fault theories that place an overriding value on autonomy or fail to see communal relationships involved in acting autonomously.[6]

Some feminists have sought to affirm autonomy but to interpret it through relationships. These conceptions of "relational autonomy" derive from the conviction that persons' identities are shaped through social relationships and complex intersecting social determinants, such as race, class, gender, ethnicity, and authority structures. These accounts see persons as interdependent, but they also caution that "oppressive socialization and oppressive social relationships" can impair autonomy, for instance, through forming an agent's desires, beliefs, emotions, and attitudes and through thwarting the development of the capacities and competencies essential for autonomy.[7] Such a relational conception of autonomy is illuminating and defensible as long as it does not neglect or obscure the main features of autonomy that we analyze in this chapter.

The Principle of Respect for Autonomy

To respect autonomous agents is to acknowledge their right to hold views, to make choices, and to take actions based on their personal values and beliefs. Such respect involves respectful *action,* not merely a respectful *attitude.* It requires more than noninterference in others' personal affairs. It includes, in some contexts, building up or maintaining others' capacities for autonomous choice while helping to allay fears and other conditions that destroy or disrupt autonomous action. Respect, in this account, involves acknowledging the value and decision-making rights of persons and enabling them to act autonomously, whereas disrespect for autonomy involves attitudes and actions that ignore, insult, demean, or are inattentive to others' rights of autonomous action.

Why is such respect owed to autonomous persons? In Chapter 9, we examine the theories of two philosophers who have powerfully influenced contemporary interpretations of respect for autonomy: Immanuel Kant and John Stuart Mill. Kant argued that respect for autonomy flows from the recognition that all persons have unconditional worth, each having the capacity to determine his or her own moral destiny.[8] To violate a person's autonomy is to treat that person merely as a means; that is, in accordance with others' goals without regard to that person's own goals. Mill concerned himself primarily with the "individuality" of autonomous agents. He argued that society should permit individuals to develop according to their own convictions, as long as they do not interfere with a like expression of freedom by others or unjustifiably harm others; but he also insisted that we sometimes have an obligation to persuade others when they have false or ill-considered views.[9] Mill's position requires both not interfering with and actively strengthening autonomous expression, whereas Kant's position entails a moral imperative of respectful treatment of persons as ends in themselves. In their different ways, these two philosophers both support a principle of respect for autonomy (although Kant is largely concerned with *morally* correct autonomous choices).

The principle of respect for autonomy can be stated as a negative obligation and as a positive obligation. As a *negative* obligation: Autonomous actions should not be subjected to controlling constraints by others. This demand asserts a broad, abstract obligation that is free of exceptive clauses such as "We must respect individuals' views and rights so long as their thoughts and actions do not seriously harm other persons." Of course, the principle of respect for autonomy needs specification in particular contexts to function as a practical guide to conduct, and appropriate specification will incorporate valid exceptions. This process of specification will affect rights and obligations of liberty, privacy, confidentiality, truthfulness, and informed consent (several of which receive sustained attention in subsequent chapters).

As a *positive* obligation, this principle requires both respectful treatment in disclosing information and actions that foster autonomous decision making. Many autonomous actions could not occur without others' material cooperation in making options available. Respect for autonomy obligates professionals in health care and research involving human subjects to disclose information, to probe for and ensure understanding and voluntariness, and to foster adequate decision making. As some contemporary Kantians declare, the demand that we treat others as ends requires that we assist them in achieving their ends and foster their capacities as agents, not merely that we avoid treating them solely as means to our ends.[10]

Temptations arise in health care for physicians and other professionals to foster or perpetuate patients' dependency, rather than to promote their autonomy. But discharging the obligation to respect patients' autonomy requires enabling patients to overcome their sense of dependence and to achieve as much control as they desire. These positive obligations of respect for autonomy derive in part from the special fiduciary obligations that health care professionals have to their patients and researchers to their subjects.

These negative and positive sides of respect for autonomy are capable of supporting many more specific moral rules. (Other principles, such as beneficence and nonmaleficence, help justify some of these same rules.) Examples include the following:

1. Tell the truth.
2. Respect the privacy of others.
3. Protect confidential information.
4. Obtain consent for interventions with patients.
5. When asked, help others make important decisions.

Respect for autonomy has only prima facie standing, and competing moral considerations sometimes can override this principle. Examples include the following: If our choices endanger the public health, potentially harm innocent others, or require a scarce resource for which no funds are available, others can justifiably restrict our exercises of autonomy. The principle of respect for autonomy does not by itself determine what a person ought to be free to know or do or what counts as a valid justification for constraining autonomy. For example, a patient with an inoperable, incurable carcinoma once asked, "I don't have cancer, do I?" The physician lied, saying, "You're as good as you were ten years ago." This lie denies the patient information that he may need to determine his future course of action, thereby infringing the principle of respect for autonomy. Although the matter is controversial, the lie may be justified (by a principle of beneficence) if we posit certain major benefits to the patient. (See our discussions of paternalism in Chapter 6 and veracity in Chapter 8.)

Our obligations to respect autonomy do not extend to persons who cannot act in a sufficiently autonomous manner (and who cannot be rendered autonomous) because they are immature, incapacitated, ignorant, coerced, or exploited. Infants, irrationally suicidal individuals, and drug-dependent patients are examples.

The Triumph or Failure of Respect for Autonomy?

Some writers lament the "triumph of autonomy" in American bioethics. They charge that autonomy's proponents sometimes disrespect patients by forcing them to make choices, even though many patients do not want to receive information about their condition or to make decisions. Carl Schneider claims that proponents of autonomy, whom he labels "autonomists," concern themselves less with what patients *do want* than with what, from the point of view of autonomy, they *should want.* He attempts to correct these views by appealing to human experience and empirical research. He concludes that, "while patients largely wish to be informed about their medical circumstances, a substantial number of them [especially the elderly and the very sick] do not want to make their own medical decisions, or perhaps even to participate in those decisions in any very significant way."[11]

The duty of respect for autonomy that we defend has a correlative *right* to choose, not a mandatory *duty* to choose. Several empirical studies of the sort cited by Schneider seem, like him, to misunderstand how autonomous choice functions in a theory such as ours and how it should function in clinical medicine. In one study, UCLA researchers examined the differences in the attitudes of elderly subjects (sixty-five years or older) from different ethnic backgrounds toward (a) disclosure of the diagnosis and prognosis of a terminal illness, and (b) decision making at the end of life. The researchers summarize their main findings, based on 800 subjects (200 from each ethnic group): "Korean Americans (47%) and Mexican Americans (65%) were significantly less likely than European Americans (87%) and African Americans (88%) to believe that a patient should be told the diagnosis of metastatic cancer. Korean Americans (35%) and Mexican Americans (48%) were less likely than African Americans (63%) to believe that a patient should be told of a terminal prognosis and less likely to believe that the patient should make decisions about the use of life-supporting technology (28% and 41% vs. 60% and 65%). Korean Americans and Mexican Americans tended to believe that the family should make decisions about the use of life support." Investigators in this study stress that "belief in the *ideal* of patient autonomy is far from universal" (italics added), and they contrast that ideal with a "family-centered model" focused on an individual's web of relationships and "the harmonious functioning of the family."[12]

However, this statement is misleading in light of the actual data. The investigators themselves conclude that "physicians should ask their patients if they wish to receive information and make decisions or if they prefer that their families handle such matters." Far from abandoning or supplanting the moral demand that we respect individual autonomy, this recommendation accepts its central condition that the choice is rightly the patient's. Even if the patient delegates that right to someone else, the choice to delegate can itself be autonomous.

In a second study, this time of Navajo values and ways of thinking regarding the disclosure of risk and medical prognoses, two researchers sought to determine how health care providers "should approach the discussion of negative information with Navajo patients" to provide "more culturally appropriate medical care." Frequent conflicts emerge, these researchers report, between autonomy and the traditional Navajo conception that "thought and language have the power to shape reality and to control events." According to the traditional conception, telling a Navajo patient who has recently been diagnosed with a disease the potential complications of that disease may actually produce those complications, because "language does not merely describe reality, language shapes reality." Traditional Navajo patients may tend to process negative information as potentially harmful to them. They expect a "positive ritual language" that promotes or restores health.

One middle-aged Navajo nurse reported that a surgeon explained the risks of bypass surgery to her father in such a way that he refused to undergo the procedure: "The surgeon told him that he may not wake up, that this is the risk of every surgery. For the surgeon it was very routine, but the way that my Dad received it, it was almost like a death sentence, and he never consented to the surgery." The researchers therefore found "ethically troublesome" those policies that, in compliance with the Patient Self-Determination Act, attempt to "expose all hospitalized Navajo patients to the idea, if not the practice, of advance care planning."[13]

These two studies and numerous others enrich our understanding of diverse cultural beliefs and values that affect what particular communities and individuals believe and do. However, several studies reflect a misinterpretation of what the principle of respect for autonomy and many laws and policies require. They mistakenly view their results as opposing rather than enriching the principle of respect for autonomy. A fundamental obligation exists to ensure that patients have the right to choose, as well as the right to accept or to decline information. Forced information and forced choice are inconsistent with this obligation. From this perspective, a tension exists between the two studies just discussed. One study recommends inquiring in advance to ascertain patients' preferences regarding information and decision making, whereas the other suggests (tenuously) that even informing certain patients of a right to decide may cause harm. The practical question is whether it is possible to inform patients of their rights to know and to decide without compromising their systems of belief and values and without otherwise disrespecting them.

Health professionals should always inquire in general terms about their patients' wishes to receive information and to make decisions, and they should never assume that because a patient belongs to a particular community or culture, he or she affirms that community's worldview and values. The fundamental requirement is to respect a particular person's autonomous choices, whatever they may be. Respect for autonomy is not a mere *ideal* in health care; it is a professional *obligation*. Autonomous choice is a *right*—not a *duty*—of patients.

Complexities in Respecting Autonomy

Varieties of autonomous consent. The basic paradigm of autonomy in health care, research, politics, and other contexts is *express* consent. However, this paradigm captures only one form of consent. Another form is *tacit* consent, which people express silently or passively by omissions. For example, if the staff of a long-term care facility asks residents whether they object to having the time of dinner changed by one hour, a uniform lack of objection constitutes consent (assuming the residents understand the proposal and the need for their consent). Similarly, *implicit* or *implied* consent is often inferable from actions. Consent to a medical procedure may be implicit in a specific consent to another procedure, and providing general consent to treatment at a teaching hospital may imply consent to various roles for physicians, nurses, and others in training. *Presumed* consent reduces to either implied or express consent if consent is presumed on the basis of what we know about a particular person's choices or values. By contrast, presuming consent on the basis of a general theory of human goods or of the rational will is morally perilous. Consent should refer to an individual's actual choices, not to presumptions about the choices the individual would or should make.

Different conceptions of consent have appeared in teaching medical students how to perform intimate examinations, especially pelvic and rectal examinations.[14] Often medical students have learned and practiced on anesthetized patients, many of whom have not given their explicit informed consent. For instance, many teaching hospitals have allowed one or two medical students to participate in the examination of women who are under anesthesia in preparation for surgery. Anesthetized patients have been considered ideal for teaching medical students how to perform a pelvic examination because the patients are relaxed and would not feel any mistakes. When questioned, some directors of obstetrics and gynecology programs have pointed to the patient's general consent provided on entering a teaching hospital. Such general consent typically authorizes medical students and residents to participate in patients' care for teaching and learning purposes. However, this consent does not specify which procedures might involve participation by medical students.

It is debatable whether general consent is sufficient or whether specific, express, informed consent is necessary in these circumstances. We often seek specific informed consent when a procedure is invasive, as in the case of surgery, or when it is risky. Although pelvic examinations are not invasive by comparison to surgery, or particularly risky, patients may object to the invasion of their bodies for others' purposes, in this case for education and training. Some women readily consent to the participation of medical students in such examinations, but others view it as a violation of their dignity and privacy. One commentator rightly stresses that "the patient must be treated as the student's teacher, not as a training tool."[15]

Determining appropriate consent in particular circumstances may require giving different weights to the different values. Using anesthetized women with general consent may be efficient, but, in view of the importance of respect for autonomy, there are ethically preferable alternatives, such as using anesthetized patients who have given informed consent or using healthy volunteers who are willing to serve as trainers or models. Either of these alternatives respects personal autonomy and avoids negative medical education. A study of medical students in the Philadelphia area found that the practice of conducting pelvic exams on anesthetized patients without specific informed consent desensitized physicians to the need for patients to give their consent before medical students undertake such procedures. For students who had finished an obstetrics/gynecology clerkship, consent was significantly less important (51%) than for students who had not completed a clerkship (70%). The authors conclude that "to avoid this decline in attitudes toward seeking consent, clerkship directors should ensure that students perform examinations only after patients have given consent explicitly."[16]

Nonexpress forms of consent are common in some contexts. In late 2006, the U.S. Centers for Disease Control and Prevention (CDC) changed its recommendations about HIV screening for patients in health care settings where various other diagnostic and screening tests are regularly performed.[17] The recommendations moved away from specific, explicit informed consent, usually in written form, to general, implicit consent as part of the acceptance of medical care. Previous policies required specific disclosure of information and a decision to accept or refuse testing. (Under the new recommendations, specific, explicit informed consent would still be expected in nonclinical settings.) Some commentators hailed this shift as an indication that so-called AIDS exceptionalism has ended.[18] "AIDS exceptionalism" is an epithet used to criticize public, institutional, and medical policies that, often on grounds of respect for autonomy and associated principles such as privacy and confidentiality, refrained from applying conventional public health measures to HIV infection and AIDS.[19] Early in the epidemic, "exceptionalism" was considered justified in HIV screening because the available treatments had only limited benefits and HIV screening involved some psychosocial risks, including stigmatization, ostracism, and discrimination. Furthermore, the argument went, everyone could take precautions in the absence of knowledge of one's own and others' HIV status.

Since the beginning of the epidemic in the early 1980s, over half a million people have died from AIDS in the United States, and many millions have died around the world. According to some estimates, over 20% of people infected with HIV in the United States do not know that they are infected. In this context, the CDC justified its new recommendations on two main grounds. First, now that HIV/AIDS are viewed as chronic conditions that can be treated, although not cured, the new screening approach will enable more people who are infected to take advantage of available therapies that can extend their lives at a higher quality. Second, the information gained from screening can enable persons who are infected with HIV to take steps to protect their sex or drug-use partners from infection.

This new approach does not eliminate patient autonomy in health care settings—patients may still refuse testing—but, by shifting the default from "opt in" to "opt out," it is expected that more people who are unaware that they are infected will be tested and will gain knowledge that can benefit themselves and others. However, compromises still could be made in the absence of a requirement for explicit informed consent in written form, making screening compulsory in some health care contexts. According to one AIDS activist, "This is not informed consent, and it is not even consent, [but rather an attempt] to ram HIV testing down people's throats without their permission."[20] Although an "opt-out" approach can be justified in some circumstances, this strategy would be ethically improved if *notification* were used. Notification provides information that people can use to opt out if they choose.

Another context in which an opt-out approach, in the form of presumed consent, could be justified is organ donation from deceased individuals. In the opt-in system in the United States, deceased organ donation requires express, explicit consent, whether by an individual while alive or by the next of kin after his or her death. Even though the information disclosed for the individual's consent is usually quite limited—for instance, in a cursory exchange in the context of obtaining a license to operate an automobile—it is arguably adequate for purposes of postmortem organ donation. In view of the tremendous gap between the number of organs donated each year and the number of patients awaiting a transplant, many propose adopting in the United States an opt-out model that exists in a number of European countries. This model shifts the default so that an individual's silence, or failure to register his or her dissent, counts as consent. Two questions arise: Is such a policy of presumed consent ethically acceptable? Could it be adopted and would it be effective in the United States?

To be ethically justifiable such a policy would require vigorous efforts to ensure public understanding of the options they face as individuals, and a clear, reliable, easy, and nonburdensome mechanism for them to use to opt out. Such a policy will not likely be adopted in the United States, and, if it were adopted, it probably would not increase the number of organs for transplantation because so many citizens would opt out.[21]

The varieties of consent we have now examined point to a fundamental question that pervades this chapter: Who should seek what kind of consent from whom for what?

Consents and refusals over time. Beliefs and choices shift over time. Ethical and interpretive problems arise when a person's present choices contradict his or her previous choices, which, in some cases, he or she explicitly designed to prevent possible future changes of mind from affecting an outcome. In one case, a twenty-eight-year-old man decided to terminate chronic renal dialysis because of his restricted lifestyle and the burdens on his family. He had diabetes, was legally blind, and could not walk because of progressive neuropathy. His wife and physician agreed to provide medication to relieve his pain and further agreed not to put him back on dialysis even if he requested this action under the influence of pain or other bodily changes. (Increased amounts of urea in the blood, which result from kidney failure, can sometimes lead to altered mental states, for example.) While dying in the hospital, the patient awoke complaining of pain and asked to be put back on dialysis. The patient's wife and physician decided to act on the patient's earlier request not to intervene, and he died four hours later.[22] Although their decision was understandable, respect for autonomy suggests that the spouse and physician should have put the patient back on dialysis to flush the urea out of his bloodstream and thereby determine if he had autonomously revoked his prior choice. If the patient later indicated that he had not revoked his prior choice, he could have refused again, thereby providing the caregivers with increased assurance about his settled preferences.

The key question is whether people are acting autonomously in revoking their prior decisions. Discerning whether particular decisions are autonomous may depend, in part, on whether they are in character or out of character. Out-of-character actions can raise caution flags that warn others to seek explanations and to probe more deeply into whether the actions are autonomous, but they often turn out to be autonomous. Consider, for example, a woman's sudden and unexpected decision to discontinue dialysis even though she has displayed considerable courage and zest for life through many years of disability. The abrupt and unexpected change provides evidence—but not decisive evidence—that her decision was not sufficiently autonomous. Actions are more likely to be substantially autonomous if they are in character (e.g., when a committed Jehovah's Witness refuses a blood transfusion), but acting in character does not necessarily show autonomy. How, then, are we to determine whether actions are autonomous?

THE CAPACITY FOR AUTONOMOUS CHOICE

Many patients and potential subjects are not competent to give a valid consent or refusal. Inquiries about competence focus on whether patients or potential subjects are capable, psychologically or legally, of adequate decision making. Competence in decision making is closely connected to autonomous decision making, as well as to the validity of consent. Several commentators distinguish judgments of capacity from judgments of competence on the grounds that health professionals assess capacity and incapacity, whereas courts determine competence and incompetence. However, this distinction breaks down in practice. As Thomas Grisso and Paul Appelbaum note, "When clinicians determine that a patient lacks decision-making capacity, the practical consequences may be the same as those attending a legal determination of incompetence."[23]

The Gatekeeping Function of Competence Judgments

Competence judgments serve a gatekeeping role in health care by distinguishing persons whose decisions should be solicited or accepted from persons whose decisions need not or should not be solicited or accepted. (We use the terms *capacity* and *competence* interchangeably.) Health professionals' judgments of a person's incompetence may lead them to override that person's decisions, to turn to informal surrogates for decision making, to ask the court to appoint a guardian to protect his or her interests, or to seek that person's involuntary institutionalization. When a court establishes legal incompetence, it appoints a surrogate decision maker with either partial or plenary (full) authority over the incompetent individual. Physicians and other health professionals do not have the authority to declare patients incompetent as a matter of law, but, within limits, they often have the de facto power to override or constrain patients' decisions about care.

Competence judgments have the distinctive *normative* role of qualifying or disqualifying persons for certain decisions or actions, but those in control sometimes incorrectly present these judgments as *empirical* findings. For example, a person who appears irrational or unreasonable to others might fail a psychiatric test, and so be declared incompetent. The test is an empirical measuring device, but normative judgments determine how to use the test to sort persons into the two classes of competent and incompetent, and, therefore, how persons ought to be or may permissibly be treated.

The Concept of Competence[24]

Some commentators hold that we lack both a single acceptable *definition* of competence and a single acceptable *standard* of competence. They also contend that no nonarbitrary *test* exists to distinguish between competent and incompetent persons. We here sharply distinguish *definitions, standards,* and *tests.* We focus first on the problem of definition.

A single core meaning of the word *competence* applies in all contexts. That meaning is "the ability to perform a task."[25] By contrast to this core meaning, the *criteria* of particular competencies vary from context to context because the criteria are relative to specific tasks. The criteria for someone's competence to stand trial, to raise dachshunds, to write checks, or to lecture to medical students are radically different. The competence to decide is therefore relative to the particular decision to be made. Rarely should we judge a person incompetent with respect to every sphere of life. We usually need to consider only some type of competence, such as the competence to decide about treatment or about participation in research. These judgments of competence and incompetence affect only a limited range of decision making. For example, a person who is incompetent to decide about financial affairs may be competent to decide to participate in medical research, or able to handle simple tasks easily while faltering before complex ones.

Competence may vary over time and may be intermittent. Many persons are incompetent to do something at one point in time but competent to perform the same task at another point in time. Judgments of competence about such persons can be complicated by the need to distinguish categories of illness that result in *chronic* changes of intellect, language, or memory from those characterized by *rapid reversibility* of these functions, as in the case of transient ischemic attack or transient global amnesia. In some of the latter cases competence varies from hour to hour. In such cases, a declaration of *specific incompetence* may prevent vague generalizations that exclude persons from all forms of decision making.

These conceptual observations have practical significance. The law has traditionally presumed that a person who is incompetent to manage his or her estate is also incompetent to vote, make medical decisions, get married, and the like. The global sweep of these laws, based on a total judgment of the person, at times has extended too far. In one classic case, a physician argued that a patient was incompetent to make decisions because of epilepsy,[26] although in fact many persons who suffer from epilepsy are competent in most contexts. Such judgments defy much that we now know about the etiology of various forms of incompetence, even in hard cases of mentally retarded individuals, psychotic patients, and patients with uncontrollably painful afflictions. In addition, persons who are incompetent by virtue of dementia, alcoholism, immaturity, and mental retardation present radically different types and problems of incompetence.

Sometimes a competent person who can usually select appropriate means to reach his or her goals will act incompetently in a particular circumstance. Consider the following actual case of a hospitalized patient with an acute disc problem whose goal is to control back pain. The patient decided to manage the problem by wearing a brace, a method she had used successfully in the past. She believes strongly that she should return to this treatment modality. This approach conflicts, however, with her physician's unwavering and insistent advocacy of surgery. When the physician, an eminent surgeon who alone in her city is suited to treat the patient, asks her to sign the surgical permit, she is psychologically unable to refuse. Her illness increases both her hopes and her fears, and, in addition, she has a passive personality. In these circumstances, it is psychologically too risky for her to act as she desires. Even though she is competent to choose in general, she is not competent to choose on this occasion because she lacks adequate capacity.

This case indicates how close the concept of competence in decision making is to the concept of autonomy. Patients or prospective subjects are competent to make a decision if they have the capacity to understand the material information, to make a judgment about this information in light of their values, to intend a certain outcome, and to communicate freely their wishes to caregivers or investigators. Law, medicine, and, to some extent, philosophy presume a context in which the characteristics of the competent person are also the properties possessed by the autonomous person. Although *autonomy* and *competence* differ in meaning (*autonomy* meaning self-governance; *competence* meaning the ability to perform a task or range of tasks), the criteria of the autonomous person and of the competent person are strikingly similar.

Persons are more and less able to perform a specific task to the extent that they possess a certain level or range of abilities, just as persons are more and less intelligent and athletic. For example, in the emergency room an experienced and knowledgeable patient is likely to be more qualified to consent to a procedure than a frightened, inexperienced patient. This ability continuum runs from full mastery through various levels of partial proficiency to complete ineptitude. Nonetheless, it is confusing to view this *continuum* in terms of degrees of *competency.* For practical and policy reasons, we need *threshold levels* below which a person with a certain level of abilities for a particular task is incompetent.[27] Not all competent persons are equally able, and not all incompetent persons are equally unable, but competence determinations sort persons into these two basic classes, and thus treat persons as either competent or incompetent for specific purposes. Above the threshold, we treat persons as equally competent; below the threshold we treat them as equally incompetent. Gatekeepers test to determine who is above and who is below the threshold. Where we draw the line should depend on the particular tasks involved.[28]

Standards of Competence

Questions about competence often center on the standards for its determination; that is, the conditions a competence judgment must satisfy. Standards of competence feature mental skills or capacities closely connected to the attributes of autonomous persons, such as cognitive skills and independence of judgment. In criminal law, civil law, and clinical medicine, standards for competence cluster around various abilities to comprehend and process information and to reason about the consequences of one's actions. In medical contexts, physicians usually consider a person competent if he or she can understand a therapeutic or research procedure, deliberate regarding its major risks and benefits, and make a decision in light of this deliberation. If a person lacks any of these capacities, then his or her competence to decide, consent, or refuse is questionable.

The following case illustrates some difficulties encountered in attempts to judge competence. A man who generally exhibits normal behavior patterns is involuntarily committed to a mental institution as the result of bizarre self-destructive behavior (pulling out an eye and cutting off a hand). This behavior results from his unusual religious beliefs. The institution judges him incompetent, despite his generally competent behavior and despite the fact that his peculiar actions coherently follow from his religious beliefs.[29] This troublesome case is not one of intermittent competence. Analysis in terms of limited competence at first appears plausible, but this analysis perilously suggests that persons with unorthodox or bizarre religious beliefs are less than competent, even if they reason coherently in light of their beliefs. This policy would not be ethically acceptable unless specific and careful qualifications spelled out the grounds of incompetence.

Rival standards of incompetence. The following schema expresses the range of *inabilities* currently required by competing standards of incompetence.[30] These standards range progressively from one requiring the least ability to the other end of the spectrum.

1. Inability to express or communicate a preference or choice
2. Inability to understand one's situation and its consequences

3. Inability to understand relevant information

4. Inability to give a reason

5. Inability to give a rational reason (although some supporting reasons may be given)

6. Inability to give risk/benefit-related reasons (although some rational supporting reasons may be given)

7. Inability to reach a reasonable decision (as judged, for example, by a reasonable person standard)

These standards cluster around three kinds of abilities or skills. Standard 1 looks for the simple ability to state a preference, a notably weak standard. Standards 2 and 3 probe for abilities to understand information and to appreciate one's situation. Standards 4 through 7 look for the ability to reason through a consequential life decision. These standards have been and still are used, either alone or in combination, to determine incompetence.[31]

Testing for incompetence. A clinical need exists to select one or more of these general standards and to turn it into an operational test of incompetence that establishes passing and failing evaluations. Dementia rating scales, mental status exams, and similar devices test for factors such as time-and-place orientation, memory, understanding, and coherence. Although these clinical assessments are empirical tests, normative judgments underlie each test. The following ingredients incorporate normative judgments:[32]

1. Choosing the relevant abilities for competence

2. Choosing a threshold level of the abilities in item 1

3. Choosing an empirical test for item 2

For any test already accepted under item 3, it is an empirical question whether someone possesses the requisite level of abilities, but this empirical question can only be addressed if normative criteria have already been fixed under items 1 and 2. Institutional rules or traditions usually establish these criteria, but decision making should be open to further review and modification.

It is beyond the scope of this volume to analyze and evaluate the numerous tests and instruments that have been developed to assess decisional capacity for clinical treatment or research. Several recent reviews[33] of these instruments—one review examined twenty-three such instruments—find that, even though these instruments can aid clinicians' and researchers' assessment of decision-making competence, they produce variable results. It is thus premature to conclude that any one of them provides a fully accurate and reliable way to assess decision-making capacity. In the final analysis, the assessment of decisional competence remains heavily a matter of clinical judgment.

The sliding-scale strategy. Properties of autonomy and of mental and psychological capacity are not the only criteria used in fashioning competence standards. Many policies use pragmatic criteria of efficiency, feasibility, and social acceptability to determine whether a person is competent to make decisions about medical care. For example, age has conventionally been used as an operational criterion of valid authorization or refusal of medical procedures. Established thresholds of age vary in accordance with a community's standards, with the degree of risk involved, and with the importance of the prospective benefits. From this perspective, standards of competence should be connected to levels of experience, maturity, responsibility, and welfare.

Some writers offer a sliding-scale strategy for how to realize this goal. They argue that, as the risks of a medical intervention increase for patients, we should raise the level of ability required for a judgment of competence to elect or refuse the intervention. As the consequences for well-being become less substantial, we should lower the level of capacity required for competence. The sliding-scale approach allows standards of competence in decision making to vary with risk. For example, Grisso and Appelbaum present a "competence balance scale." An "autonomy" cup is suspended from the end of one arm of a measuring scale, and a "protection" cup is suspended from the other; the fulcrum is set initially to give more weight to the "autonomy" cup. The balancing judgment depends "on the balance of (1) the patient's mental abilities in the face of the decisional demands, weighed against (2) the probable gain-risk status of the patient's treatment choice."[34] If a serious risk such as death is present, then we need a correspondingly stringent standard of competence; if a low or insignificant risk is present, then we may use a relaxed or lower standard of competence. Thus, the same person—a child, for example—might be competent to decide whether to take a tranquilizer but incompetent to decide whether to authorize surgery.[35]

Such a sliding-scale strategy is attractive. A decision about which standard to use to determine competence depends on several factors, often risk-related. The sliding-scale strategy rightly recognizes that our interests in ensuring good outcomes legitimately contribute to the way we inquire about and create standards for judging persons competent or incompetent. If the consequences for welfare are grave, our need to certify that the patient possesses the requisite capacities increases; but if little in the way of welfare is at stake, we might lower the level of capacity required for decision making. For example, if a patient with a reversible dementia needs enteral nutrition to recover, a powerful reason exists for protecting that patient against rash or imprudent decision making and thus for adopting a rigid standard of competence.

The sliding-scale strategy is generally a sound protective device. However, it creates confusion about the nature of both competence judgments and competence itself because of certain conceptual and moral difficulties. This strategy suggests that a person's *competence* to decide is contingent on the decision's importance or on some harm that might follow from the decision. This thesis is dubious. A person's competence to decide whether to participate in cancer research does not depend on the decision's consequences. As risks increase or decrease, we can legitimately increase or reduce the rules, procedures, or measures we use to *ascertain* whether someone is competent; but in formulating what we are doing, we need to distinguish between a person's *competence* and the *modes of ascertaining* that person's competence.[36] Leading proponents of the sliding-scale strategy hold the reverse, namely, that *competence itself* varies with risk. According to the most meticulous and convincing proponents of this strategy, Allen Buchanan and Dan Brock, "Because the appropriate level of competence properly required for a particular decision must be adjusted to the consequences of acting on that decision, no single standard of decision-making competence is adequate. Instead, the level of competence appropriately required for decision making varies along a full range from low/minimum to high/maximal."[37]

This account is conceptually and morally perilous. It is correct to say that the level of demonstrated skill to decide will rise as the *complexity or difficulty* of a task increases (deciding about spinal fusion, say, as contrasted with deciding whether to take a minor tranquilizer), but the level of *competence to decide* does not rise as the risk of an outcome increases. It is confusing to blend a decision's complexity or difficulty with the risk at stake. No basis exists for believing that risky decisions require more ability at decision making than less risky decisions. To the contrary, many nonrisky decisions appear to require more ability at decision making than many risky decisions.

We can sidestep these problems by recognizing that (to assure good outcomes) the level of *evidence* for determining competence should vary according to risk. For instance, some statutes have required a higher standard of evidence for competence in making than in revoking advance directives, and the National Bioethics Advisory Commission recommended a higher standard of evidence of competence to *consent* to participate in most research than to *object* to participation.[38] These are counsels of prudence that protect patient-subjects. Whereas Brock and Buchanan propose that the level of decision-making *competence itself* belongs on a sliding scale from low to high in accordance with risk, we recommend placing only the required *standards of evidence* for determining decision-making competence on a sliding scale.

THE MEANING AND JUSTIFICATION OF INFORMED CONSENT

Since the Nuremberg trials, which exposed horrifying medical experimentation in concentration camps, biomedical ethics has placed consent at the forefront of its concerns. The term *informed consent* did not appear until a decade after these trials (held in the late 1940s). It did not receive detailed examination until the early 1970s. In recent years the focus has shifted from the physician's or researcher's obligation to *disclose* information to the quality of a patient's or subject's *understanding* and *consent*. The forces behind this shift of emphasis were autonomy driven. In this section, we treat standards of informed consent as they have evolved through the regulation of research, case law governing medical practice, changes in the patient–physician relationship, and ethical analysis.

The Justification of Informed Consent Requirements

Virtually all prominent medical and research codes and institutional rules of ethics now hold that physicians and investigators must obtain the informed consent of patients and subjects prior to a substantial intervention. Throughout the early history of concern about research subjects, consent requirements were proposed primarily as a way to minimize the potential for harm. However, since the mid-1970s the primary justification advanced for requirements of informed consent has been to protect autonomous choice, a loosely defined goal that institutions often bury in broad statements about protecting the rights of patients and research subjects.

In a series of books and articles on informed consent and autonomy, British philosopher Onora O'Neill has argued against the view that informed consent is justified in terms of respect for personal autonomy.[39] She is suspicious of contemporary conceptions of autonomy and respect for autonomy, which she finds variable, vague, and difficult to tailor to acceptable requirements of informed consent that match them. We agree that valid consent needs specification and that it is not justifiable to impose a model of explicit, specific, informed consent on all transactions in research, medicine, and health care. However, in contrast to O'Neill, we hold that respect for autonomy does provide the primary justification of rules, policies, and practices of informed consent.

O'Neill argues that rules and practices, or rituals, of informed consent are best understood as ways to prevent deception and coercion; the process of informed consent "provides reasonable assurance that a patient (research subject, tissue donor) has not been deceived or coerced."[40] However, respect for autonomy requires much more than avoiding deception and coercion. It requires an attempt to instill relevant understanding and to avoid many forms of manipulation, as we will now see.

The Meaning and Elements of Informed Consent

Some commentators have attempted to reduce the idea of informed consent to shared decision making between doctor and patient, thus rendering *informed consent* and *mutual decision making* synonymous.[41] However, informed consent cannot be reduced to shared decision making. Professionals obtain and will continue to obtain informed consent in many contexts of research and medicine in which shared decision making is a misleading model. It is critically important to distinguish informational exchanges through which patients elect medical interventions from acts of approving and authorizing those interventions. Shared decision making is a worthy ideal in medicine, but it neither defines nor displaces informed consent.[42]

Two meanings of "informed consent."[43] Two different senses of "informed consent" appear in current literature and practices. In the first sense, informed consent is analyzable through the account of autonomous choice presented earlier in this chapter: An informed consent is an individual's *autonomous authorization* of a medical intervention or of participation in research. In this first sense, a person must do more than express agreement or comply with a proposal. He or she must *authorize* something through an act of informed and voluntary consent. In a classic case, *Mohr v. Williams,* a physician obtained Anna Mohr's consent to an operation on her right ear. While operating, the surgeon determined that the left ear actually needed surgery. A court found that the physician should have obtained the patient's consent to the surgery on the left ear: "If a physician advises a patient to submit to a particular operation, and the patient weighs the dangers and risks incident to its performance, and finally consents, the patient thereby, in effect, enters into a contract authorizing the physician to operate to the extent of the consent given, but no further."[44] An informed consent in this first sense occurs if and only if a patient or subject, with substantial understanding and in absence of substantial control by others, intentionally authorizes a professional to do something quite specific.

In the second sense, informed consent is analyzable in terms of *the social rules of consent* that maintain that one must obtain legally or institutionally valid consent from patients or subjects before proceeding with diagnostic, therapeutic, or research procedures. Informed consents are not necessarily autonomous acts under these rules and sometimes are not even meaningful authorizations. *Informed consent* refers here only to an institutionally or legally effective authorization, as determined by prevailing social rules. For example, if a mature minor cannot legally authorize or consent, he or she still may autonomously authorize an intervention, even if this authorization is not an effective consent under existing rules. Thus, a patient or subject can *autonomously* authorize an intervention, and so give an informed consent in the first sense, without *effectively* authorizing the intervention (because of some set of rules), and thus without giving an informed consent in the second sense.

Institutional rules of informed consent have generally not been judged by the demanding standard of autonomous authorization. Only rarely have they been so judged. As a result, institutions, laws, or courts may impose on physicians and hospitals nothing more than an obligation to warn of risks of proposed interventions. "Consent" under these circumstances is not bona fide informed consent.[45] This problem arises from the gap between the two senses of informed consent: Physicians who obtain consent under institutional criteria can fail and often do fail to meet the more rigorous standards of an autonomy-based model.

Although it is easy to criticize institutional rules as superficial, health care professionals cannot reasonably be expected to obtain a consent that satisfies the demands of rigorous autonomy-protecting rules in all circumstances. Autonomy-protecting rules may turn out to be excessively difficult or even impossible to implement. We should evaluate institutional rules not only in terms of respect for autonomy but also in terms of the probable consequences of imposing burdensome requirements on institutions and on professionals. Policies may legitimately take account of what is fair and reasonable to require of health care professionals and researchers. Nevertheless, we take it as axiomatic that *the model of autonomous choice* (following the first sense of "informed consent") ought to serve as the benchmark for the moral adequacy of institutional rules.

The elements of informed consent. Some commentators have attempted to define *informed consent* by specifying the elements of the concept, in particular by dividing the elements into an information component and a consent component. The information component refers to the disclosure of information and the comprehension of what is disclosed. The consent component refers to both a voluntary decision and an authorization to proceed. Legal, regulatory, philosophical, medical, and psychological literatures tend to favor the following elements as the components of informed consent:[46] (1) competence, (2) disclosure, (3) understanding, (4) voluntariness, and (5) consent. Some writers present these elements as the building blocks for a definition of *informed consent:* One gives an informed consent to an intervention if (and perhaps only if) one is competent to act, receives a thorough disclosure, comprehends the disclosure, acts voluntarily, and consents to the intervention.

This five-element definition is superior to the one-element definition in terms of *disclosure* that courts and medical literature have often proposed.[47] Many patients regard the disclosure of information as less vital in clinical medicine than a health professional's *recommendation* of one or more actions. This is typically the case in direct exchanges between physicians and patients regarding surgery, medications, and the like; but it is also true, for example, of notifications to employees after a study of hazardous chemicals.

In this chapter we accept and treat each of the following seven elements:

I. Threshold elements (preconditions)
   1. Competence (to understand and decide)
   2. Voluntariness (in deciding)

II. Tnformation elements
   3. Disclosure (of material information)
   4. Recommendation (of a plan)
   5. Understanding (of 3 and 4)

III. Consent elements

   6. Decision (in favor of a plan)

   7. Authorization (of the chosen plan)

This list requires a brief explanation and augmentation. First, *an informed refusal* entails a modification of items under III, thereby turning the categories into refusal elements; for example, 6. "Decision (against a plan)." Whenever we use the phrase "informed consent," we always allow for the possibility of informed refusal. Second, consent for research involving human subjects does not necessarily involve a recommendation. Third, competence is more of a presupposition of obtaining informed consent than an element.

Having examined competence previously, we now concentrate on disclosure, understanding, and voluntariness, beginning with disclosure.

DISCLOSURE

Disclosure is the third of our seven elements of informed consent. Some institutions or authorities have presented the obligation to disclose information to patients as the only major condition of informed consent. The legal doctrine of informed consent in the United States primarily has focused on disclosure because of a physician's general obligation to exercise reasonable care in providing information. Civil litigation has emerged over informed consent because of injury (measured in terms of monetary damages) that a physician intentionally or negligently caused by his or her failure to disclose. The term *informed consent* was born in this legal context. However, from the moral viewpoint, informed consent has less to do with the liability of professionals as agents of disclosure and more to do with the autonomous choices of patients and subjects.

Nevertheless, disclosure still plays a pivotal role. Without an adequate way for professionals to deliver information, many patients and subjects will have an inadequate basis for decision making. Professionals are generally obligated to disclose a core set of information, including (1) those facts or descriptions that patients or subjects usually consider material in deciding whether to refuse or consent to the proposed intervention or research, (2) information the professional believes to be material, (3) the professional's recommendation, (4) the purpose of seeking consent, and (5) the nature and limits of consent as an act of authorization. If research is involved, disclosures should generally cover the aims and methods of the research, anticipated benefits and risks, any anticipated inconvenience or discomfort, and the subjects' right to withdraw, without penalty, from the research.

We could easily expand the list of basic information. For example, in one controversial decision, the California Supreme Court held that, when seeking an informed consent, "a physician must disclose personal interests unrelated to the patient's health, whether research or economic, that may affect the physician's professional judgment."[48] Such a disclosure requirement has acquired increased moral significance as conflicts of interest have become more pronounced and problematic in research and managed care. Researchers for example, may hold stock in a pharmaceutical company that sponsors the research, or physicians may have an investment in a radiological center to which he or she refers the patient. (We examine conflicts of interest in Chapter 8.)

Standards of Disclosure

Courts in the United States have struggled to determine which norms should govern the disclosure of information. Two competing standards of disclosure have emerged: the professional practice standard and the reasonable person standard. A third, the subjective standard, has also received some support, although courts have generally avoided it. These standards are as morally relevant as they are legally prominent.

The professional practice standard. The first standard holds that a professional community's customary practices determine adequate disclosure. That is, professional custom establishes the amount and kinds of information to be disclosed. Disclosure, like treatment, is a responsibility of physicians because of their professional expertise and commitment to the patient's welfare. As a result, only expert testimony from members of this profession could count as evidence that a physician violated a patient's right to information.

Several difficulties affect this standard, which some call a *reasonable doctor standard.* First, it is uncertain in many situations whether a customary standard exists for the communication of information in medicine. Second, if custom alone were conclusive, pervasive negligence could be perpetuated with impunity. The majority of professionals could offer the same inadequate level of information or have total discretion to determine the scope of disclosure. Third, it is questionable whether many physicians have developed the skills to determine the information that serves their patients' best interests. Empirical studies cast doubt on this claim.[49] The weighing of risks in the context of a person's subjective beliefs, fears, and hopes is not an expert skill, and information provided to patients and subjects sometimes needs to be freed from the entrenched values and goals of medical professionals. Finally, and perhaps most compellingly, the professional practice standard subverts the right of autonomous choice. Professional standards in medicine are fashioned for medical judgments, but decisions for or against medical care, which are nonmedical decisions, are rightly the province of the patient.

The reasonable person standard. Although many legal jurisdictions rely on the traditional professional practice standard, a reasonable person standard has gained acceptance in over half of the states in the United States. According to this standard, the information to be disclosed should be determined by reference to a hypothetical reasonable person. Whether information is pertinent or material is to be measured by the significance a reasonable person would attach to it in deciding whether to undergo a procedure. Hence, the authoritative determination of informational needs shifts from the physician to the patient, and physicians may be found guilty of negligent disclosures even if their behavior conforms to recognized professional practice.

Whatever its merits, the reasonable person standard encounters conceptual, moral, and practical difficulties. No one has carefully defined the concepts of "material information" and "reasonable person," and questions arise about whether and how physicians and other health care professionals can employ the reasonable person standard in practice. Its abstract and hypothetical character makes it difficult for them to use because they have to project what a reasonable patient would need to know.

A related problem emerges from empirical studies regarding whether patients use disclosed information in reaching their decisions. Data collected in one study indicate that although 93% of the patients surveyed believed they benefited from the information disclosed, only 12% used the information in their decisions to consent.[50] This study, involving family-planning patients, reached conclusions similar to an earlier study of kidney donors.[51] In both studies the data indicate that patients generally make their decisions prior to and independent of the process of receiving information. Other studies indicate that patients often deferentially accept physicians' recommendations without carefully weighing risks and benefits,[52] and that many patients agree to a procedure during their first meeting with a physician (82% of candidates for breast cancer adjuvant therapy in one study[53]).

The subjective standard. Finally, the subjective model judges adequacy of information by reference to the specific informational needs of the individual person, rather than by the hypothetical "reasonable person." Individual needs can differ: Persons may have unconventional beliefs, unusual health problems, or unique family histories that require a different informational base than the reasonable person needs. For example, a person with a family history of reproductive problems might desire information that other persons would not need or want before becoming involved in research on sexual and familial relations or accepting employment in certain industries. If a physician knows or has reason to believe that a person wants such information, then withholding it may undermine autonomy. At issue is the extent to which a standard should be tailored to the individual patient—that is, made subjective. The subjective standard requires the physician to disclose the information a particular patient needs to know, if it is reasonable to expect the physician to know that patient's informational needs.[54]

The subjective standard is the preferable *moral* standard of disclosure, because it alone meets persons' specific informational needs. Nevertheless, exclusive reliance on a subjective standard does not suffice for either law or ethics because patients often do not know what information is relevant for their deliberations, and we cannot reasonably expect a doctor to do an exhaustive background and character analysis of each patient to determine the relevant information.

Intentional Nondisclosure

Some types of research are incompatible with complete disclosure, and in certain clinical situations physicians claim that nondisclosures benefit the patient. Are such intentional nondisclosures justifiable?

The therapeutic privilege. Legal exceptions to the rule of informed consent allow the health professional to proceed without consent in cases of emergency, incompetence, and waiver. These three exceptive conditions are not controversial. However, one controversial exception is the therapeutic privilege, which states that a physician may legitimately withhold information, based on a sound medical judgment that divulging the information would potentially harm a depressed, emotionally drained, or unstable patient. Several possible and harmful outcomes include endangering life, causing irrational decisions, and producing anxiety or stress.[55] Despite the protected status this doctrine traditionally has enjoyed, U.S. Supreme Court Justice Byron White once vigorously attacked the idea that possibly increasing a person's anxiety about a procedure provides grounds for an exception to rules of informed consent.[56] White suggested that the legal status of the doctrine of therapeutic privilege lacks the security it once had.

The precise formulation of this therapeutic privilege varies across legal jurisdictions. Some formulations permit physicians to withhold information if disclosure would cause *any* countertherapeutic deterioration in the patient's condition. Other formulations permit the physician to withhold information if and only if the patient's knowledge of the information would have serious health-related consequences, for example, by jeopardizing the treatment's success or by critically impairing relevant decision-making processes. The narrowest formulation appeals to a circumstance of incompetence: A physician may only invoke the therapeutic privilege if he or she has sufficient reason to believe that disclosure would render the patient incompetent to consent to or refuse the treatment. To invoke the therapeutic privilege under this condition does not in principle conflict with respect for autonomy, because the patient would not be capable of an autonomous decision at the point consent would be needed.

Therapeutic use of placebos. The therapeutic use of placebos typically involves incomplete disclosure or even intentional deception. A placebo is a substance or intervention that the clinician believes to be pharmacologically or biomedically inert for the condition being treated. Studies indicate that placebos relieve some symptoms in approximately 35% of patients who suffer from conditions such as angina pectoris, cough, anxiety, depression, hypertension, headache, and the common cold.[57]

Arguments against therapeutic uses of placebos without full disclosure focus on the possible negative consequences, such as damage to a specific clinical relationship or to clinical relationships more generally because of the loss of trust, and on the failure to respect patient autonomy through deceptive nondisclosure. Some defenses of the use of placebos without full disclosure appeal to the patient's consent to an unspecified generic treatment, such as "an effective pill" or "a powerful medicine." A related defense of the use of placebos appeals to the patient's prior general consent to the goals of treatment. However, this "consent" clearly is not an adequately informed consent. Such an appeal to the patient's consent would be acceptable if, prior to the initiation of the patient's care, the patient were informed that a placebo might be used at some point in the treatment and he or she consented to this arrangement.[58]

Evidence suggests that the placebo response or placebo effect, an improvement in the patient after the use of a placebo, can sometimes be produced without nondisclosure or deception. For example, the placebo response sometimes occurs even if patients have been informed that a particular substance is pharmacologically inert and still consent to its use. The mechanisms of placebo responses are poorly understood, but several hypotheses have been proposed. These hypotheses center on the healing context, with its symbolic significance, and the professional's care, compassion, and skill in fostering trust and hope.[59]

Withholding information from research subjects. Problems of intentional nondisclosure in clinical practice have parallels in research in which investigators sometimes need to withhold some information from subjects. Occasionally, good reasons support nondisclosure. Scientists could not conduct vital research in fields such as epidemiology if they always had to obtain consent from subjects for access to medical records. Officials often justify using those records without consent to establish the prevalence of a particular disease. Such research is sometimes only the first phase of an investigation intended to determine whether a need exists to trace and contact particular individuals who are at risk of disease, and often the researchers must obtain their permission for further participation in research. Occasionally, researchers need not contact individuals at all; for example, when hospitals strip personal identifiers from their records so that epidemiologists cannot identify the patients. In other circumstances, researchers only need to notify persons in advance about how they will use data and to offer these persons the opportunity to refuse to participate in the research. In short, disclosures, warnings, and opportunities to decline involvement are sometimes legitimately substituted for an informed consent.

However, many other forms of intentional nondisclosure in research are difficult to justify. For instance, debate arose about a study, designed and conducted by two physicians at the Emory University School of Medicine, to determine the prevalence of cocaine use among patients and the reliability of their self-reports about drug use. Controversy centered on the questions that would most likely elicit accurate answers from a group of men in an Atlanta walk-in, inner-city hospital clinic that serves low-income, predominantly black residents. In this study, which the institutional human investigations committee approved, researchers asked weekday outpatients at Grady Memorial Hospital to participate in a study about asymptomatic carriage of sexually transmitted diseases (STDs). The participants provided informed consent for the STD study, but not for an *unmentioned* piggy-back study of recent cocaine use and the reliability of self-reports of such use. More specifically, researchers informed patients that their urine would be tested for STDs, but they did not inform the participants that they would also analyze the urine for cocaine metabolites. Of the 415 eligible men who agreed to participate, 39% tested positive for a major cocaine metabolite, although 72% of those with positive urinary assays denied any illicit drug use in the three days prior to sampling. Researchers concluded: "Our findings underscore the magnitude of the cocaine abuse problem for young men seeking care in inner-city, walk-in clinics. Health care providers need to be aware of the unreliability of patient self-reports of illicit drug use."[60]

The researchers deceived the subjects about some aims and purposes of the research and did not disclose the means that would be used. Investigators thought they faced a dilemma: On the one hand, they needed accurate information about illicit drug use for health care and public policy. On the other hand, obtaining adequate informed consent would be difficult, because many potential subjects would either refuse to participate or would offer false information to researchers.

Nonetheless, rules requiring consent have been designed specifically to protect subjects from manipulation and abuse during the research process. Reports of this cocaine study could increase suspicion of medical institutions and professionals and could make patients' self-reports of illegal activities less reliable.[61] Although informed consent is sometimes unnecessary, this study of cocaine use is not a legitimate exceptive case. Investigators should have resolved their dilemma by developing alternative research designs, including sophisticated methods of using questions that can either reduce or eliminate response errors without abridging informed consent.

In general, research cannot be justified if significant risk is involved and subjects are not informed that they are being placed at risk. This conclusion does not imply that researchers can never justifiably undertake studies involving deception. Professionals often conduct relatively risk-free research that requires deception or incomplete disclosure in fields such as behavioral and physiological psychology. However, researchers should permit deception in their work only if it is essential to obtain vital information, it involves no substantial risk, they inform subjects that deception or incomplete disclosure is part of the study, and subjects consent to participate under these conditions. We will return, in Chapter 8, to a broader examination of the ethics of randomized clinical trials.

UNDERSTANDING

Understanding is the fifth element of informed consent listed earlier. Clinical experience and empirical data indicate that patients and research subjects exhibit wide variation in their understanding of information about diagnoses, procedures, risks, probable benefits, and prognoses.[62] For instance, in a study of participants in cancer clinical trials, 90% indicated they were satisfied with the informed consent process and most of them thought they were well informed. However, approximately three-fourths of them did not recognize nonstandard and unproven treatment, and approximately one-fourth did not appreciate that the primary purpose of the trials was to benefit future patients and that the benefits to them personally were uncertain.[63]

There are many reasons for such limited understanding in the informed consent process. Some patients and subjects are calm, attentive, and eager for dialogue, whereas others are nervous or distracted in ways that impair or block understanding. Many conditions limit their understanding, including illness, irrationality, and immaturity. Furthermore, deficiencies in the communication process may hamper understanding. Some barriers to understanding can be addressed, but debate continues about how best to do so and about the level of understanding that is essential for valid consent.

The Nature of Understanding

No consensus exists about the nature of understanding, but an analysis sufficient for our purposes is that persons understand if they have acquired pertinent information and have relevant beliefs about the nature and consequences of their actions. Such understanding need not be *complete,* because a grasp of central facts is generally sufficient. Some facts are irrelevant or trivial; others are vital, perhaps decisive. In some cases, a person's lack of awareness of even a single risk or missing fact can deprive him or her of adequate understanding. Consider, for example, the case of *Bang v. Miller Hospital,* in which patient Bang did not intend to consent to a sterilization entailed in prostate surgery.[64] Bang did, in fact, consent to prostate surgery, but without being told that sterilization was an inevitable outcome. (Although sterilization is not necessarily an outcome of prostate surgery, it is inevitable in the specific procedure recommended in this case.) Bang's failure to understand this one surgical consequence compromised what was otherwise an adequate understanding and invalidated what otherwise would have been a valid consent.

Patients and subjects usually should understand at least what an attentive health care professional or researcher believes a patient or subject needs to understand to authorize an intervention. Diagnoses, prognoses, the nature and purpose of the intervention, alternatives, risks and benefits, and recommendations typically are essential. Patients or subjects also need to share an understanding with professionals about the terms of the authorization before proceeding. Unless agreement exists about the essential features of what is authorized, there can be no assurance that a patient or subject has made an autonomous decision and provided a valid consent. Even if physician and patient both use a word such as *stroke* or *hernia,* their interpretations will be different if standard medical definitions and conceptions have no meaning for the patient.

Some argue that many patients and subjects cannot comprehend enough information or sufficiently appreciate its relevance to make decisions about medical care or participation in research. Such statements are overgeneralizations based partially on an improper ideal of full disclosure and full understanding. If we replace this ideal standard with a more acceptable account of understanding relevant information, we can thwart such skepticism. From the fact that actions are never *fully* informed, voluntary, or autonomous, it does not follow that they are never *adequately* informed, voluntary, or autonomous.[65]

However, some patients have such limited knowledge bases that communication about alien or novel situations is exceedingly difficult, especially if physicians introduce new concepts and cognitive constructs. Studies indicate that these patients likely will have an impoverished and distorted understanding of scientific goals and procedures.[66] But even in these difficult situations, enhanced understanding and adequate decision making are often possible. For instance, professionals may be able to communicate novel and specialized information to lay persons by drawing analogies between this information and more ordinary events familiar to the patient or subject. Similarly, professionals can express risks in both numeric and nonnumeric probabilities, while helping the patient or subject to assign meanings to the probabilities through comparison with more familiar risks and prior experiences, such as risks involved in driving automobiles or using power tools.[67]

However, even with these strategies, enabling a patient not only to comprehend but also to appreciate risks and benefits can be a formidable task. For example, patients confronted with various forms of surgery understand that they will suffer postoperative pain. Nevertheless, their projected expectations of the pain are often inadequate. Many patients cannot, in advance, adequately appreciate the nature of the pain, and many ill patients reach a point at which they can no longer balance with clear judgment the threat of pain against the benefits of surgery. At this point, they find the benefits of surgery overwhelmingly attractive, while discounting the risks. In one respect, these patients correctly understand basic facts about procedures that involve pain, but in other respects their understanding is inadequate.

Special concerns about adequate understanding for valid consent arise in the context of research, which is designed not to benefit the subject or participant but to generate generalizable knowledge. Several interventions have been proposed and studied as possible ways to enhance research participants' understanding as part of the consent process. One review of dozens of trials of such interventions notes the limited success of uses of multimedia and enhanced consent forms and the greater success of lengthy one-on-one conversations between a member of the research team or a neutral educator and the research participant.[68] Another proposal is to conduct a postdecision consent evaluation, by using a questionnaire and then addressing points that the individual did not adequately understand, even though he or she consented to participate.[69]

One misunderstanding that such interventions have to address is the "therapeutic misconception": Subjects in research fail to distinguish between clinical care and research and to understand the purpose and aim of research, thereby misconceiving their participation as therapeutic in nature.[70] We have already seen examples of this misconception. In a stringent interpretation of the standard of adequate understanding, the "therapeutic misconception" would invalidate the subject's consent because he or she is not consenting to participation in research. This could undermine some clinical trials. A partial solution is twofold: first, to recognize that the label "therapeutic misconception" is too broad, and, second, to find interventions to address the different misunderstandings under that rubric.

Sam Horng and Christine Grady have distinguished therapeutic misconception in the strict sense from therapeutic misestimation and therapeutic optimism.[71] The therapeutic misconception, if it cannot be corrected, invalidates subjects' consent because they do not have the facts straight enough to truly consent to participate in research. However, some participants who clearly understand that they are involved in research, and not clinical care, may still overestimate the therapeutic possibilities and probabilities, that is, the odds that any participants will benefit. Such a therapeutic misestimation, Horng and Grady argue, should be tolerated if "modest misestimates do not compromise a reasonable awareness of possible outcomes." By contrast, in therapeutic optimism, participants accurately understand the odds that any participants will benefit but are overly optimistic about their own chances of beating those odds. This therapeutic optimism generally does not compromise or invalidate the individual's informed consent. The optimism is more like a legitimate hope than an informational bias.

Problems of Information Processing

With the exception of a few limited studies of comprehension, studies of patients' decision making often pay too little attention to information processing. Too much information can cause just as much of a problem as too little.

Information overload may prevent adequate understanding, and physicians exacerbate these problems if they use unfamiliar terms or if patients cannot meaningfully organize information. Patients and potential subjects also may rely on modes of selective perception, and it is often difficult to determine when words have special meanings for them, when preconceptions distort their processing of the information, and when other biases intrude.

Some studies have uncovered difficulties in processing information about risks, indicating that risk disclosures commonly lead subjects to distort information and promote inferential errors and disproportionate fears of some risks. Some ways of framing information are so misleading that both health professionals and patients regularly misconstrue the content. For example, choices between risky alternatives can be heavily influenced by whether the same risk information is presented as providing a gain or an opportunity for a patient, or as constituting a loss or a reduction of opportunity.[72] One study asked radiologists, outpatients with chronic medical problems, and graduate business students to make a hypothetical choice between two alternative therapies for lung cancer: surgery and radiation therapy.[73] Whether researchers framed the information about outcomes in terms of survival or death affected the preferences of all three groups. When faced with outcomes framed in terms of probability of *survival,* 25% chose radiation over surgery. However, when the identical outcomes were presented in terms of probability of *death,* 42% preferred radiation. The mode of presenting the risk of immediate death from surgical complications, which has no counterpart in radiation therapy, appears to have made the decisive difference.

These framing effects reduce understanding, with direct implications for autonomous choice. If a misperception prevents a person from adequately understanding the risk of death and this risk is material to the person's decision, then the person's choice of a procedure does not reflect a substantial understanding and does not qualify as an autonomous authorization. The lesson to be learned is the need for better understanding of techniques that will enable professionals to communicate both the positive and the negative sides of information—for example, both the survival and the mortality probabilities.

Problems of Nonacceptance and False Belief

A breakdown in a person's ability to *accept* information as true or untainted, even if he or she adequately *comprehends* the information, can also compromise decision making. A single false belief can invalidate a patient's or subject's consent, even when there has been a suitable disclosure and comprehension. For example, a seriously ill patient who has been thoroughly informed about the nature of the illness and has been asked to make a treatment decision might refuse under the false belief that he or she is not ill. Even if the physician recognizes the patient's false belief and adduces conclusive evidence to prove to the patient that the belief is mistaken, and the patient comprehends the information provided, the patient may go on believing that what has been (truthfully) reported is false.

When certain beliefs are demonstrably false, the question arises whether professionals should force patients and subjects to abandon those beliefs to enable them to reach an informed decision. If ignorance prevents an informed choice, it may be permissible or possibly even obligatory to promote autonomy by attempting to impose unwelcome information. Consider the following case in which a false belief played a major role in a patient's refusal of treatment:[74]

> A 57-year-old woman was admitted to the hospital because of a fractured hip....During the course of the hospitalization, a Papanicolaou test and biopsy revealed stage 1A carcinoma of the cervix.... Surgery was strongly recommended, since the cancer was almost certainly curable by a hysterectomy.... The patient refused the procedure. The patient's treating physicians at this point felt that she was mentally incompetent. Psychiatric and neurological consultations were requested to determine the possibility of dementia and/or mental incompetency. The psychiatric consultant felt that the patient was demented and not mentally competent to make decisions regarding her own care. This determination was based in large measure on the patient's steadfast "unreasonable" refusal to undergo surgery. The neurologist disagreed, finding no evidence of dementia. On questioning, the patient stated that she was refusing the hysterectomy because she *did not believe* she had cancer. "Anyone knows," she said, "that people with cancer are sick, feel bad and lose weight," while she felt quite well. The patient continued to hold this view despite the results of the biopsy and her physicians' persistent arguments to the contrary.

The physician seriously considered overriding the patient's refusal, because solid medical evidence demonstrated that she was unjustified in believing she did not have cancer. As long as this patient continues to hold a false belief that is material to her decision, her refusal is not an *informed* refusal. This case illustrates the complexities involved in effective communication: The patient was a poor white woman from Appalachia with a third-grade education. The fact that her treating physician was black was the major reason for her false belief that she did not have cancer. She would not believe what a black physician told her. However, intense and sometimes forced discussions with a white physician and with her daughter eventually corrected her belief and led her to consent to a successful hysterectomy.

The Problem of Waivers

A further problem about understanding arises in waivers of informed consent. In the exercise of a waiver, a patient voluntarily relinquishes the right to an informed consent and relieves the physician of the obligation to obtain informed consent.[75] The patient delegates decision-making authority to the physician—or to someone else—or asks not to be informed. The patient makes a decision not to make an informed decision.

Some courts have held that "a medical doctor need not make disclosures of risks when the patient requests that he not be so informed,"[76] and some prominent writers in biomedical ethics hold that "rights are always waivable."[77] It is usually appropriate to recognize waivers of rights because we enjoy discretion over whether to exercise our rights. Contexts of consent are no exception. For example, if a committed Jehovah's Witness informed a doctor that he wished to have everything possible done for him, but did not want to know if the hospital utilized transfusions or similar procedures, it is difficult to construct a moral argument to support the conclusion that he must give a specific informed consent to the transfusions. Nevertheless, a general practice of allowing waivers is dangerous. Many patients have an inordinate trust in physicians, and the general acceptance of waivers of consent in research and therapeutic settings could make patients more vulnerable to those who omit consent procedures for convenience, already a serious problem in health care.

No general solution to these problems about waivers is likely to emerge. Each case or situation of waiver needs to be considered separately. There may, however, be appropriate *procedural* responses. For example, institutions could develop rules that disallow waivers except when they have been approved by deliberative bodies, such as institutional review committees and hospital ethics committees. If a committee determined that recognizing a waiver would best protect a person's interest in a particular case, then the waiver could be sustained. This procedural solution could effectively eliminate the problem because good committee review could respond to appropriate requests, while disallowing inappropriate ones.

VOLUNTARINESS

Voluntariness is the second element of informed consent in our list of elements. We concentrate in this section on a person's voluntariness in acting. We use the term *voluntariness* more narrowly than some writers do to distinguish it from broader uses that make it synonymous with autonomy. Some have analyzed voluntariness in terms of the presence of adequate knowledge, the absence of psychological compulsion, and the absence of external constraints.[78] If we were to adopt this broad meaning, we would be equating voluntariness with autonomous action. We therefore hold only that a person acts voluntarily if he or she wills the action without being under the control of another's influence. We consider only the condition of control by other individuals, although conditions such as debilitating disease, psychiatric disorders, and drug addiction can also diminish or void voluntariness.

Not all influences exerted on another person are controlling. If a physician orders a reluctant patient to undergo cardiac catheterization and coerces the patient into compliance through a threat of abandonment, then the physician's influence controls the patient. If, by contrast, a physician persuades the patient to undergo the procedure when the patient is at first reluctant to do so, then the physician's actions influence, but do not control, the patient. Many influences are resistible, and some are welcomed rather than resisted. The broad category of influence includes acts of love, threats, education, lies, manipulative suggestions, and emotional appeals, all of which can vary dramatically in their impact on persons.

Forms of Influence

Our analysis focuses on three categories of influence: coercion, persuasion, and manipulation. Coercion occurs if and only if one person intentionally uses a credible and severe threat of harm or force to control another.[79] The threat of force used by some police, courts, and hospitals in acts of involuntary commitment for psychiatric treatment is coercive. Some threats will coerce virtually all persons (e.g., a credible threat to kill the person), whereas others will coerce only a few persons (e.g., an employee's threat to an employer to quit a job unless a raise is offered). Whether coercion occurs depends on the subjective responses of the coercion's intended target. However, a subjective response in which persons comply because they *feel* threatened (although no threat has been issued) does not qualify as coercion. Coercion occurs only if a credible and intended threat displaces a person's self-directed course of action. Coercion renders even intentional and well-informed behavior nonautonomous.

There is a tendency in debates in biomedical ethics for "coercion" to become an all-purpose term of ethical criticism and thus to obscure the relevant and important ethical concerns in particular cases in health care and research. For instance, it does not apply to all dire situations in which individuals have to make hard and even tragic choices. This point about the limits of the concept of coercion does not imply that it is ethically acceptable to take advantage of a person in dire straits.[80]

In *persuasion* a person must come to believe in something through the merit of reasons another person advances. Appeal to reason—i.e., attempted persuasion—is distinguishable from influence by appeal to emotion. In health care, the problem is to distinguish emotional responses from cognitive responses and to determine which are likely to be evoked. Disclosures or approaches that might rationally persuade one patient might overwhelm another whose fear or panic would short-circuit reason.

Manipulation is a generic term for several forms of influence that are neither persuasive nor coercive. The essence of manipulation is swaying people to do what the manipulator wants by means other than coercion or persuasion. In health care, the most likely form of manipulation is informational manipulation, a deliberate act of managing information that nonpersuasively alters a person's understanding of a situation and motivates him or her to do what the agent of influence intends. Many forms of informational manipulation are incompatible with autonomous decision making. For example, lying, withholding information, and misleading exaggeration with the intent to lead persons to believe what is false all compromise autonomous choice. The manner in which a health care professional presents information—by tone of voice, by forceful gesture, and by framing information positively ("we succeed most of the time with this therapy") rather than negatively ("we fail with this therapy in 35% of the cases")—can also manipulate a patient's perception and response, thereby affecting understanding and voluntariness.

Nevertheless, it is easy to inflate the threat of control by manipulation beyond its actual significance in health care. We typically make decisions in a context of competing influences, such as personal desires, familial constraints, legal obligations, and institutional pressures. These influences usually do not control decisions to a morally worrisome degree. In biomedical ethics we need only establish general criteria for the point at which influence threatens autonomous choice, while recognizing that in many cases no sharp boundary separates controlling and noncontrolling influences.

The Obligation to Abstain from Controlling Influence

Coercion and controlling manipulation are occasionally justified—infrequently in medicine, more often in public health, and even more often in law enforcement. If a physician taking care of a disruptive and childishly noncompliant patient threatens to discontinue treatment unless the patient alters certain behaviors, the physician's mandate may be justified, even if it is coercive. The most difficult problems about manipulation do not involve threat and punishment, which are almost always unjustified in health care and research, but rather involve the effect of rewards, offers, and encouragement.

A classic example of an unjustified offer occurred during the Tuskegee syphilis study. Researchers used various offers to stimulate and sustain the subjects' interest in continued participation. These offers included free burial assistance and insurance, free transportation to and from the examinations, and a free stop in town on the return trip. Subjects received free medicines and free hot meals on the days of the examination. The subjects' socioeconomic deprivation made them vulnerable to these overt and unjustified forms of manipulation.[81]

The conditions under which an influence both controls persons and lacks moral justification may be clear in theory, but are often unclear in concrete situations. For example, many patients report feeling severe pressure to enroll in clinical trials, even though their enrollment is voluntary.[82] Some difficult cases in health care involve manipulation-like situations in which patients or subjects are in desperate need of a given medication or a source of income. Attractive offers such as free medication or extra money can leave a person without any meaningful choice. A threatening situation can constrain a person even in the absence of another's intentional manipulation. Influences that persons ordinarily find resistible can control abnormally weak, dependent, and surrender-prone patients.[83]

The threat of exploitation is substantial in institutions where populations are admitted involuntarily, yet the fact that a person is coercively institutionalized or lives in a coercive institution does not automatically entail that each of that person's decisions is coerced. No reason exists why prisoners, for example, cannot validly consent to some research if researchers do not use coercive tactics in recruitment or make manipulative offers, such as unduly large payments for excessive risk taking.[84]

Even if persons voluntarily admit themselves to institutions, rules, policies, and practices can work to compromise autonomous choice. Perhaps nowhere is this compromise more evident than in long-term care. For example, the elderly in nursing homes frequently experience constricted choices, particularly in routine or everyday matters. Many people in nursing homes have already suffered a decline in their ability to carry out personal choices because of physical impairments. This decline in *executional* autonomy need not be accompanied by a decline in *decisional* autonomy, but caregivers in nursing homes often neglect, misunderstand, or override residents' autonomous decisions.[85] Everyday decisions range over food (when, what kind, how it is prepared, and how much), roommates (who selects them and how to resolve conflicts), possessions (which to keep and how to protect them), exercise (when, what kind, and with what supervision), sleep (when and how much), clothes (what to wear and when to wash), and baths, medications, and restraints.

A FRAMEWORK OF STANDARDS FOR SURROGATE DECISION MAKING

We shift now from the conditions of consent to problems of consent when surrogate decision makers are involved. Surrogate decision makers are authorized to reach decisions for doubtfully autonomous or nonautonomous patients. If a patient is not competent to choose or to refuse treatment, a hospital, a physician, or a family member may justifiably exercise a decision-making role or go before a court or other authority to resolve the issues before implementing a decision. Since the Quinlan decision in New Jersey in 1976, courts and legislatures in the United States have established many procedures and standards for surrogate decision making. However, much remains unresolved. Many surrogates daily make decisions to terminate or continue treatment for incompetent patients, for example, those suffering from stroke, Alzheimer's disease, Parkinson's disease, chronic depression affecting cognitive function, senility, and psychosis.

In this section, we consider three general standards that surrogate decision makers might use: *substituted judgment,* which is sometimes presented as an autonomy-based standard; *pure autonomy;* and *the patient's best interests.* Our objective is to restructure and to integrate this set of standards for surrogate decision making into a coherent framework. Although we evaluate these standards for law and policy, our underlying argument is a moral argument that extends our earlier discussions of the value of protecting autonomy. Only in Chapter 5 do we consider *who* should be the surrogate decision maker.

The Substituted Judgment Standard

The standard of substituted judgment is constructed on the premise that decisions about treatment properly belong to the incompetent or nonautonomous patient, by virtue of his or her rights of autonomy and privacy. In this conception, the patient has the right to decide and the right to have his or her values and preferences taken seriously, but is incompetent to exercise these rights, and it would be unfair to deprive such an incompetent patient of decision-making rights merely because he or she is no longer (or has never been) autonomous.

This standard is a weak standard of autonomy. It requires the surrogate decision maker to "don the mental mantle of the incompetent," as a classic court case (*Saikewicz*) put it—that is, to make the decision the incompetent person would have made if competent. In this case, the court invoked the standard of substituted judgment to decide that Joseph Saikewicz, a never-competent patient, would not have chosen treatment had he been competent. Asserting that what the majority of reasonable people would choose could differ from what a particular incompetent person would choose, the court said that,

> [T]he decision in many cases such as this should be that which would be made by the incompetent person, if that person were competent, but taking into account the present and future incompetency of the individual as one of the factors which would necessarily enter into the decision-making process of the competent person.[86]

The basic premise of the substituted judgment standard here rests on a fiction. An incompetent person cannot literally have the right to make medical decisions when other competent persons in fact exercise that right. The standard of substituted judgment should be used for once-competent patients only if reason exists to believe that the surrogate decision maker can make a judgment as the patient would have made it. In such cases, the surrogate should have such a deep and relevant familiarity with the patient that the particular judgment made reflects the patient's views and values. Merely knowing something in general about the patient's personal values is not adequate. Accordingly, if the surrogate can reliably answer the question, "What would *the patient* want in this circumstance?" substituted judgment is an appropriate standard that approximates first-person consent. But if the surrogate can only answer the question, "What do *you* want for the patient?" then this standard is inappropriate, because all connection to the patient's former autonomy has vanished. Similarly, we should reject the standard of substituted judgment for never-competent patients. No basis exists for a judgment of autonomous choice if a person has never been autonomous.

The standard of substituted judgment helps us understand what we should do for once-competent patients whose relevant prior preferences can be discerned; but, so interpreted, it collapses into a pure autonomy standard that respects previous autonomous choices.

The Pure Autonomy Standard

The second standard therefore eliminates the dubious autonomy reflected in substituted judgment and replaces it with a correct account of the role of autonomy. The pure autonomy standard applies exclusively to formerly autonomous, now-incompetent patients who expressed a relevant, autonomous treatment preference. The principle of respect for autonomy compels us to respect such preferences, even if the person can no longer express the preference for himself or herself. This standard asserts that, whether or not a formal advance directive exists, caretakers should accept prior autonomous judgments. This form of autonomy is sometimes referred to as "precedent autonomy." It has been invoked for a wide range of circumstances.[87]

The classic Claire Conroy case, in which the New Jersey Supreme Court grappled with several standards of surrogate decision making, sheds light on some of the moral issues surrounding this standard.[88] Conroy, an eighty-three-year-old nursing home resident, suffered from irreversible physical and mental impairments, including organic brain syndrome, arteriosclerotic heart disease, hypertension, diabetes, necrotic ulcers on her left foot, and a gangrenous left leg. She was awake enough to track persons with her eyes, but was severely demented, lay in a fetal position, and was unable to speak. She had no discernible cognitive or volitional functioning. Conroy's nephew (Thomas Whittemore), who was her guardian and only surviving blood relative, sought court permission to remove his aunt's nasogastric tube, an action that would result in her dehydration and death in about a week. He appealed to two of her expressed values and preferences: her general fear of doctors and her refusal to have her gangrenous leg amputated. He argued that his request for tube removal would conform to her wishes. Conroy's physician opposed Whittemore's petition as a violation of medical ethics. The trial court authorized removal of Conroy's feeding tube, even though she might die painfully, but a court-appointed guardian ad litem appealed the court's order. The New Jersey Supreme Court ultimately held that physicians could withhold or withdraw any medical treatment, including artificial nutrition and hydration, from an incompetent patient under certain conditions. More specifically, it held that physicians can legitimately withhold or withdraw life-sustaining treatment from an incompetent patient when a "subjective test"—meaning that there is a demonstrable basis in the patient's former autonomous choices—shows that this particular patient, when autonomous, would have preferred withdrawal. The court reasoned that a written document (such as a living will); an oral directive to family member, friend, or health care provider; a durable power of attorney; the patient's convictions about medical treatment administered to others; religious beliefs and tenets; or the "patient's consistent pattern of conduct with respect to prior decisions about medical care" can in principle, satisfy the autonomy-based standard. The court further noted that "in the absence of adequate proof of the patient's wishes, it is naive to pretend that the right to self-determination serves as the basis for substituted decision-making."

Although we too commend a pure autonomy standard, problems are evident in *Conroy* and similar legal decisions regarding satisfactory *evidence* for action under this standard. In the absence of explicit instructions, a surrogate decision maker might, for example, selectively choose from the patient's life history those values that accord with the surrogate's own values, and then use only those selected values in reaching decisions. The surrogate might also base his or her findings on values of the patient that are only distantly relevant to the immediate decision (e.g., the patient's expressed dislike of hospitals). One can reasonably ask what a decision maker could legitimately infer from Conroy's prior conduct, especially her fear and avoidance of doctors and her earlier refusal to consent to amputation of a gangrenous leg. A recurrent problem is that surrogates often assume an explicitness in a patient's directive about the future that does not directly show an autonomous preference with regard to the decision at hand.[89]

The Best Interests Standard

Sometimes the patient's relevant preferences cannot be known. Under the best interests standard a surrogate decision maker must determine the highest net benefit among the available options, assigning different weights to interests the patient has in each option and discounting or subtracting inherent risks or costs. The term *best* is used because the surrogate's obligation is to maximize benefit through a comparative assessment that locates the highest net benefit. The best interests standard protects an incompetent person's well-being by requiring surrogates to assess the risks and benefits of various treatments and alternatives to treatment. It is therefore inescapably a quality-of-life criterion. Those applying the best interests standard should consider the formerly autonomous patient's preferences, values, and perspectives only as far as they affect interpretations of quality of life, direct benefit, and the like.

We believe that the best interests standard can in some circumstances validly override advance directives executed by now incompetent but once autonomous patients, as well as refusals by minors and by other incompetent patients. This overriding can occur, for example, in a case in which a person has designated another by a durable power of attorney to make medical decisions on his or her behalf. If the designated surrogate makes a decision that threatens the patient's best interests, the decision should be overridden unless there is a clearly worded second document executed by the patient that specifically supports the surrogate's decision.

Problems of a person's ability to anticipate a future state often challenge reliance on advance directives. Much discussed are cases of apparently contented, nonsuffering, incompetent patients who can be expected to survive if treated against their advance directive, but who otherwise would die. Several discussions have focused on "Margo," a patient with Alzheimer's, who, according to the medical student who visited her regularly, is "one of the happiest people I have ever known."[90] Some discussants of her situation ask us to imagine what should be done if Margo had a living will, executed just at the onset of her Alzheimer's, stating that she did not want life-sustaining treatment if she developed another life-threatening illness. In that circumstance caregivers would have to determine whether to honor her advance directive, and thereby to respect her precedent autonomy by not using antibiotics to treat her pneumonia, or to act in accord with what may appear to be her current best interests given her overall happiness.

The challenge is serious. As persons slip into incompetence, their condition can be very different from, and better than, they had anticipated. If so, it seems unfair to the now happily situated incompetent person to be bound by a prior decision that may have been ill informed. In Margo's case, not using antibiotics would arguably harm what Ronald Dworkin called, in discussing this case, "experiential interests"—her contentment with her current life. However, providing antibiotics would violate her living will, which articulates her "critical interests"—her interests in a mode of living and dying that expresses her considered values, her life story and commitments, and the like. Dworkin argues that Margo should not be treated in these circumstances.[91] By contrast, the President's Council on Bioethics concludes that "Margo's apparent happiness would seem to make the argument for overriding the living will morally compelling in this particular case."[92]

Except in rare cases we are obligated to respect the previously expressed autonomous wishes of the now nonautonomous person precisely because of the force of the principle of respect for the autonomy of the person who made the decision. However, there are complicated issues about advance directives that we return to in Chapter 5.

Finally, best interests judgments are meant to focus attention entirely on the value of the life for the person who must live it, not on the value the person's life has for others. "Quality-of-life judgments" also concern only the individual's best interests, not his or her worth to enhance another's quality of life. Unfortunately, the best interests standard has sometimes been interpreted in highly malleable ways, thereby permitting consideration of values irrelevant to the individual's benefits or burdens. For example, when parents have sought court permission for a kidney transplant from an incompetent minor child to a sibling, parental judgments about the "donor's best interests" have on occasion taken into account projected psychological trauma from the death of the sibling and the psychological benefits of the unselfish act of "donation."[93] Such considerations should be greeted with skepticism and call attention to the need for additional procedural protections such as committee review. (We examine a range of concerns about the best interests standard in Chapters 5 and 6.)

In summary, it has been popular, although by no means universal, in biomedical ethics to hold that an ordered set of standards for surrogate decision making runs from (1) autonomously executed advance directives to (2) substituted judgment to (3) best interests, with the first having priority over the second and the first and second having priority over the third in a circumstance of conflict. We have argued that previously competent patients who autonomously expressed their preferences in an oral or written advance directive should be treated under the pure autonomy standard, and we have suggested an *economy of standards*; that is, we have determined that the first and second positions are essentially identical. The principle of respect for autonomy provides the only foundation, and it applies if and only if either a prior autonomous judgment itself constitutes an authorization or such a judgment supports a reasonable basis of inference for a surrogate. If the previously competent person left no reliable traces of his or her preferences, surrogate decision makers should adhere only to the best interests standard.

CONCLUSION

The intimate connection between autonomy and decision making in health care and research, especially in various circumstances of consent and refusal, unifies this chapter's several sections. Although we justified the obligation to solicit decisions from patients and potential research subjects by the principle of respect for autonomy, we also acknowledged that the principle's precise demands remain unsettled and open to interpretation and specification. We also maintained that construing respect for autonomy as a principle with priority over all other moral principles, rather than as one principle in a framework of prima facie principles, is indefensible. The human moral community, indeed morality itself, is rooted no less deeply in the three clusters of principles to be discussed in the next three chapters.

NOTES

1. Generally we refer to those who enroll in research as *subjects*, but sometimes as *participants*. Traditionally, the term *subject* was used to indicate that the enrollee was being experimented on, but it also reflected a distinction between object and subject and identified enrollees as partners and collaborators with investigators. In recent years, the term *subject* has been thought to reflect an unequal power relationship between researchers and enrollees that calls for significant safeguards. Many find "subject" also to suggest passivity on the part of enrollees, and to appear disrespectful or offensive. Although various terms, such as *volunteer, respondent,* and *interviewee,* have also been used, depending in part on the method of research being employed, the term *participant* is now widely used. However, *participant* is overly inclusive. The investigator and the research team are participants, and not all humans enrolled in research have chosen to enroll. In many cases others have enrolled them. Clearly, there is no perfect term. See the discussion in National Bioethics Advisory Commission (NBAC), *Ethical and Policy Issues in Research Involving Human Participants, Vol. I: Report and Recommendations* (Bethesda, MD: NBAC, August 2001), pp. 32–33.

2. The core idea of autonomy is treated by Joel Feinberg, *Harm to Self,* vol. III in *The Moral Limits of Criminal Law* (New York: Oxford University Press, 1986), chaps. 18–19; Thomas E. Hill, Jr., *Autonomy and Self-Respect* (Cambridge: Cambridge University Press, 1991), chaps. 1–4; and several essays in James Stacey Taylor, ed., *Personal Autonomy: New Essays on Personal Autonomy and Its Role in Contemporary Moral Philosophy* (Cambridge: Cambridge University Press, 2005). For a critical analysis and assessment of the conceptions of autonomy in previous editions of *Principles of Biomedical Ethics,* see Merle Spriggs, *Autonomy and Patients' Decisions* (Lanham, MD: Lexington Books, 2004). For a combination of empirical research and theory development in relation to patient autonomy, see Maartje Schermer, *The Different Faces of Autonomy: Patient Autonomy in Ethical Theory and Hospital Practice* (Dordrecht, Netherlands: Kluwer Academic, 2002). Several British and European scholars in bioethics have published rich analyses and critiques of autonomy and respect for autonomy. See, for example, the work of Onora O'Neill, briefly discussed later in this volume, and Francesc Torralba Rosselló, "The Limits of the Autonomy Principle: Philosophical Considerations," in *Basic Ethical Principles in European Bioethics and Biolaw, Vol. II: Partners' Research,* ed. Jacob Dahl Rendtorff and Peter Kemp (Copenhagen, Denmark: Centre for Ethics and Law, and Barcelona, Spain: Institut Borja de Bioètica, 2000), pp. 217–36.

3. For a rich theory that points to the importance of a broader theory of the autonomous person than we provide, see Rebecca Kukla, "Conscientious Autonomy: Displacing Decisions in Health Care," *Hastings Center Report* 35 (March–April 2005): 34–44.

4. Gerald Dworkin, *The Theory and Practice of Autonomy* (New York: Cambridge University Press, 1988), chaps. 1–4; Harry G. Frankfurt, "Freedom of the Will and the Concept of a Person," *Journal of Philosophy* 68 (1971): 5–20, as reprinted in *The Importance of What We Care About* (Cambridge: Cambridge University Press, 1988), pp. 11–25. Although it is not clear that Frankfurt holds a theory *of autonomy,* he uses the language of "autonomy" in his *Necessity, Volition, and Love* (Cambridge: Cambridge University Press, 1999), chaps. 9, 11, especially pp. 95–110, 137.

5. See Robert Paul Wolff, *In Defense of Anarchism* (New York: Harper & Row, 1970), pp. 4–6, 13ff; and Arthur Kuflik, "The Inalienability of Autonomy," *Philosophy and Public Affairs* 13 (1984): 271–98. See also Joseph Raz, "Authority and Justification," *Philosophy and Public Affairs* 14 (1985): 3–29; and Christopher McMahon, "Autonomy and Authority," *Philosophy and Public Affairs* 16 (1987): 303–28.

6. See several essays in *Relational Autonomy: Feminist Perspectives on Autonomy, Agency, and the Social Self,* ed. Catriona Mackenzie and Natalie Stoljar (New York: Oxford University Press, 2000); Susan Sherwin, *No Longer Patient: Feminist Ethics and Health Care* (Philadelphia: Temple University Press, 1992), esp. p. 138; Marilyn Friedman, *Autonomy, Gender, and Politics* (New York: Oxford University Press, 2003); John Christman, "Feminism and Autonomy," in *Nagging Questions: Feminist Ethics in Everyday Life,* ed. Dana Bushnell (Lanham, MD: Rowman & Littlefield, 1995).

7. See, further, Carolyn Ells, "Shifting the Autonomy Debate to Theory as Ideology," *Journal of Medicine and Philosophy* 26 (2001): 417–30; Mackenzie and Stoljar, "Introduction: Autonomy

Refigured," in *Relational Autonomy,* ed. Mackenzie and Stoljar, pp. 3–31, and see the chapters by Susan Dodds, Anne Donchin, Carolyn McLeod and Susan Sherwin. See also Susan Sherwin, "A Relational Approach to Autonomy in Health-Care," in *The Politics of Women's Health: Exploring Agency and Autonomy,* The Feminist Health Care Ethics Research Network (Philadelphia: Temple University Press, 1998); and Anne Donchin, "Understanding Autonomy Relationally," *Journal of Medicine and Philosophy* 23, No. 4 (1998).

8. Kant, *Foundations of the Metaphysics of Morals,* trans. Lewis White Beck (Indianapolis, IN: Bobbs-Merrill, 1959); *The Doctrine of Virtue,* part II of the *Metaphysics of Morals,* trans. Mary Gregor (Philadelphia: University of Pennsylvania Press, 1964), esp. p. 127. A probing treatment of Kant's theory that connects it to his ideas about moral practice is Paul Guyer, "Kant on the Theory and Practice of Autonomy," *Social Philosophy and Policy* 20 (2003): 70–98.

9. Mill, *On Liberty,* in *Collected Works of John Stuart Mill,* vol. 18 (Toronto: University of Toronto Press, 1977), chaps. I, III.

10. See Barbara Herman, "Mutual Aid and Respect for Persons," *Ethics* 94 (July 1984): 577–602, esp. 600–02; and Onora O'Neill, "Universal Laws and Ends-in-Themselves," *Monist* 72 (1989): 341–61.

11. See Carl E. Schneider, *The Practice of Autonomy: Patients, Doctors, and Medical Decisions* (New York: Oxford University Press, 1998), p. xi. See, similarly, Paul Root Wolpe, "The Triumph of Autonomy in American Bioethics: A Sociological View," in *Bioethics and Society: Constructing the Ethical Enterprise,* ed. Raymond DeVries and Janardan Subedi (Upper Saddle River, NJ: Prentice Hall, 1998), pp. 38–59; the essays in *The Right to Know and the Right Not to Know,* ed. Ruth Chadwick (Brookfield, MA: Avebury, 1997); Daniel Callahan, "Autonomy: A Moral Good, Not a Moral Obsession," *Hastings Center Report* 14 (October 1984): 40–42; Robert M. Veatch, "Autonomy's Temporary Triumph," *Hastings Center Report* 14 (October 1984): 38–40; James F. Childress, "The Place of Autonomy in Bioethics," *Hastings Center Report* 20 (January–February 1990): 12–16; and Thomas May, "The Concept of Autonomy in Bioethics: An Unwarranted Fall from Grace," in *Personal Autonomy,* ed. Taylor, pp. 299–309.

12. Leslie J. Blackhall, Sheila T. Murphy, Gelya Frank, et al., "Ethnicity and Attitudes toward Patient Autonomy," *Journal of the American Medical Association* 274 (September 13, 1995): 820–25.

13. Joseph A. Carrese and Lorna A. Rhodes, "Western Bioethics on the Navajo Reservation: Benefit or Harm?" *Journal of the American Medical Association* 274 (September 13, 1995): 826–29.

14. See Avram Goldstein, "Practice vs. Privacy on Pelvic Exams: Med Students' Training Intrusive and Needs Patient Consent, Activists Say," *Washington Post,* May 10, 2003, p. A1. For a larger discussion about informed consent for various medical students' interactions with patients, see Daniel L. Cohen et al., "Informed Consent Policies Governing Medical Students' Interactions with Patients," *Journal of Medical Education* 62 (October 1987): 789–829.

15. Britt-Ingjerd Nesheim, "Commentary: Respecting the Patient's Integrity Is the Key," *British Medical Journal* 326 (January 11, 2003): 100.

16. Peter A. Ubel, Christopher Jepson, and Ari Silver-Isenstadt, "Don't Ask, Don't Tell: A Change in Medical Student Attitudes after Obstetrics/Gynecology Clerkships toward Seeking Consent for Pelvic Examinations on an Anesthetized Patient," *American Journal of Obstetrics and Gynecology* 188 (February 2003): 575–79.

17. Bernard M. Branson, H. Hunter Handsfield, Margaret A. Lampe, et al., "Revised Recommendations for HIV Testing of Adults, Adolescents, and Pregnant Women in Health-Care Settings," *Morbidity and Mortality Weekly Report, Recommendations and Report* 55 (RR-14) (September 22, 2006): 1–17.

18. See Ronald Bayer and Amy L. Fairchild, "Changing the Paradigm for HIV Testing—The End of Exceptionalism," *New England Journal of Medicine* 355 (August 17, 2006): 647–49; Lawrence O. Gostin, "HIV Screening in Health Care Setting: Public Health and Civil Liberties in Conflict?" *Journal*

of the American Medical Association 296 (October 25, 2006): 2023–25. For a cost-effectiveness analysis, see Gillian D. Sanders et al., "Cost-Effectiveness of Screening for HIV in the Era of Highly Active Antiretroviral Therapy," *New England Journal of Medicine* 352 (February 10, 2005): 570–85.

19. Thomas R. Frieden et al., "Applying Public Health Principles to the HIV Epidemic," *New England Journal of Medicine* 353 (December 1, 2005): 2397–402.

20. See Bayer and Fairchild, "Changing the Paradigm for HIV Testing," p. 649.

21. For a fuller discussion of these issues, see the report of a committee for the Institute of Medicine on increasing the rates of organ donation, in James F. Childress and Catharyn Liverman, eds., *Organ Donation: Opportunities for Action* (Washington, DC: National Academies Press, 2006), chap. 7.

22. This case was provided by Gail Povar, M.D.

23. Thomas Grisso and Paul S. Appelbaum, *Assessing Competence to Consent to Treatment: A Guide for Physicians and Other Health Professionals* (New York: Oxford University Press, 1998), p. 11.

24. The analysis in this section has profited from discussions with Ruth R. Faden, Nancy M. P. King, and Dan Brock.

25. See the analysis of the core meaning in Charles M. Culver and Bernard Gert, *Philosophy in Medicine* (New York: Oxford University Press, 1982), pp. 123–26.

26. *Pratt v. Davis,* 118 Ill. App. 161 (1905), aff'd, 224 Ill. 300, 79 N.E. 562 (1906).

27. See Daniel Wikler, "Paternalism and the Mildly Retarded," *Philosophy and Public Affairs* 8 (1979): 377–92.

28. Subtleties and needed qualifications in this analysis are discussed by Kenneth F. Schaffner, "Competency: A Triaxial Concept," in *Competency,* ed. M. A. G. Cutter and E. E. Shelp (Dordrecht, Netherlands: Kluwer Academic, 1991), pp. 253–81.

29. This case was prepared by P. Browning Hoffman, M.D., for presentation in the series of "Medicine and Society" conferences at the University of Virginia. This case and our analysis have been challenged by Adrienne M. Martin, in "Tales Publicly Allowed: Competence, Capacity, and Religious Belief," *Hastings Center Report* 37 (2007): 33–40. However, her challenge is marred by conceptual confusions and misinterpretations of our position. See James F. Childress, "Must We Always Respect Religious Belief?" *Hastings Center Report* 37 (2007): 3.

30. This schema is indebted to Paul S. Appelbaum, Charles W. Lidz, and Alan Meisel, *Informed Consent: Legal Theory and Clinical Practice* (New York: Oxford University Press, 1987), chap. 5; and Paul S. Appelbaum and Thomas Grisso, "Assessing Patients' Capacities to Consent to Treatment," *New England Journal of Medicine* 319 (December 22, 1988): 1635–38. A later edition of the first work cited is Jessica W. Berg, Paul S. Appelbaum, Charles W. Lidz, and Lisa S. Parker, *Informed Consent: Legal Theory and Clinical Practice,* 2nd ed. (New York: Oxford University Press, 2001).

31. Grisso and Appelbaum focus on four functional abilities in assessments of competence to consent to treatment: ability to express a choice, ability to understand information relevant to treatment decision making, ability to appreciate the significance of that information for one's own situation, and ability to reason logically using relevant information. *Assessing Competence to Consent to Treatment,* chap. 3. Our list here does not include "appreciation," which we treat later as part of understanding.

32. For additional ways in which values are incorporated, see Loretta M. Kopelman, "On the Evaluative Nature of Competency and Capacity Judgments," *International Journal of Law and Psychiatry* 13 (1990): 309–29. For conceptual and epistemic problems in available tests, see E. Haavi Morreim, "Competence: At the Intersection of Law, Medicine, and Philosophy," in *Competency,* pp. 93–125, esp. pp. 105–08.

33. See Sander P. K. Welie, "Criteria for Patient Decision Making (In)competence: A Review of and Commentary on Some Empirical Approaches," *Medicine, Health Care and Philosophy* 4 (2001): 139–51; Jennifer Moye, Ronald J. Guerrera, Michele J. Karel et al., "Empirical Advances in the Assessment of the Capacity to Consent to Medical Treatment: Clinical Implications and Medical Needs," *Clinical Psychology Review* 26 (2006): 1054–77; and Laura B. Dunn, Milap A. Nowrangi, Barton W. Palmer et al., "Assessing Decisional Capacity for Clinical Research or Treatment: A Review of Instruments," *American Journal of Psychiatry* 163 (2006): 1323–34.

34. Grisso and Appelbaum, *Assessing Competence to Consent to Treatment,* p. 139.

35. See Willard Gaylin, "The Competence of Children: No Longer All or None," *Hastings Center Report* 12 (April 1982): 33–38, esp. 35; Allen Buchanan and Dan Brock, *Deciding for Others* (Cambridge: Cambridge University Press, 1989), pp. 51–70; and Brock, "Children's Competence for Health Care Decision Making," in *Children and Health Care,* ed. Loretta Kopelman and John Moskop (Boston: Kluwer Academic, 1989), pp. 181–212; and Eric Kodish, "Children's Competence for Assent and Consent: A Review of Empirical Findings," *Ethics & Behavior* 14 (2004): 255–95.

36. We also need to distinguish two senses of *standard of competence.* In one sense, *criteria of competence* are at stake; that is, the conditions under which a person is competent. In a second sense, *standard of competence* refers to the *pragmatic guidelines* we use to determine competence. For example, a mature teenager could be competent to decide about a kidney transplant (satisfying criteria of competence) but could also be legally incompetent by virtue of age (failing pragmatic guidelines). To avoid this problem of a dual meaning of *standard of competence* we use the term only to mean a criterion for determining competence.

37. Buchanan and Brock, *Deciding for Others,* pp. 52–55. For elaboration and defense, see Brock, "Decisionmaking Competence and Risk," *Bioethics* 5 (1991): 105–12.

38. *Report and Recommendations of the National Bioethics Advisory Commission, Research Involving Persons with Mental Disorders That May Affect Decision Making Capacity,* Vol. I (Rockville, MD: National Bioethics Advisory Commission, December 1998), p. 58.

39. Onora O'Neill, *Autonomy and Trust in Bioethics* (Cambridge: Cambridge University Press, 2002); O'Neill, "Autonomy: The Emperor's New Clothes," *Proceedings of the Aristotelian Society,* supp. Vol. 77 (2003): 1–21; O'Neill, "Some Limits of Informed Consent," *Journal of Medical Ethics* 29 (2003): 4–7; Neil C. Manson and Onora O'Neill, *Rethinking Informed Consent in Bioethics* (Cambridge: Cambridge University Press, 2007).

40. O'Neill, "Some Limits of Informed Consent," p. 5.

41. See Jay Katz, *The Silent World of Doctor and Patient* (New York: Free Press, 1984), pp. 86–87 [Reprint ed. (Baltimore, MD: The Johns Hopkins University Press, 2002)]; and President's Commission for the Study of Ethical Problems in Medicine and Biomedical and Behavioral Research, *Making Health Care Decisions,* vol. I (Washington, DC: U.S. Government Printing Office, 1982), p. 15.

42. For extensions of this thesis, see Simon Whitney, Amy McGuire, and Laurence McCullough, "A Typology of Shared Decision Making, Informed Consent, and Simple Consent," *Annals of Internal Medicine* 140 (2003): 54–59.

43. The analysis in this subsection is based in part on Faden and Beauchamp, *A History and Theory of Informed Consent,* chap. 8.

44. *Mohr v. Williams,* 95 Minn. 261, 265; 104 N.W. 12, 15 (1905).

45. See Jay Katz, "Disclosure and Consent," in *Genetics and the Law II,* ed. A. Milunsky and G. Annas (New York: Plenum, 1980), pp. 122, 128.

46. See, for example, Alan Meisel and Loren Roth, "What We Do and Do Not Know about Informed Consent," *Journal of the American Medical Association* 246 (1981): 2473–77; President's Commission,

Making Health Care Decisions, vol. II, pp. 317–410, esp. 318, and vol. I, chap. 1, esp. pp. 38–39; National Commission for the Protection of Human Subjects of Biomedical and Behavioral Research, *The Belmont Report* (Washington, DC: DHEW Publication OS 78–0012, 1978), p. 10.

47. See, for a classic case, *Planned Parenthood of Central Missouri v. Danforth,* 428 U.S. 52 at 67 n.8 (1976) (U.S. Supreme Court).

48. *Moore v. Regents of the University of California,* 793 P.2d 479 (Cal. 1990) at 483.

49. See, for example, Clarence H. Braddock et al., "How Doctors and Patients Discuss Routine Clinical Decisions: Informed Decision Making in the Outpatient Setting," *Journal of General Internal Medicine* 12 (1997): 339–45; John Briguglio et al., "Development of a Model Angiography Informed Consent Form Based on a Multiinstitutional Survey of Current Forms," *Journal of Vascular and Interventional Radiology* 6 (1995): 971–78; and Charles Keown, Paul Slovic, and Sarah Lichtenstein, "Attitudes of Physicians, Pharmacists, and Laypersons toward Seriousness and Need for Disclosure of Prescription Drug Side Effects," *Health Psychology* 3 (1984): 1–11.

50. Ruth R. Faden and Tom L. Beauchamp, "Decision-Making and Informed Consent: A Study of the Impact of Disclosed Information," *Social Indicators Research* 7 (1980): 313–36.

51. Carl H. Fellner and John R. Marshall, "Kidney Donors—The Myth of Informed Consent," *American Journal of Psychiatry* 126 (1970): 1245–50, and "Twelve Kidney Donors," *Journal of the American Medical Association* 206 (1968): 2703–07. See also Roberta G. Simmons, Susan Klein Marine, and Richard L. Simmons, *Gift of Life: The Effect of Organ Transplantation on Individual, Family, and Societal Dynamics* (New Brunswick, NJ: Transaction Books, 1987), esp. chap. 8.

52. See L. A. Siminoff and J. H. Fetting, "Factors Affecting Treatment Decisions for a Life-Threatening Illness: The Case of Medical Treatment of Breast Cancer," *Social Science and Medicine* 32 (1991): 813–18; Jennifer S. Mark and Howard Spiro, "Informed Consent for Colonoscopy: A Prospective Study," *Archives of Internal Medicine* 150 (1990): 777–80; and Christina G. Blanchard et al., "Information and Decision-Making Preferences of Hospitalized Adult Cancer Patients," *Social Science and Medicine* 27 (1988): 1139–45.

53. L. A. Siminoff, J. H. Fetting, and M. D. Abeloff, "Doctor–Patient Communication about Breast Cancer Adjuvant Therapy," *Journal of Clinical Oncology* 7 (1989): 1192–1200; and J. H. Fetting, L. A. Siminoff et al., "Effect of Patients' Expectations of Benefit with Standard Breast Cancer Adjuvant Chemotherapy on Participation in Randomized Clinical Trial," *Journal of Clinical Oncology* 8 (1990): 1476–82.

54. The Oklahoma Supreme Court has supported this standard. See *Scott v. Bradford,* 606 P.2d 554 (Okla. 1979) at 559 (together with *Masquat v. Maguire,* 638 P.2d 1105, Okla. 1981).

55. *Canterbury v. Spence,* 464 F.2d 772 (1977), at 785–89. For studies of levels of anxiety and stress produced by informed consent disclosures, see Jeffrey Goldberger et al., "Effect of Informed Consent on Anxiety in Patients Undergoing Diagnostic Electrophysiology Studies," *American Heart Journal* 134 (1997): 119–26; Kenneth D. Hopper et al., "The Effect of Informed Consent on the Level of Anxiety in Patients Given IV Contrast Material," *American Journal of Roentgenology* 162 (1994): 531–35; and S. Inglis and D. Farnill, "The Effects of Providing Preoperative Statistical Anaesthetic-Risk Information," *Anaesthesia and Intensive Care* 21 (1993): 799–805.

56. *Thornburgh v. American College of Obstetricians,* 106 S.Ct. 2169, at 2199–2200 (1986) (White, J., dissenting).

57. See Howard Brody, *Placebos and the Philosophy of Medicine: Clinical, Conceptual, and Ethical Issues* (Chicago: University of Chicago Press, 1980), pp. 10–11.

58. For a similar proposal, see Armand Lione, "Ethics of Placebo Use in Clinical Care" (Correspondence), *The Lancet* 362 (September 20, 2003): 999. For cases involving the different appeals to "consent," along

with analysis and assessment, see P. Lichtenberg, U. Heresco-Levy, and U. Nitzan, "The Ethics of the Placebo in Clinical Practice," *Journal of Medical Ethics* 30 (2004): 551–54; "Case Vignette: Placebos and Informed Consent," *Ethics and Behavior* 8 (1998): 89–90, with commentaries by Jeffrey Blustein, Walter Robinson, and Gregory S. Loeben and Benjamin S. Wilfond; and Philip Levendusky and Loren Pankratz, "Self-Control Techniques as an Alternative to Pain Medication," *Journal of Abnormal Psychology* 84 (1975): 165–68.

59. Brody, *Placebos and the Philosophy of Medicine,* pp. 110, 113, et passim; Brody, "The Placebo Response: Recent Research and Implications for Family Medicine," *The Journal of Family Practice* 49, No. 7 (July 2000): 649–54; Katz, *The Silent World,* pp. 189–95. For a broader defense of placebos, see Howard Spiro, *Doctors, Patients, and Placebos* (New Haven, CT: Yale University Press, 1986). See also Arthur K. Shapiro and Elaine Shapiro, *The Powerful Placebo: From Ancient Priest to Modern Physician* (Baltimore: The Johns Hopkins University Press, 1997).

60. Sally E. McNagy and Ruth M. Parker, "High Prevalence of Recent Cocaine Use and the Unreliability of Patient Self-Report in an Inner-City Walk-in Clinic," *Journal of the American Medical Association* 267 (February 26, 1992): 1106–08.

61. Sissela Bok, "Informed Consent in Tests of Patient Reliability," *Journal of the American Medical Association* 267 (February 26, 1992): 1118–19.

62. Barbara A. Bernhardt et al., "Educating Patients about Cystic Fibrosis Carrier Screening in a Primary Care Setting," *Archives of Family Medicine* 5 (1996): 336–40.

63. Steven Joffe et al., "Quality of Informed Consent in Cancer Clinical Trials: A Cross-Sectional Survey," *The Lancet* 358 (November 24, 2001): 1772–77.

64. *Bang v. Charles T. Miller Hospital,* 251 Minn. 427, 88 N.W. 2d 186 (1958).

65. See also Gopal Sreenivasan, "Does Informed Consent to Research Require Comprehension?" *The Lancet* 362 (December 13, 2003): 2016–18.

66. C. K. Dougherty et al., "Perceptions of Cancer Patients and Their Physicians Involved in Phase I Clinical Trials," *Journal of Clinical Oncology* 13 (1995): 1062–72; Paul R. Benson et al., "Information Disclosure, Subject Understanding, and Informed Consent in Psychiatric Research," *Law and Human Behavior* 12 (1988): 455–75.

67. See further Edmund G. Howe, "Approaches (and Possible Contraindications) to Enhancing Patients' Autonomy," *Journal of Clinical Ethics* 5 (1994): 179–88.

68. James Flory and Ezekiel Emanuel, "Interventions to Improve Research Participants' Understanding in Informed Consent for Research," *Journal of the American Medical Association* 292 (October 6, 2004): 1593–1601.

69. David Wendler, "Can We Ensure that All Research Subjects Give Valid Consent?" *Archives of Internal Medicine* 164 (November 8, 2004): 2201–04.

70. This label was apparently coined by Paul S. Appelbaum, Loren Roth, and Charles W. Lidz in "The Therapeutic Misconception: Informed Consent in Psychiatric Research," *International Journal of Law and Psychiatry* 5 (1982): 319–29. For an indication that the misconception is still widespread, see Appelbaum, Lidz, and Thomas Grisso, "Therapeutic Misconception in Clinical Research: Frequency and Risk Factors," *IRB: Ethics and Human Research* 26 (2004): 1–8. See also W. Glannon, "Phase I Oncology Trials: Why the Therapeutic Misconception Will Not Go Away," *Journal of Medical Ethics* 32 (2006): 252–55.

71. Sam Horng and Christine Grady, "Misunderstanding in Clinical Research: Distinguishing Therapeutic Misconception, Therapeutic Misestimation, & Therapeutic Optimism," *IRB: Ethics and Human Research* 25 (January–February 2003): 11–16.

72. The pioneering work was done by Amos Tversky and Daniel Kahneman. See "Choices, Values and Frames," *American Psychologist* 39 (1984): 341–50; and "The Framing of Decisions and the Psychology of Choice," *Science* 211 (1981): 453–58. See also Daniel Kahneman and Amos Tversky, eds., *Choices, Values, and Frames* (Cambridge: Cambridge University Press, 2000). On informed consent specifically, see Dennis J. Mazur and Jon F. Merz, "How Age, Outcome Severity, and Scale Influence General Medicine Clinic Patients' Interpretations of Verbal Probability Terms," *Journal of General Internal Medicine* 9 (1994): 268–71.

73. S. E. Eraker and H. C. Sox, "Assessment of Patients' Preferences for Therapeutic Outcome," *Medical Decision Making* 1 (1981): 29–39; Barbara McNeil et al., "On the Elicitation of Preferences for Alternative Therapies," *New England Journal of Medicine* 306 (May 27, 1982): 1259–62.

74. Ruth Faden and Alan Faden, "False Belief and the Refusal of Medical Treatment," *Journal of Medical Ethics* 3 (1977): 133–36.

75. Neil Manson and Onora O'Neill interpret all consent as a waiver of rights. Although this account is not incorrect, it is generally more illuminating to describe informed consent as an exercise of rights rather than a waiver of rights. See Manson and O'Neill, *Rethinking Informed Consent in Bioethics,* esp. pp. 72–77, 187–89.

76. *Cobbs v. Grant,* 502 P.2d 1, 12 (1972).

77. Baruch Brody, *Life and Death Decision Making* (New York: Oxford University Press, 1988), p. 22.

78. See Joel Feinberg, *Social Philosophy* (Englewood Cliffs, NJ: Prentice Hall, 1973), p. 48; *Harm to Self,* pp. 112–18. Our theory of autonomy has been accused of harboring a "voluntariness bias." See Anne Donchin, "Reworking Autonomy: Toward a Feminist Perspective," *Cambridge Quarterly* of *Health Care Ethics* 4 (1995): 44–55, esp. 46–47.

79. Our formulation is indebted to Robert Nozick, "Coercion," in *Philosophy, Science and Method: Essays in Honor of Ernest Nagel,* ed. Sidney Morgenbesser, Patrick Suppes, and Morton White (New York: St. Martin's, 1969), pp. 440–72; and Bernard Gert, "Coercion and Freedom," in *Coercion: Nomos XIV,* ed. J. Roland Pennock and John W. Chapman (Chicago: Aldine, Atherton, 1972), pp. 36–37. See also Alan Wertheimer, *Coercion* (Princeton, NJ: Princeton University Press, 1987).

80. For a discussion of coercion in relation to exploitation and undue inducement, which we consider later, see Jennifer S. Hawkins and Ezekiel J. Emanuel, "Clarifying Confusions about Coercion," *Hastings Center Report* 35 (September–October 2005): 16–19.

81. See James H. Jones, *Bad Blood,* rev. ed. (New York: Free Press, 1993); David J. Rothman, "Were Tuskegee & Willowbrook 'Studies in Nature'?" *Hastings Center Report* 12 (April 1982): 5–7; and Susan M. Reverby, ed., *Tuskegee's Truths: Rethinking the Tuskegee Syphilis Study* (Chapel Hill, NC: University of North Carolina Press, 2000).

82. See Sarah E. Hewlett, "Is Consent to Participate in Research Voluntary?" *Arthritis Care and Research* 9 (1996): 400–04; and Nancy E. Kass et al., "Trust: The Fragile Foundation of Contemporary Biomedical Research," *Hastings Center Report* 25 (September–October 1996): 25–29.

83. See Charles W. Lidz et al., *Informed Consent: A Study of Decision Making in Psychiatry* (New York: Guilford, 1984), chap. 7, esp. pp. 110–11, 117–23.

84. Little research has been conducted on prisoners in the United States since the 1970s, as a result of the work, and stringent interpretations of the work, of the National Commission for the Protection of Human Subjects of Biomedical and Behavioral Research, which focused on the implications of the principles of respect for persons and justice. For an ethical framework that would allow more research involving prisoners, see an Institute of Medicine Committee report: Lawrence O. Gostin,

Cori Vanchieri, and Andrew Pope, eds., *Ethical Considerations for Research Involving Prisoners* (Washington, DC: National Academies Press, 2007), esp. chap. 5.

85. For the distinction between decisional autonomy and executional autonomy, see Bart J. Collopy, "Autonomy in Long Term Care," *The Gerontologist* 28, Supplementary Issue (June 1988): 10–17. On failures to appreciate both capacity and incapacity to consent in nursing homes, see C. Dennis Barton et al., "Clinicians' Judgement of Capacity of Nursing Home Patients to Give Informed Consent," *Psychiatric Services* 47 (1996): 956–60; and Meghan B. Gerety et al., "Medical Treatment Preferences of Nursing Home Residents," *Journal of the American Geriatrics Society* 41 (1993): 953–60.

86. *Superintendent of Belchertown State School v. Saikewicz,* Mass. 370 N.E. 2d 417 (1977).

87. See John K. Davis, "The Concept of Precedent Autonomy," *Bioethics* 16 (2002): 114–33.

88. In re *Conroy,* 486 A.2d 1209 (N.J. 1985). All quotations that follow are from this source.

89. See, for example, *In the Matter of the Application of John Evans against Bellevue Hospital,* Supreme Court of the State of New York, Index No. 16536/87 (1987).

90. A. D. Firlik, "Margo's Logo" (Letter), *Journal of the American Medical Association* 265 (1991): 201.

91. Ronald Dworkin, *Life's Dominion: An Argument about Abortion, Euthanasia, and Individual Freedom* (New York: Knopf, 1993), pp. 221–29. He admits that we might have reasons other than respect for autonomy for not wanting to live in a community that fails to provide life-prolonging care to such a patient if she now wants it (even though she lacks autonomous capacity to revoke her prior living will) (pp. 228–29).

92. President's Council on Bioethics, *Taking Care: Ethical Caregiving in Our Aging Society* (Washington, DC: The President's Council on Bioethics, September 2005), p. 84. The President's Council draws in part on the work of one of its members, Rebecca Dresser, "Dworkin on Dementia: Elegant Theory, Questionable Policy," *Hastings Center Report* 25 (1995): 32–38; and Dresser and John Robertson, "Quality of Life and Non-Treatment Decisions for Incompetent Patients: A Critique of the Orthodox Approach," *Law, Medicine, and Health Care* 17 (1989): 234–44. For other discussions, see Jeffrey Blustein, "Choosing for Others as Continuing a Life Story: The Problem of Personal Identity Revisited," *Journal of Law, Medicine and Ethics* 27 (Spring 1999): 20–31; Helga Kuhse, "Some Reflections on the Problem of Advance Directives, Personhood and Personal Identity," *Kennedy Institute of Ethics Journal* 9 (December 1999): 347–64.

93. The classic case is *Strunk v. Strunk,* 445 S.W.2d 145 (Ky 1969), which considered these benefits in terms of a standard of substituted judgment.

5
Nonmaleficence

The principle of nonmaleficence imposes an obligation not to inflict harm on others. In medical ethics it has been closely associated with the maxim *Primum non nocere:* "Above all [or first] do no harm." Health care professionals frequently invoke this maxim, despite its obscure origins and implications. Often proclaimed the fundamental principle in the Hippocratic tradition of medical ethics, the principle of nonmaleficence does not appear in the Hippocratic corpus, and a venerable statement sometimes confused with it—"at least, do no harm"—is a strained translation of a single Hippocratic passage.[1] Nonetheless, the Hippocratic oath clearly expresses an obligation of nonmaleficence and an obligation of beneficence: "I will use treatment to help the sick according to my ability and judgment, but I will never use it to injure or wrong them."

This chapter explores the principle of nonmaleficence and its implications for several areas of biomedical ethics. For example, we examine distinctions between killing and letting die, intending and foreseeing harmful outcomes, withholding and withdrawing life-sustaining treatments, and extraordinary and ordinary treatments. Several issues center on the terminally ill and the seriously ill and injured. The framework for decision making about life-sustaining procedures and assistance in dying that we defend would alter current medical practice for both competent and incompetent patients. Central to this framework is an interpretation of the commitments of the principle of nonmaleficence that strongly supports, rather than suppresses, quality-of-life judgments.

THE CONCEPT OF NONMALEFICENCE

The Distinction between Nonmaleficence and Beneficence

Many types of ethical theory recognize a principle of nonmaleficence.[2] Some philosophers combine nonmaleficence with beneficence to form a single principle. William Frankena, for example, divides the principle of beneficence into four general obligations, the first of which we identify as the obligation of nonmaleficence and the other three of which we refer to as principles and obligations of beneficence:

1. One ought not to inflict evil or harm.
2. One ought to prevent evil or harm.
3. One ought to remove evil or harm.
4. One ought to do or promote good.[3]

If we bring the ideas of benefiting others and not injuring them under a single principle, we will be forced to note, as does Frankena, the several distinct obligations embedded in this general principle. In our view, conflating nonmaleficence and beneficence into a single principle obscures important distinctions. Obligations not to harm others (e.g., those prohibiting theft, disablement, and killing) are distinct from obligations to help others (e.g., those prescribing the provision of benefits, protection of interests, and promotion of welfare).

Obligations not to harm others are sometimes more stringent than obligations to help them, but the reverse is also true. If in a particular case a health care provider inflicts a very minor injury (swelling from a needlestick, say), but simultaneously provides a major benefit (a life-saving intervention, say), then we consider the obligation of beneficence to take priority over the obligation of nonmaleficence.[4] The point is that causing some risks of surgical harm, introducing social costs to protect the public health, and placing burdens on some research subjects can all be justified by the benefits of the actions.

One might try to reformulate the idea of nonmaleficence's increased stringency as follows: Generally, obligations of nonmaleficence are more stringent than obligations of beneficence, and, in some cases, nonmaleficence overrides beneficence, even if the best utilitarian outcome would be obtained by acting beneficently. If a surgeon, for example, could save two innocent lives by killing a prisoner on death row to retrieve his heart and liver for transplantation, this outcome would have the highest net utility (in the circumstances), but the surgeon's action would be morally indefensible. This formulation of the stringency of nonmaleficence has an initial ring of plausibility, especially if the act of benefiting involves committing a moral wrong. Again, however, we should be cautious about constructing axioms of priority. A beneficial action does not necessarily take second place to an act of not causing harm. Nonmaleficence typically overrides other principles, but the weights of these moral principles vary in different circumstances. In our view, no rule in ethics favors avoiding harm over providing benefit in *all* circumstances. The claim that an order of priority exists among elements 1 through 4 in Frankena's scheme mentioned earlier is therefore unsustainable.

Rather than attempting to structure a hierarchical ordering, we group the principles of nonmaleficence and beneficence into four norms that (a priori) lack hierarchical ordering:

Nonmaleficence

1. One ought not to inflict evil or harm.

Beneficence

2. One ought to prevent evil or harm.
3. One ought to remove evil or harm.
4. One ought to do or promote good.

Each of the three principles of beneficence requires taking action by *helping*—preventing harm, removing harm, and promoting good—whereas nonmaleficence requires only *intentionally refraining* from actions that cause harm. Rules of nonmaleficence therefore take the form "Do not do X." Some philosophers accept only principles or rules that take this proscriptive form. They even limit rules of respect for autonomy to rules of the form "Do not interfere with a person's autonomous choices." These philosophers reject all principles or rules that require helping, assisting, or rescuing other persons (although they recognize these norms as legitimate *moral ideals*). Mainstream moral philosophy, however, does not accept such a *sharp* distinction between obligations of refraining from harming and obligations of helping and, instead, recognizes and preserves the relevant distinctions in other ways. We take this same path, and in Chapter 6 we explain further the nature of the distinction.

Legitimate disagreements arise about how to classify actions under categories 1 through 4, as well as about the nature and stringency of the obligations that arise from them. Consider the following case: Robert McFall was dying of aplastic anemia, and his physicians recommended a bone marrow transplant from a genetically compatible donor to increase his chances of living one additional year from twenty-five percent to a range of forty to sixty percent. The patient's cousin, David Shimp, agreed to undergo tests to determine his suitability as a donor. After completing the test for tissue compatibility, he refused to undergo the test for genetic compatibility. He had changed his mind about donation. Robert McFall's lawyer asked a court to compel Shimp to undergo the second test and donate his bone marrow if the test indicated a good match.[5]

Public discussion focused on whether Shimp had an obligation of beneficence toward McFall in the form of an obligation to prevent harm, to remove harm, or to promote McFall's welfare. McFall's lawyer contended (unsuccessfully) that even if Shimp did not have a legal obligation of beneficence to rescue his cousin, he did have a legal obligation of nonmaleficence, which required that he not make McFall's situation worse. The lawyer argued that when Shimp agreed to undergo the first test and then backed out, he caused a "delay of critical proportions" that constituted a violation of the obligation of nonmaleficence. The judge ruled that Shimp did not violate any legal obligations but also held that his actions were "morally indefensible."[6]

This case illustrates difficulties of identifying specific obligations under the principles of beneficence and nonmaleficence. Again we see the importance of *specifying* these principles to handle circumstances such as donating organs or tissues, withholding life-sustaining treatments, hastening the death of a dying patient, and biomedical research involving both human and animal subjects.

The Concept of Harm

The concept of nonmaleficence has been explicated by the concepts of *harm* and *injury,* but we confine our analysis to harm. This term has both a normative and a nonnormative use. "X harmed Y" sometimes means that X wronged Y or treated Y unjustly, but it sometimes means only that X's action had an adverse effect on Y's interests. As we use these notions, *wronging* involves violating someone's rights, but *harming* need not signify such a violation. People are harmed without being wronged in attacks by disease, natural disasters, bad luck, and acts by others to which the harmed person has consented.[7] People can also be wronged without being harmed. For example, if an insurance company improperly refuses to pay a patient's hospital bill and the hospital shoulders the full bill, the insurance company wronged the patient without harming him or her.

We construe harm exclusively in the second and nonnormative sense of thwarting, defeating, or setting back some party's interests. Therefore, a *harmful* action by one party may not be wrong or unjustified, although acts of harming in general are prima facie wrong. The reason for their prima facie wrongness is that they set back the interests of the persons affected. Harmful actions that involve *justifiable* setbacks to another's interests are not wrong. They include cases of justified punishment of physicians for incompetence or negligence, justified demotion of an employee for poor performance in a job, and some forms of research involving animals.

Some definitions of harm are so broad that they include setbacks to interests in reputation, property, privacy, and liberty. So broad is the term *harm* in some writings that it seems to include causing discomfort, humiliation, offense, and annoyance. Such a broad conception can still distinguish trivial harms from serious harms by the magnitude of the interests affected. Other accounts with a narrower focus view harms exclusively as setbacks to physical and psychological interests, such as those in health and survival.

Whether a broad or a narrow construal is preferable is not a matter we need to decide. Although *harm* is a contested concept, everyone agrees that significant bodily harms and other setbacks to significant interests are paradigm instances of harm. We concentrate on physical harms, especially pain, disability, suffering, and death, while still affirming the importance of mental harms and other setbacks to one's interests. In particular, we concentrate on intending, causing, and permitting death or the risk of death.

Rules Specifying the Principle of Nonmaleficence

The principle of nonmaleficence supports several more specific moral rules (although principles other than nonmaleficence help justify some of these rules).[8] Examples of more specific rules include the following:[9]

1. Do not kill.
2. Do not cause pain or suffering.
3. Do not incapacitate.
4. Do not cause offense.
5. Do not deprive others of the goods of life.

Both the principle of nonmaleficence and its specifications in these moral rules are prima facie, not absolute (see pp. 14–16).

Negligence and the Standard of Due Care

Obligations of nonmaleficence include not only obligations not to inflict harms, but also obligations not to impose *risks* of harm. A person can harm or place another person at risk without malicious or harmful intent, and the agent of harm may or may not be morally or legally responsible for the harms. In some cases agents are causally responsible for a harm that they did not intend or know about. For example, if cancer rates are elevated at a chemical plant as the result of exposure to a chemical not previously suspected as a carcinogen, the employer has placed its workers at risk by its actions or decisions, although the employer did not intentionally or knowingly cause the harm.

In cases of risk imposition, both law and morality recognize a standard of due care that determines whether the agent who is causally responsible for the risk is legally or morally responsible as well. This standard is a specification of the principle of nonmaleficence. Due care is taking sufficient and appropriate care to avoid causing harm, as the circumstances demand of a reasonable and prudent person. This standard requires that the goals pursued justify the risks that must be imposed to achieve those goals. Grave risks require commensurately momentous goals for their justification. Serious emergencies justify risks that many nonemergency situations do not justify. For example, attempting to save lives after a major accident justifies, within limits, the dangers created by speeding emergency vehicles. A person who takes due care in this sense does not violate moral or legal rules, even in imposing great risk on other parties.

Negligence is the absence of due care. In the professions negligence involves a departure from the professional standards that determine due care in given

circumstances. The term *negligence* covers two types of situations: (1) intentionally imposing unreasonable risks of harm (advertent negligence or recklessness)
and (2) unintentionally but carelessly imposing risks of harm (inadvertent negligence). In the first type, an agent knowingly imposes an unwarranted risk. For
example, a nurse knowingly fails to change a bandage as scheduled, creating an
increased risk of infection. In the second type, an agent unknowingly performs a
harmful act that he or she should have known to avoid. For example, a physician
acts negligently if he or she forgets that a patient does not want to receive certain
types of information and discloses that information, causing fear and shame in
the patient. Both types of negligence are morally blameworthy, although some
conditions may mitigate the blameworthiness. Subtle forms of such judgments
pervade morality and medical ethics, as well as criminal and civil law.[10]

In treating negligence, we concentrate on conduct that falls below a standard
of due care that law or morality establishes to protect others from the care-
less imposition of risks. Courts must determine responsibility and liability for
harm, because a patient, client, or customer seeks compensation for setbacks to
interests or punishment of a responsible party, or both. We do not here consider
legal liability, but the legal model of responsibility for harmful action suggests a
framework that we can adapt to express moral responsibility for harm caused by
health care professionals. The following are essential elements in a professional
model of due care:

1. The professional must have a duty to the affected party.
2. The professional must breach that duty.
3. The affected party must experience a harm.
4. The harm must be caused by the breach of duty.

Professional malpractice is an instance of negligence that involves not following professional standards of care.[11] By entering into the profession of medicine,
physicians accept a responsibility to observe the standards specific to their
profession. If their conduct falls below these standards, they act negligently.
Conversely, even if the therapeutic relationship proves harmful or unhelpful,
malpractice occurs if and only if physicians do not meet professional standards
of care. For example, in *Adkins v. Ropp* the Supreme Court of Indiana considered
a patient's claim that a physician acted negligently in removing foreign matter
from the patient's eye:

> When a physician and surgeon assumes to treat and care for a patient, in
> the absence of a special agreement, he is held in law to have impliedly
> contracted that he possesses the reasonable and ordinary qualifications of
> his profession and that he will exercise at least reasonable skill, care and
> diligence in his treatment of him. This implied contract on the part of the
> physician does not include a promise to effect a cure and negligence cannot
> be imputed because a cure is not effected, but he does impliedly promise

that he will use due diligence and ordinary skill in his treatment of the patient so that a cure may follow such care and skill. This degree of care and skill is required of him, not only in performing an operation or administering first treatments, but he is held to the same degree of care and skill in the necessary subsequent treatments unless he is excused from further service by the patient himself, or the physician or surgeon upon due notice refuses to further treat the case.[12]

The line between due care and inadequate care (that which falls below what is due) is often difficult to draw. Increased safety measures in epidemiological and toxicological studies, educational or health promotional programs, and other training programs can sometimes reduce health risks. A substantial question, however, remains about the lengths to which physicians, employers, and others must go to avoid or lower risks—a problem in determining the scope of obligations of nonmaleficence.

DISTINCTIONS AND RULES GOVERNING NONTREATMENT

Religious traditions, philosophical discourse, professional codes, and the law have developed several guidelines to specify the requirements of nonmaleficence in health care, particularly with regard to treatment and nontreatment decisions. Some of these guidelines are helpful, but others need revision or replacement. Many draw heavily on at least one of the following distinctions:

1. *Withholding* and *withdrawing* life-sustaining treatment
2. *Extraordinary* (or heroic) and *ordinary* treatment
3. Sustenance technologies and medical treatments
4. *Intended* effects and *merely foreseen* effects
5. *Killing* and *letting die*

Although at times influential in medicine and law, these distinctions are all outmoded and untenable. The venerable position that these traditional distinctions have occupied in professional codes, institutional policies, and writings in biomedical ethics provides no warrant for retaining them, and some of these distinctions are morally dangerous.

Withholding and Withdrawing Treatments

Debate about the principle of nonmaleficence and forgoing life-sustaining treatments has centered on the omission–commission distinction, especially the distinction between withholding (not starting) and withdrawing (stopping) treatments. Many professionals and family members feel justified in withholding treatments they never started, but not in withdrawing treatments already initiated. They sense that decisions to stop treatments are more momentous and consequential than decisions not to start them. Stopping a respirator, for example, seems, to some, to cause a person's death, whereas not starting the respirator does not seem to have this same causal role.

In one case, an elderly man suffered from several major medical problems with no reasonable chance of recovery. He was comatose and unable to communicate. Antibiotics to fight infection and an intravenous (IV) line to provide nutrition and hydration kept him alive. No evidence indicated that he had expressed his wishes about life-sustaining treatments while competent, and he had no family member to serve as a surrogate decision maker. The staff quickly agreed on a "no code" or "do not resuscitate" (DNR) order, a signed order not to attempt cardiopulmonary resuscitation if a cardiac or respiratory arrest occurred. In the event of such an arrest, the physicians would allow the patient to die. The staff felt comfortable with this decision because of the patient's overall condition and prognosis, and because they could view not resuscitating the patient as withholding rather than withdrawing treatment.

Questions arose about whether to continue the interventions in place. Some members of the health care team thought that they should stop all medical treatments, including antibiotics and artificial nutrition and hydration, because they were "extraordinary" or "heroic measures." Others thought it wrong to stop these treatments once they had been started. A disagreement erupted about whether it would be permissible not to insert the IV line again if it became infiltrated; that is, if it broke through the blood vessel and began leaking fluid into surrounding tissue. Some who had opposed stopping treatments were comfortable with not inserting the IV line again, because they viewed the action as withholding rather than withdrawing. They emphatically opposed reinsertion if it required a cutdown (an incision to gain access to the deep large blood vessels) or a central line. Others viewed the provision of artificial nutrition and hydration as a single process and felt that inserting the IV line again was simply continuing what had been interrupted. For them, not restarting was equivalent to withdrawing and thus (unlike withholding) morally wrong.[13]

In many similar cases caregivers' discomfort about withdrawing life-sustaining treatments appears to reflect the view that such actions render them causally responsible for a patient's death, whereas they are not responsible if they never initiate a life-sustaining treatment. The conviction that starting a treatment often creates valid claims or expectations for its continuation frequently serves as another source of caregiver discomfort. Only if patients waive the claim for continued treatment does it seem legitimate to many caregivers to stop procedures. Otherwise stopping procedures appears to breach expectations, promises, or contractual obligations to the patient, family, or surrogate decision maker. Patients for whom physicians have not initiated treatments seem to hold no parallel claim.[14]

Feelings of reluctance about withdrawing treatments are understandable, but the distinction between withdrawing and withholding treatments is morally irrelevant, and can be dangerous. The distinction is unclear, inasmuch as withdrawing can happen through an omission (withholding) such as not recharging batteries that power respirators or not putting the infusion into a feeding tube. In multistaged treatments, decisions not to start the next stage of a treatment plan can be tantamount to stopping treatment, even if the early phases of the treatment continue.

Even if the distinction were clear, both not starting and stopping can be justified, depending on the circumstances. Both can be instances of allowing to die, and both can be instances of killing. Courts recognize that individuals can commit a crime by omission if they have an obligation to act, just as physicians can commit a wrong by omission in medical practice. Such a judgment depends on whether a physician has an obligation either not to withhold or not to withdraw treatment. In these cases if a physician has a duty to treat, omission of treatment breaches this duty, whether or not withholding or withdrawing is involved. However, if a physician does not have a duty to treat or has a duty not to treat, omission of either type involves no moral violation. Indeed, if the physician has a duty not to treat, it would be a moral violation not to withdraw the treatment if it has already begun.

In the classic case of Earle Spring, a court raised a legal problem about continuing kidney dialysis as follows: "The question presented by ... modern technology is, once undertaken, at what point does it cease to perform its intended function?" The court held that "a physician has no duty to continue treatment, once it has proven to be ineffective." The court emphasized the need to balance benefits and burdens to determine overall effectiveness.[15] Although legal responsibility cannot be equated with moral responsibility in such cases, the court's conclusion is consistent with the moral conclusions about justified withdrawal for which we are presently arguing. Today, approximately one in four deaths of patients with end-stage renal disease occurs after decisions to withdraw dialysis.[16] The practice is common, and there is no reason to believe that the decisions are not usually justified.

Giving priority to withholding over withdrawing treatment can lead to *overtreatment* in some cases; that is, the continuation of no longer beneficial or desirable treatment for the patient. Less obviously, the distinction can lead to *undertreatment*. Patients and families worry about being trapped by biomedical technology that, once begun, cannot be stopped. To circumvent this problem, they become reluctant to authorize the technology, even when it could possibly benefit the patient. Health care professionals often exhibit the same reluctance. In one case, a seriously ill newborn died after several months of treatment, much of it against the parents' wishes, because a physician was unwilling to stop the respirator once it had been connected. Later this physician reportedly felt "less eager to attach babies to respirators now."[17]

This example illustrates that the moral burden of proof often is heavier when the decision is to withhold than when it is to withdraw treatments. Only after starting treatments will it be possible, in many cases, to make a proper diagnosis and prognosis as well as to balance prospective benefits and burdens. This trial period can reduce uncertainty about outcomes. Patients and surrogates often feel less stress and more in control if they can reverse or otherwise change a decision to treat after the treatment has started. Accordingly, responsible health care may require proposing a trial with periodic reevaluation. Caregivers then have time to judge the effectiveness of the treatment, and the patient or surrogate has time to evaluate its benefits and burdens. Not to propose or allow the test at all is morally worse than not trying. Hence, withholding might be worse than withdrawing in such cases.

We conclude that the distinction between withholding and withdrawing is morally untenable and possibly morally dangerous. If a caregiver makes decisions about treatment using this irrelevant distinction, or allows a surrogate (without efforts at dissuasion) to make such a decision, the caregiver is morally blameworthy for negative outcomes. The felt importance of the distinction between not starting and stopping procedures undoubtedly accounts for, but does not justify, the ease with which hospitals and health care professionals have accepted no code or DNR orders and formed hospital policies regarding cardiopulmonary resuscitation (CPR). Policies regarding CPR often stand independent of other policies regarding life-sustaining technologies, such as respirators, in part because many health care professionals view not providing CPR as withholding rather than withdrawing treatment. Their decisions are especially problematic when made without advance consultation with patients or their families.[18]

Ordinary and Extraordinary Treatments

The distinction between ordinary and extraordinary treatments was once widely invoked both to justify and to condemn decisions to use or to forgo life-sustaining treatments. The rule was that extraordinary treatments can legitimately be forgone, whereas ordinary treatments cannot legitimately be forgone. The distinction has a prominent history in medical practice, judicial decisions, and Roman Catholic casuistry. It has also been used to determine whether an act that results in death counts as killing. As developed by Roman Catholic theologians to deal with problems of surgery (prior to the development of antisepsis and anesthesia), this distinction was used to determine whether a patient's refusal of treatment should be classified as suicide. More specifically, refusal of ordinary means of life-sustaining treatment was long considered suicide, but refusal of extraordinary means was not. Likewise, families and physicians did not commit homicide if they withheld or withdrew extraordinary means of treatment from patients.

Unfortunately, neither a long history nor precedent guarantees clarity or acceptability. The distinction between ordinary and extraordinary means of treatment is unacceptably vague and morally misleading. Throughout its history, the distinction has acquired a confusing array of meanings and functions. Interpreters have often taken *ordinary* to mean "usual" or "customary" and *extraordinary* to mean "unusual" or "uncustomary"—under either the professional practice standard discussed in Chapter 3 or the due care standard discussed earlier in this chapter. According to this interpretation, treatments are extraordinary if they are unusual or uncustomary for physicians to use in the relevant contexts. Over time, the terms thus became attached to particular technologies and alterable standards of practice.

Criteria other than usual and unusual medical practice have also been proposed for classifying procedures as extraordinary. These criteria include whether the treatment is simple or complex, natural or artificial, noninvasive or highly invasive, inexpensive or expensive, and routine or heroic. These substitutions, classifications, or distinctions have rarely been analyzed with care and offer no improvement over *usual* and *unusual.* A treatment that is simple, natural, noninvasive, inexpensive, or routine is more likely to be viewed as ordinary (and thus obligatory) than a treatment that is complex, artificial, invasive, expensive, or heroic (and thus optional). However, these criteria are relevant only if some deeper moral considerations make them relevant.

More consequential than these conceptual problems is whether such distinctions give sound moral guidance for treatment and nontreatment decisions. The principal consideration should always be whether a treatment is beneficial or burdensome, not what its classification is. All of these distinctions are irrelevant except insofar as they point to a quality-of-life criterion that requires balancing benefits against burdens. We conclude that the distinction between ordinary and extraordinary treatment is morally irrelevant. The distinction between optional and obligatory treatment, as determined by the balance of benefits and burdens to the patient, is the pertinent distinction.

Sustenance Technologies and Medical Treatments

Widespread debate has occurred about whether health care institutions can legitimately use the distinction between *medical* technologies and *sustenance* technologies to distinguish between justified and unjustified forgoing of life-sustaining treatments. Some argue that technologies for dispensing sustenance (those that supply nutrition and hydration using needles, tubes, catheters, and the like) are *nonmedical* means of maintaining life that are unlike optional forms of medical life-sustaining technologies, such as respirators and dialysis machines.

To help determine whether this distinction is more acceptable than the previous distinctions, we examine some cases, beginning with a case of a seventy-nine-year-old widow who had resided in a nursing home for several years. In the past she experienced repeated transient ischemic attacks (caused by reductions or stoppages of blood flow to the brain). Because of progressive organic brain syndrome, she had lost most of her mental abilities and had become disoriented. She also had thrombophlebitis (inflammation of a vein associated with clotting) and congestive heart failure. Her daughter and grandchildren visited her frequently and loved her deeply. One day she suffered a massive stroke. She made no recovery, remained nonverbal, manifested a withdrawal reaction to painful stimuli, and exhibited a limited range of purposeful behaviors. She strongly resisted a nasogastric tube being placed into her stomach to introduce nutritional formulas and water. At each attempt she thrashed about violently and pushed the tube away. When the tube was finally placed, she managed to remove it. After several days the staff could not find new sites for inserting IV lines, and debated whether to take further "extraordinary" measures to maintain fluid and nutritional intake for this elderly patient, who did not improve and was largely unaware and unresponsive. After lengthy discussions with nurses on the floor and with the patient's family, the physicians in charge concluded that they should not provide further IVs, cutdowns, or a feeding tube. The patient had minimal oral intake and died quietly the following week.[19]

Second, in a groundbreaking case in 1976, the New Jersey Supreme Court ruled it permissible for a guardian to disconnect Karen Ann Quinlan's respirator and allow her to die.[20] After the respirator was removed, Quinlan lived for almost ten years, protected by antibiotics and sustained by nutrition and hydration provided through a nasogastric tube. Unable to communicate, she lay comatose in a fetal position, with increasing respiratory problems, bedsores, and weight loss (from 115 to 70 pounds). A moral issue developed over those ten years. If it is permissible to remove the respirator, is it permissible to remove the feeding tube? Several Roman Catholic moral theologians advised the parents that they were not morally required to continue medically administered nutrition and hydration (MN&H) or antibiotics to fight infections. Nevertheless, the Quinlans continued MN&H because they believed that the feeding tube did not cause pain, whereas the respirator did.

While Karen Quinlan lingered, the same state supreme court faced another case involving artificial nutrition and hydration in which a guardian requested withdrawal of MN&H for an eighty-four-year-old nursing home resident. The court held that the provision of nutrition and hydration through nasogastric tubes and other medical means is not always legally required.[21] A Massachusetts court soon reached a similar decision in the *Brophy* case, involving a forty-nine-year-old man who had been in a persistent vegetative state for more than three years.[22] Courts have since increasingly maintained that no relevant difference distinguishes MN&H from other life-support measures. They have viewed MN&H as a medical procedure subject to the same standards of evaluation as other medical procedures and thus sometimes unjustifiably burdensome.[23]

In the preceding cases, the same moral question is present: Should MN&H be construed as obligatory or as optional? And, if either, under which circumstances?[24] We maintain that caregivers may justifiably forego MN&H for patients in some circumstances, as holds true for other life-sustaining technologies. No morally relevant difference exists between the various life-sustaining technologies, and the right to refuse medical treatment for oneself or others is not contingent on the type of treatment. There is no reason to believe that MN&H is always an essential part of palliative care or that it necessarily constitutes a beneficial medical treatment.

Although our view is consistent with many court decisions, professional codes, and philosophical arguments, it remains controversial. Three arguments have been advanced to challenge the position we take. The first argument holds that MN&H is required because it is necessary for the patient's comfort and dignity. A second argument focuses on symbolic significance. Medical professionals generally find it intuitively devastating to "starve" someone. Provision of nutrition and hydration symbolizes the essence of care and compassion. As Daniel Callahan puts it, to feed the hungry and to nurse those in need of nourishment are "rudimentary healing gesture[s]" and "the perfect symbol[s] of the fact that human life is inescapably social and communal."[25] The third argument is a version of the wedge or slippery-slope argument considered later in this chapter. The controlling idea is that policies of not providing MN&H will lead to adverse consequences because society will lose its ability to limit decisions about MN&H to legitimate cases, especially under pressures of cost containment in health care. Whereas "death with dignity" first emerged as a compassionate response to the threat of overtreatment, patients now face the threat of undertreatment because of pressures to contain the escalating costs of health care. Such concerns about psychological and social barriers focus on a slide from considering the patient's quality of life (the patient's interest) to considering the patient's value for society (society's interest), from decisions about terminally ill patients to decisions about nondying patients, from letting die to killing, and from cessation of artificial feeding to cessation of natural feeding. Some fear that the "right to die" will be transformed into the "obligation to die," perhaps against the patient's wishes and interests.[26]

These arguments merit serious consideration, but they are not entirely persuasive. Procedures of MN&H themselves sometimes involve risks of harm, discomfort, and indignity, such as pain from a central IV and physical restraints that prevent patients from removing the lines or tubes. Evidence indicates that patients who are allowed to die without artificial hydration sometimes die more comfortably than patients who receive hydration. It is also misleading to project the common experience of hunger and thirst on a dying patient who is malnourished and dehydrated. Malnutrition is not identical with hunger, dehydration is not identical with thirst, and starvation is very different from acute dehydration in a medical setting. Caregivers can alleviate feelings of hunger, thirst, dryness of the mouth, and related problems by other means, such as ice on the lips, without introducing MN&H.[27] Finally, in response to concerns about a slippery slope, no evidence exists to support the claim that protecting patients, the elderly, and other vulnerable populations from undertreatment requires the provision of MN&H in all circumstances.

We conclude that health care providers may legitimately withhold or withdraw MN&H under some conditions.

Intended Effects and Merely Foreseen Effects

Another venerable attempt to specify the principle of nonmaleficence appears in the rule of double effect (RDE), often called the principle or doctrine of double effect. This rule incorporates a very influential distinction between intended effects and merely foreseen effects.

Functions and conditions of the RDE. The RDE is invoked to justify claims that a single act having two foreseen effects, one good and one harmful (such as death), is not always morally prohibited.[28] As an example of the use of the RDE, consider a patient experiencing terrible pain and suffering who asks a physician for help in ending his life. If the physician injects the patient with a chemical to end the patient's pain and suffering, he or she intentionally causes the patient's death as a means to end pain and suffering. In contrast, suppose the physician could provide medication to relieve the patient's pain and suffering at a substantial risk that the patient would die as a result of the medication. If the physician refuses to administer the medication, the patient will endure continuing pain and suffering; if the physician provides the medication, it may hasten the patient's death. If the physician intended, through the provision of medication, to relieve grave pain and suffering and did not intend to cause death, then the act of indirectly hastening death is not wrong, according to the RDE.

Classical formulations of the RDE identify four conditions or elements that must be satisfied for an act with a double effect to be justified. Each is a necessary condition, and together they form sufficient conditions of morally permissible action:[29]

1. *The nature of the act.* The act must be good, or at least morally neutral, independent of its consequences.
2. *The agent's intention.* The agent intends only the good effect, not the bad effect. The bad effect can be foreseen, tolerated, and permitted, but it must not be intended.
3. *The distinction between means and effects.* The bad effect must not be a means to the good effect. If the good effect were the causal result of the bad effect, the agent would intend the bad effect in pursuit of the good effect.

4. *Proportionality between the good effect and the bad effect.* The good effect must outweigh the bad effect. That is, the bad effect is permissible only if a proportionate reason compensates for permitting the foreseen bad effect.

Controversy has surrounded all four of these conditions. We begin to investigate the cogency of the RDE by considering four cases of what many call therapeutic abortion (limited to protecting maternal life in these examples): (1) A pregnant woman has cervical cancer; she needs a hysterectomy to save her life, but this procedure will result in the death of the fetus. (2) A pregnant woman has an ectopic pregnancy—the nonviable fetus is in the fallopian tube—and physicians must remove the tube to prevent hemorrhage, which will result in the death of the fetus. (3) A pregnant woman has a serious heart disease that probably will result in her death if she attempts to carry the pregnancy to term. (4) A pregnant woman in difficult labor will die unless the physician performs a craniotomy (crushing the head of the unborn fetus). Some interpretations of Roman Catholic teaching hold that actions that produce fetal deaths in the first two cases sometimes satisfy the four conditions of the RDE and therefore can be morally acceptable, whereas the actions that produce fetal deaths in the latter two cases never meet the conditions of the RDE and therefore are always morally unacceptable.[30]

In the first two cases, according to proponents of the RDE, a physician undertakes a legitimate medical procedure aimed at saving the pregnant woman's life with the foreseen, but unintended, result of fetal death. Viewed as unintended side effects (rather than as ends or means), these fetal deaths are said to be justified by a proportionately grave reason, namely, saving the pregnant woman. In both of the latter two cases, the action of terminating fetal life is a means to save the pregnant woman's life. As such, it requires intending the fetus's death (even if the death is not desired). Therefore, in those cases, criteria 2 and 3 are violated and the act cannot be justified by proportionality (criterion 4).

However, it is not likely that a morally relevant difference can be established between cases such as a hysterectomy or a craniotomy in terms of the abstract conditions that comprise the RDE. In neither case does the agent want or desire the death of the fetus, and the descriptions of the acts in these cases do not indicate morally relevant differences between intending, on the one hand, and foreseeing but not intending, on the other. More specifically, it remains unclear why advocates of RDE conceptualize craniotomy as killing the fetus rather than as the act of crushing the skull of the fetus with the unintended result that the fetus dies. Similarly, it remains unclear why in the hysterectomy case the death of the fetus is foreseen but not intended. Proponents of the RDE must have a practicable way to distinguish the intended from the merely foreseen, but they face major difficulties in providing a theory of intention precise enough to draw defensible moral lines between the hysterectomy and craniotomy cases.

A problematic conception of intention. Adherents of the RDE need an account of intentional actions and intended effects of action to distinguish them from nonintentional actions and unintended effects. The literature on intentional action is itself controversial and focuses on diverse conditions such as volition, deliberation, willing, reasoning, and planning. One of the few widely shared views in this literature is that intentional actions require that an agent have a plan—a blueprint, map, or representation of the means and ends proposed for the execution of an action.[31] For an action to be intentional, it must correspond to the agent's plan for its performance.

Alvin Goldman uses the following example in an attempt to prove that agents do not intend merely foreseen effects.[32] Imagine that Mr. G takes a driver's test to prove competence. He comes to an intersection that requires a right turn and extends his arm to signal for a turn, although he knows it is raining and that he will get his hand wet. According to Goldman, Mr. G's signaling for a turn is an intentional act. By contrast, his getting a wet hand is an unintended effect or "incidental by-product" of his hand-signaling. A defender of the RDE must elect a similarly narrow conception of what is intended to avoid the conclusion that an agent intentionally brings about all the consequences of an action that the agent foresees. The defender distinguishes between acts and effects, and then between effects that are desired or wanted and effects that are foreseen but not desired or wanted. The RDE views the latter effects as foreseen, but not intended.

It is more suitable in these contexts to discard the language of "wanting" and to say that foreseen but not desired effects are "tolerated."[33] These effects are not so undesirable that the actor would choose not to perform the act that results in them; the actor includes them as a part of his or her plan of intentional action. To account for this point, let us use a model of intentionality based on what is *willed* rather than what is *wanted.* On this model intentional actions and intentional effects include any action and any effect specifically willed in accordance with a plan, including tolerated as well as wanted effects.[34] In this conception a physician can desire not to do what he intends to do, in the same way that one can be willing to do something but, at the same time, reluctant to do it or even detest doing it.

Under this conception of intentional acts and intended effects, the distinction between what agents intend and what they merely foresee in a planned action is not viable.[35] For example, if a man enters a room and flips a switch that he knows turns on both a light and a fan, but desires only to activate the light, he cannot say that he activates the fan unintentionally. Even if the fan made an obnoxious whirring sound that he is aware of and wants to avoid, it would be mistaken to say that he unintentionally brought about the obnoxious noise by flipping the switch. More generally, a person who knowingly and voluntarily acts to bring about an effect brings about that effect intentionally. The person intends the effect, although he or she did not desire it, did not will it for its own sake, and did not intend it as the goal of the action.

Now we can reconsider the moral relevance of the RDE and its distinctions. Is it plausible to distinguish morally between intentionally causing the death of a fetus by craniotomy and intentionally removing a cancerous uterus that causes the death of a fetus? In both actions the intention is to save the woman's life with knowledge that the fetus will die. No agent in either scenario desires the negative result (the fetus's death) for its own sake, and none would have tolerated the negative result if its avoidance were morally preferable to the alternative outcome. All parties accept the bad effect only because they cannot eliminate it without sacrificing the good effect.

In the standard interpretation of the RDE, the fetus's death is a *means* to saving a woman's life in the unacceptable case, but merely a *side effect* in the acceptable case. That is, an agent intends a means, but does not intend a side effect. This approach seems to allow persons to foresee almost anything as a side effect rather than as an intended means. It does not follow, however, that people can create or direct intentions as they please. For example, in the craniotomy case, the surgeon might not intend the death of the fetus but only intend to remove it from the birth canal. The fetus will die, but is this outcome more than an unwanted and (in double effect theory) unintended consequence?[36]

The RDE might appear to fare better in care of dying patients, where there is no conflict between different parties. It is often invoked to justify a physician's administration of medication to relieve pain and suffering (the primary intention and effect) even though it will probably hasten the patient's death (the unintended, secondary effect). A related practice, terminal sedation, challenges the boundaries and use of the RDE. In cases of terminal sedation, physicians induce a deep sleep or unconsciousness to relieve pain and suffering in the expectation that this state will continue until the patient dies. Some commentators contend that some cases of terminal sedation can be justified under the RDE, whereas others argue that terminal sedation directly, although slowly, kills the patient and thus is a form of active euthanasia.[37] Much depends on the description of terminal sedation in a particular set of circumstances, including the patient's overall condition, the proximity of death, the availability of alternative means to relieve pain and suffering, and so on, as well as the intention of the physician and other parties. Interpretations of the RDE to cover some cases of terminal sedation allow compassionate acts of relieving pain, suffering, and discomfort that foreseeably will hasten death. Such acts can be accommodated within legal frameworks in many countries, including the United States. However, the concentrated efforts to stay within the boundaries of the RDE, and even stretch those boundaries, may also direct attention away from and preclude the most respectful care for some patients.

Often in dispute is whether death is good or bad for a particular person, and nothing in the RDE settles this dispute. The RDE applies only in cases with both a bad and a good effect, but determining the goodness and badness of different effects is a separate judgment. Accordingly, the goodness or badness of death for a particular person, whether it occurs directly or indirectly, must be determined and defended on independent grounds.[38]

Defenders of the RDE eventually may solve the puzzles and problems that critics have identified, but they have not succeeded thus far. One constructive effort to retain an emphasis on intention without entirely abandoning the larger point of the RDE focuses on the way actions display a person's motives and character. In the case of performing a craniotomy to save a pregnant woman's life, a physician may not *want* or *desire* the death of the fetus and may regret performing a craniotomy just as much as he or she would in the case of removing a cancerous uterus. Such facts about the physician's motivation and character can make a decisive difference to a moral assessment of the action and the agent. But this moral conclusion also can be reached independently of the RDE. In effect, we are proposing to focus on motivation in a way that will transform the RDE into the moral framework of character judgments that we established in Chapter 2.

Some parts of the RDE are perfectly acceptable; for example, that we justifiably allow a harmful effect only if we will probably bring about a proportionately weighty good one. But, as we will now see, biomedical ethics can put this same general requirement to many uses beyond those permitted by the RDE itself.

Optional Treatments and Obligatory Treatments

We have now rejected several common distinctions and rules about forgoing life-sustaining treatment and causing harm that are accepted in some traditions of medical ethics. In place of them we propose a distinction between obligatory and optional treatments. We rely heavily on an analysis of quality of life that is generally incompatible with the distinctions and rules that we have already rejected. The following categories are basic to our arguments:

  I.   Obligatory to Treat (Wrong Not to Treat)
  II. Obligatory Not to Treat (Wrong to Treat)
  III. Optional Whether to Treat (Neither Required nor Prohibited)

Under III, the question is whether it is morally neutral and therefore optional to provide or not to provide a treatment.

The principles of nonmaleficence and beneficence have often been specified to establish a presumption in favor of providing life-sustaining treatments for sick and injured patients. This presumption does not entail that it is always obligatory to provide the treatments. The use of life-sustaining treatments occasionally violates patients' interests. For example, pain can be so severe and physical restraints so burdensome that these factors outweigh anticipated benefits, such as brief prolongation of life. In these circumstances, providing the treatment is sometimes inhumane or cruel. Even for the incompetent patient, the burdens can so outweigh the benefits that the treatment is wrong rather than optional, just as it would be in the case of a competent patient who refuses treatment.

Conditions for Overriding the Prima Facie Obligation to Treat

Several conditions justify decisions by patients, surrogates, or health care professionals to withhold or withdraw treatment. We introduce these conditions (other than valid refusal of treatment) in this section.

Futile or pointless treatment. Physicians have no obligation to provide pointless and futile or contraindicated treatment. In a radical example, if a patient has died but remains on a respirator, cessation of treatment cannot harm him or her, and a physician has no obligation to treat. However, some religious and personal belief systems do not consider a patient dead according to the same criteria health care institutions recognize. For example, if there is heart and lung function, some religious traditions hold that the person is not dead, and the treatment is, from this perspective, not futile even if health care professionals deem it useless and wasteful. This is the tip of an iceberg of controversies that underlie the notion of futility.

Typically the term *futile* refers to a situation in which irreversibly dying patients have reached a point at which further treatment provides no physiological benefit or is hopeless and becomes optional. Palliative interventions may still be continued. This model, however, covers only a narrow range of treatments that have been labeled futile in the literature on the subject. All of the following have been referred to as "futile": (1) whatever physicians cannot perform, (2) whatever will not produce a physiological effect, (3) whatever is highly unlikely to be efficacious (i.e., statistically, the odds of success are exceedingly small), (4) whatever probably will produce only a low-grade, insignificant outcome (i.e., qualitatively, the results are expected to be exceedingly poor), (5) whatever is highly likely to be more burdensome than beneficial, (6) whatever is completely speculative because it is an untried "treatment," and (7) whatever—in balancing effectiveness, potential benefit, and potential burden—warrants withdrawing or withholding treatment.[39] Thus, the term *futility* is used to cover many situations of predicted improbable outcomes, improbable success, and unacceptable benefit–burden ratios. This situation of competing conceptions and ambiguity suggests that we should generally avoid the term *futility* in favor of more precise language.

Ideally, health care providers will focus on objective medical factors in decisions involving either the dead or the irreversibly dying. Realistically, though, this ideal is difficult to satisfy. Disagreement often exists among health professionals, and conflicts may arise from a family's belief in a possible miracle, a religious tradition's insistence on doing everything in such circumstances, and so forth. It is sometimes difficult to know whether a judgment of futility is based on a probabilistic prediction of failure or on something closer to medical certainty. If an elderly patient has a 1% chance of surviving an arduous and painful regimen, one physician may call the procedure futile while another may view survival as an unlikely outcome but still a possibility that should be considered. We here encounter a value judgment about what is worth the effort, as well as a judgment based on scientific knowledge. Decision makers typically use "futility" to express a combined value judgment and scientific judgment.

Writings in biomedical ethics that discuss futility often focus on the patient's or surrogate's right to refuse futile treatment. However, compelling medical circumstances and new legislation have raised the question whether the physician may or even must refuse to provide certain treatments. The fact that a treatment is futile is often said to change the physician's moral relationship to patients or surrogates. The physician is not morally required to provide a futile or contraindicated treatment (and in some cases is required not to provide the treatment at all) and may not even be required to discuss the treatment.[40] These circumstances often involve incompetent persons, especially patients in a persistent vegetative state (PVS), where physicians or hospital policies sometimes impose decisions to forgo life support on patients or surrogates. Hospitals are increasingly adopting policies aimed at denying therapies that physicians judge to be futile, especially after trying them for a reasonable period of time.

The possibility of judgmental error by physicians should lead to caution in formulating these policies, but, at the same time, unreasonable demands by patients and families should not preclude reasonable policies by health care institutions. Respect for the autonomy of patients or authorized surrogates is not a trump that allows them alone to determine whether a treatment is required or is futile.

The upshot is that a pointless or futile treatment—one that has no chance of being efficacious—is morally optional and in many cases ought not be used. However, some *putatively* futile treatments must be handled differently because they involve conflicts about values.[41]

Burdens of treatment outweigh benefits. Medical codes and institutional policies often mistakenly assume that physicians may terminate life-sustaining treatments for persons not able to consent or refuse the treatments only if the patient is terminally ill. However, even if the patient is not terminally ill, life-sustaining medical treatment is still not obligatory if its burdens outweigh its benefits to the patient. Medical treatment for those not terminally ill is sometimes optional even if it could prolong life for an indefinite period and the patient is incompetent and has left no advance directive. The principle of nonmaleficence does not imply the maintenance of biological life, nor does it require the initiation or continuation of treatment without regard to the patient's pain, suffering, and discomfort.

For example, seventy-eight-year-old Earle Spring developed numerous medical problems, including chronic organic brain syndrome and kidney failure. Hemodialysis controlled the latter problem. Although several aspects of this case were never resolved—such as whether Spring was aware of his surroundings and able to express his wishes—a plausible argument exists that the family and health care professionals were not morally obligated to continue hemodialysis because of the balance of benefits and burdens to a patient whose compromised mental condition and kidney function would gradually worsen regardless of what was done. However, in this case, as in so many others, a family conflict of interest complicated the situation: The family had to pay mounting health care costs while attempting to make judgments in the patient's best interests. (We return later in this chapter to procedures designed to protect incompetent patients.)

The Centrality of Quality-of-Life Judgments

Controversies about quality-of-life judgments. Our arguments thus far give considerable weight to quality-of-life judgments in determining whether treatments are optional or obligatory. We have relied on the premise that when quality of life is sufficiently low and an intervention produces more harm than benefit for the patient, caregivers may justifiably withhold or withdraw treatment. Such judgments require defensible criteria of benefits and burdens in order to not reduce quality of life to arbitrary judgments of personal preference and the patient's social worth.

In a landmark case involving quality-of-life judgments, sixty-eight-year-old Joseph Saikewicz, who had an IQ of 10 and a mental age of approximately two years and eight months, suffered from acute myeloblastic monocytic leukemia. Chemotherapy would have produced extensive suffering and possibly serious side effects. Remission under chemotherapy occurs in only 30% to 50% of such cases and typically only for between two and thirteen months. Without chemotherapy, doctors expected Saikewicz to live for several weeks or perhaps several months, during which time he would not experience severe pain or suffering. In not ordering treatment, the lower court considered "the quality of life available to him [Saikewicz] even if the treatment does bring about remission." The supreme judicial court of Massachusetts, however, rejected the lower court's judgment that the value of life could be equated with one measure of the quality of life—in particular, Saikewicz's lower quality of life because of mental retardation. Instead, the court interpreted "the vague, and perhaps ill-chosen, term 'quality of life'... as a reference to the continuing state of pain and disorientation precipitated by the chemotherapy treatment."[42] It thus balanced prospective benefit against pain and suffering, finally determining that the patient's interests supported a decision not to provide chemotherapy. From a moral standpoint, we agree with the reasoning and the conclusion reached in this legal opinion.

"Quality of life," however, needs further qualification. Some writers have argued that we should reject *moral* or otherwise *evaluative* judgments about quality of life and rely exclusively on *medical* indications for treatment decisions. Paul Ramsey, in a classic attempt, argues that, for incompetent patients, we need only determine which treatment is medically indicated to know which treatment is obligatory and which is optional. For imminently dying patients, responsibilities are not fixed by obligations to provide treatments that serve only to extend the dying process, but rather by obligations to provide appropriate care in dying. Ramsey argues that, unless we use these guidelines, we will gradually move toward a policy of active, involuntary euthanasia for unconscious or incompetent, nondying patients, based on uncontrollable quality-of-life judgments.[43]

However, putatively objective medical factors, such as criteria used to determine medical indications for treatment, cannot provide the objectivity that Ramsey seeks. These criteria undermine his fundamental distinction between the medical and the moral (or evaluative). It is impossible to determine what will benefit a patient without presupposing some quality-of-life standard and some conception of the life the patient will live after a medical intervention. Accurate medical diagnosis and prognosis are indispensable, but a judgment about whether to use life-prolonging measures rests unavoidably on the anticipated quality of life of the patient, not merely on a standard of what is medically indicated.[44]

Ramsey maintains that a quality-of-life approach improperly shifts the focus from whether treatments benefit patients to whether patients' lives are beneficial to them—a shift that opens the door to active, involuntary euthanasia.[45] The real issue is whether we can state criteria of quality of life with sufficient precision and cogency to avoid such dangers. We think we can, although the vagueness surrounding terms such as *dignity* and *meaningful life* is a cause for concern, and cases in which seriously ill or disabled newborn infants have been "allowed to die" under questionable justifications do provide a reason for caution.

We should exclude several conditions of patients from consideration altogether. For example, mental retardation is irrelevant in determining whether treatment is in the patient's best interest. Proxies should not confuse quality of life for the patient with the value of the patient's life for others. Furthermore, criteria focused on the incompetent patient's best interests should be decisive for a proxy, even if the patient's interests conflict with familial or societal interests in avoiding burdens or costs.

This position contrasts with that of the President's Commission for the Study of Ethical Problems in Medicine and Biomedical and Behavioral Research. It recognizes a broader conception of "best interests" that includes the welfare of the family: "The impact of a decision on an incapacitated patient's loved ones may be taken into account in determining someone's best interests, for most people do have an important interest in the well-being of their families or close associates."[46] It is true that a patient often has an interest in his or her family's welfare, but it is a long step from this premise to a conclusion about whose interests should be overriding (unless the patient explicitly so states). When the incompetent patient has never been competent or never expressed his or her wishes while competent, it is not proper to impute altruism or any other motive to that patient against his or her medical best interests.

Children with serious illnesses or disabilities.
Endangered near-term fetuses, seriously ill newborns, and young children present difficult questions about quality of life and treatment omission. Prenatal obstetric management and neonatal intensive care can now salvage the lives of many anomalous fetuses and disabled newborns with physical conditions that would have been fatal four decades ago. However, the resultant quality of life is sometimes so low that it becomes questionable whether aggressive obstetric management or intensive care has produced more harm than benefit for the patient. Some commentators argue that avoidance of harm (including iatrogenic harm) is the best guide to decisions on behalf of near-term fetuses and infants in neonatal nurseries,[47] and others argue that aggressive intervention violates the obligation of nonmaleficence if any one of three conditions is present: (1) inability to survive infancy, (2) inability to live without severe pain, and (3) inability to minimally participate in human experience.[48]

Managing high-risk pregnancies nonaggressively and allowing seriously disabled newborns to die are, under some conditions, morally permissible actions that do not violate obligations of nonmaleficence. When a patient has such a low quality of life that aggressive intervention or intensive care produces more harm than benefit, physicians justifiably may withhold or withdraw treatment from near-term fetuses, newborns, or infants, just as they do with persons of older ages. The conditions that would lead to a sufficiently poor quality of life include a number of antenatal conditions that commonly eventuate in stillbirth; severe brain damage caused by birth asphyxia; Tay–Sachs disease, which involves increasing spasticity and dementia and usually results in death by age three or four; and Lesch–Nyhan disease, which involves uncontrollable spasms, mental retardation, compulsive self-mutilation, and early death. Severe cases of neural tube defects in which newborns lack all or most of the brain and will inevitably die also occasion a justifiable decision not to treat.

Consistent with our arguments at the end of Chapter 4, the most appropriate standard in cases of never-competent patients, including seriously ill newborns, is that of best interests, as judged by the best estimate of what reasonable persons would consider the highest net benefit among the available options. Competent patients and authorized surrogates can use controlled quality-of-life considerations with medical input to legitimately determine whether treatments are optional or obligatory (or even, in extreme cases, wrong). These categories of optional and obligatory should replace the traditional distinctions and rules examined earlier in this chapter. However, we now consider the most difficult of all the distinctions that have been used to determine acceptable decisions about treatment and acceptable forms of professional conduct with seriously ill or injured patients, namely the distinction between killing and letting die.

KILLING AND LETTING DIE

The distinction between killing and letting die (or allowing to die) has long been the most critical one in law, medicine, and moral philosophy to distinguish appropriate from inappropriate ways to death. A large body of distinctions and rules about life-sustaining treatments derives from the killing–letting die distinction, which in turn draws on the act–omission and active–passive distinctions.[49] The killing–letting die distinction has also affected distinctions between suicide and forgoing treatment and between homicide and natural death. Similarly, the putative difference between killing and letting die often provides the grounds for a distinction between overseeing a refusal of treatment and assisting in a "suicide."[50] Withdrawals and withholdings of treatment, particularly of so-called extraordinary means, have generally been classified as "letting die."[51] In short, the killing–letting die distinction has been widely used to separate permissible practices from condemnable practices. We need to examine whether this distinction is coherent, defensible, and useful for moral guidance.

This section addresses three questions. (1) A *conceptual question:* What conceptually is the difference between killing and letting die? (2) A *moral question:* Is killing in itself morally wrong, whereas allowing to die is not in itself morally wrong? (3) A *conceptual and causal question:* Is forgoing life-sustaining treatment sometimes a form of killing? If so, is it sometimes suicide and sometimes homicide?

Conceptual Questions about the Nature of Killing and Letting Die

Can we define *killing* and *letting die* so that they are conceptually distinct and do not overlap? The following two cases suggest that we cannot: (1) A newborn with Down syndrome needed an operation to correct a tracheoesophageal fistula (a congenital deformity in which a connection exists between the trachea and the esophagus, thereby allowing food or milk to get into the lungs). The parents and physicians maintained that survival was not in this infant's best interests and decided to let the infant die rather than perform the operation. However, a public outcry erupted over the case, and critics charged that the parents and physicians had killed the child by negligently allowing the child to die. (2) Dr. Gregory Messenger, a dermatologist, was charged with manslaughter after he unilaterally terminated his premature (twenty-five weeks gestation, 750 g.) son's life-support system in a Lansing, Michigan, neonatal intensive care unit. He thought he had merely acted compassionately in letting his son die after a neonatologist had failed to fulfill a promise not to resuscitate the infant.[52]

Can we legitimately describe actions that involve intentionally not treating a patient as "allowing to die" or "letting die," rather than "killing"? Do at least some of these actions involve both killing and allowing to die? Is "allowing to die" a euphemism in some cases for "acceptable killing" or "acceptable taking of life"? These conceptual questions have moral implications. Unfortunately, both ordinary discourse and legal concepts are vague and equivocal. In ordinary language, *killing* is a causal action that brings about death, whereas *letting die* is an intentional avoidance of causal intervention so that disease, system failure, or injury causes death. Killing extends to animal and plant life. Neither in ordinary language nor in law does the word "killing" entail a wrongful act or a crime, or even an intentional action. For example, we can say properly that, in automobile accidents, one driver killed another even when no awareness, intent, or negligence was present.

Conventional definitions are unsatisfactory for drawing any sharp distinction between killing and letting die. They allow many acts of letting die to count as killing, thereby defeating the very point of the distinction. For example, under these definitions, health professionals kill patients when they intentionally let them die in circumstances in which they have a duty to keep the patients alive. It is unclear in literature on the subject how to distinguish killing from letting die so as to avoid even simple cases that satisfy the conditions of both killing and letting die. The meanings of "killing" and "letting die" clearly are vague and inherently contestable. Attempts to refine their meanings likely will produce controversy without closure. We use these terms because they are prominent in mainstream literature, but we avoid them insofar as possible.

Connecting Right and Wrong to Killing and Letting Die

"Letting die" is (prima facie) acceptable in medicine under one of two conditions: (1) a medical technology is *useless* (in the strict sense of medical futility), or (2) patients (or their authorized surrogates) have *validly refused* a medical technology. That is, letting a patient die is acceptable if and only if it satisfies the condition of futility or the condition of a valid refusal of treatment. If neither of these two conditions is satisfied, then letting a patient die usually involves negligence and may constitute a form of killing.

In medicine and health care, "killing" has traditionally been conceptually and morally connected to *unacceptable* acts. The conditions of medical practice make this connection understandable, but the absolute unacceptability of killing is not assumed outside of medical circles. In general, the term "killing" does not necessarily entail a wrongful act or a crime, and the rule "Do not kill" is not an absolute rule. Standard justifications of killing, such as killing in self-defense, killing to rescue a person endangered by other persons' wrongful acts, and killing by misadventure (accidental, nonnegligent killing while engaged in a lawful act) prevent us from prejudging an action as wrong merely because it is a killing. To correctly apply the label "killing" or the label "letting die" to a set of events (outside of traditional assumptions in medicine) will therefore fail to determine whether an action is acceptable or unacceptable.[53]

Killing may generally be wrong and letting die only rarely wrong, but, if so, this conclusion is contingent on the features of particular cases. The general wrongness of killing and the general rightness of letting die are not surprising features of the moral world inasmuch as killings are *rarely authorized* by appropriate parties (excepting contexts of warfare and capital punishment), and cases of letting die generally are *validly authorized*. Be that as it may, the *frequency* with which one kind of act is justified, by contrast to the other kind of act, should not determine whether either kind of act is legally or morally justified. Forgoing treatment to allow patients to die can be both as intentional and as immoral as actions that in some more direct manner take their lives, and both can be forms of killing.

Correctly labeling an act as "killing" or as "letting die," therefore, does not determine that one form of action is better or worse, or more or less justified, than the other. Some particular instance of killing (a brutal murder, say) may be worse than some particular instance of allowing to die (forgoing treatment for a PVS patient, say); but some particular instance of letting die (not resuscitating a patient whom physicians could potentially save, say) also may be worse than some particular instance of killing (mercy killing at the patient's request, say). Nothing about either killing or allowing to die entails judgments about actual wrongness or rightness. Rightness and wrongness depend on the merit of the justification underlying the action, not on whether it is an instance of killing or of letting die. Neither killing nor letting die is per se wrong; in this regard, we can distinguish them from murder, which is per se wrongful.

Accordingly, judging whether an act of either killing or letting die is justified or unjustified requires that we know something else about the act besides these characteristics. We need to know about the actor's motive (e.g., whether it is benevolent or malicious), the patient's preferences, and the act's consequences. These additional factors will allow us to place the act on a moral map and make a normative judgment.

Forgoing Life-Sustaining Treatment: Killing or Allowing to Die?

Many writers in medicine, law, and ethics have construed a physician's intentionally forgoing a medical technology as letting die, rather than killing, if and only if an underlying disease or injury causes death. When physicians withhold or withdraw medical technology, according to this doctrine, a natural death occurs, because natural conditions do what they would have done if the physicians had never initiated the technology. By contrast, killings occur when acts of persons rather than natural conditions cause death.[54] From this perspective, one acts nonmaleficently in allowing to die and maleficently in killing.

Although this view is influential in law and medicine, it is flawed. To obtain a satisfactory account, we must add that the forgoing of the medical technology is *validly authorized* and for this reason *justified*. If the physician's forgoing of technology were unjustified and a person died from "natural" causes of injury or disease, the result would be unjustified killing, not justified allowing to die. The validity of the authorization—not some independent assessment of causation—determines the morality of the action.

The distinction between "killing" and "letting die" is unsatisfactory for a number of reasons, not least because it tends to mask, rather than promote, consideration of the relevant factors that ought to be considered in determining permissible conduct. For example, withdrawing treatment from a competent patient is not morally justifiable unless the patient has made an informed decision authorizing this withdrawal. If a physician removes a respirator from a patient who needs it and wants to continue its use, the action is wrong, even though the physician has only removed artificial life support and let nature take its course.[55] Absent the patient's authorization, such "letting die" is morally unacceptable. The lack of authorization by the patient is the relevant consideration in assessing the act as unacceptable, not the distinction between letting die and killing.

A physician's nonintervention that leads to the patient's death is appropriate where the physician is following the patient's instruction and thus has valid authorization not to intervene. The physician is not the relevant cause of death and does not act wrongly if he or she has valid authorization for withholding or withdrawing treatment. By contrast, comparable action or inaction is inappropriate in medicine if a physician has a duty to treat. A physician is the relevant cause of death, and thereby acts wrongly, if he or she has no valid authorization from the patient to withhold or withdraw treatment.

Even from a legal perspective, we can provide a better account than "the preexisting disease caused the death." The better account is that legal liability should not be imposed on physicians and surrogates unless they have an obligation to provide or continue the treatment. If no obligation to treat exists, then questions of causation and liability do not arise. If the categories of obligatory and optional are primary, we have a reason for avoiding discussions about killing and letting die altogether and for focusing instead on health care professionals' obligations and problems of moral and legal responsibility.

We conclude that the distinction between killing and letting die suffers from vagueness and moral confusion. The language of killing is so confusing—causally, legally, and morally—that it can provide little, if any, help in discussions of assistance in dying. In the next section we add further support to this conclusion.

THE JUSTIFICATION OF INTENTIONALLY ARRANGED DEATHS

We now address a set of moral questions that builds on the conceptual, causal, and moral conclusions reached in the previous section. We formulate the issues largely free of the language of "killing." The general question we address is, "Under what conditions, if any, is it permissible for a patient and a health professional to arrange for assistance in intentionally ending the patient's life?"

Withholding or withdrawing treatment will hasten death only for those individuals who could be or are being sustained by a technology. Many other individuals, including some patients with cancer, face a protracted period of dying when respirators and other life-preserving technology are not being utilized. Great improvements in and extensions of palliative care adequately address the needs of many, perhaps most, of these patients.[56] However, for some of these patients, palliative care and the ability to refuse treatment do not adequately address all their concerns. During their prolonged period of dying, they may endure a loss of functional capacity, unremitting pain and suffering, an inability to experience the simplest of pleasures, and long hours aware of the hopelessness of their condition. Some patients find this prospect unbearable and desire a painless means to hasten their deaths.

Physicians also may use a so-called active means to bring about death. Some argue that the use of an active means in medicine constitutes an inappropriate killing. But there are several problems inherent in the idea that we can determine appropriate and inappropriate conduct by considering whether an active means to death was involved. This is especially true (but true not only) in the context of the Oregon Death with Dignity Act (ODWDA),[57] where the distinction between "letting die" and "killing" is not helpful. Physicians who act under the ODWDA do not "kill" patients in any meaningful sense. A physician who prescribes a lethal medication at a patient's request is writing a prescription. Under the ODWDA, the patient must make a conscious decision to use the drug. About one-third of the patients who fill a prescription under the ODWDA never ingest the lethal drug. For those who take the drug, the physician's writing of the prescription is a necessary step in the process that leads to the patient's death, but it is not the determinative or even the final step. Under any reasonable interpretation of the term, the Oregon physician does not "kill" the patient. Nor, however, does this physician "let the patient die." The terms "letting die" and "killing" do not illuminate what happens when a physician helps a person seeking to escape the ravages of a fatal illness.

Literature often treats issues about active physician assistance under the umbrella of the legal protection of a "right to die,"[58] but underlying the legal issues is a powerful struggle in law, medicine, and ethics over the nature, scope, and foundations of the right to choose the manner of one's death. We here offer a few judgments about legalization, public policy, and institutional policy, but our primary interest is in moral questions about whether these acts of assistance by health professionals are justified—chiefly whether autonomy rights justify requests for active forms of aid-in-dying. We begin with the importance of the distinction between acts and policies. We then work back to more foundational moral issues.

Acts, Practices, and Slippery-Slope Problems

Justifying an act is distinct from justifying a practice or a policy that permits or even legitimates the act's performance. A rule of practice or a public policy or a law that prohibits various forms of assistance in dying in medicine may be justified even if it excludes some acts of causing a person's death that in themselves are *morally* justifiable. For example, there may be sufficient reasons that a law might not permit physicians to use a drug overdose to cause death for a patient who suffers from terrible pain, who will probably die within a few weeks, and who requests a merciful assisted death. However, this same act might be morally justified in an individual case.

The problem is that a practice or policy that allows physicians to intervene to cause deaths or help cause deaths runs risks of abuse and might cause more harm than benefit. The argument is not that serious abuses will occur immediately, but that they will grow incrementally over time. Society could start by severely restricting the number of patients who qualify for assistance in dying, but might later loosen these restrictions so that cases of unjustified killing begin to occur. Unscrupulous persons would learn how to abuse the system, just as they do now with methods of tax evasion on the margins of the system of legitimate tax avoidance. In short, the slope of the trail toward the unjustified taking of life will be so slippery and precipitous that we ought never to embark on it.

Many dismiss such slippery-slope, or wedge, arguments because of a lack of empirical evidence to support their claims, as well as because of their heavily metaphorical character ("the thin edge of the wedge," "the first step on the slippery slope," "the foot in the door," and "the camel's nose under the tent"). However, some slippery-slope arguments should be taken with the utmost seriousness.[59] They force us to think carefully about whether unacceptable harm is likely to result from attractive and apparently innocent first steps. If society removes certain restraints against interventions that cause death, various psychological and social forces would likely make it more difficult to maintain the relevant distinctions in practice.

Opponents of legalization of physician-assisted dying have generally maintained that the practice inevitably would be expanded to include euthanasia, that the quality of palliative care for all patients would deteriorate, that patients would be manipulated or coerced into requesting assistance in hastening death, that patients whose judgment was impaired would be allowed to request such assistance, and that members of allegedly vulnerable groups (the elderly, women, members of racial and ethnic minorities, etc.) would be adversely affected in disproportionate numbers. Such slippery-slope claims are enhanced when we consider the effects of social discrimination based on disability, the increasing number of newborns with disabilities who survive at heavy cost to the public, and the growing number of aging persons with medical problems that require larger and larger proportions of the public's financial resources. If permissive rules became public policy, the risk would increase that persons in these populations will be harmed. For example, the risk would increase that families and health professionals may abandon treatments for disabled newborns and adults with severe brain damage to avoid social and familial burdens. Moreover, if decision makers reach judgments that some newborns and adults have overly burdensome conditions or lives with no value, the same logic can be extended to other populations of feeble, debilitated, and seriously ill patients who are financial and emotional burdens on families and society.

Rules in our moral code against passively or actively causing the death of another person are not isolated fragments. They are threads in a fabric of rules that uphold respect for human life. The more threads we remove, the weaker the fabric may become. If we focus on the modification of *attitudes* and *beliefs,* not merely on *rules,* shifts in public policy may also erode the general attitude of respect for life. Prohibitions are often both instrumentally and symbolically important, and their removal could weaken a set of attitudes, as well as practices and restraints that we cannot replace.

Rules against bringing about another's death also provide a basis of trust between patients and health care professionals. We expect health care professionals to promote our welfare under all circumstances. We may risk a loss of public trust if physicians become agents of intentionally causing death in addition to being healers and caregivers. We may also risk a loss of trust if patients and families believe that physicians abandon them in their suffering because the physicians lack the courage to offer the assistance needed in the darkest hours of their lives.[60]

The success or failure of slippery-slope arguments that oppose assistance in dying ultimately depends on speculative predictions of a progressive erosion of moral restraints. If dire consequences will flow from the legalization of physician-assisted dying, then these arguments are cogent and such practices are justifiably prohibited. But how good is the evidence that dire consequences will occur? Does the evidence indicate that we cannot maintain firm distinctions in public policies between, for example, patient-requested death and involuntary euthanasia?[61]

Scant evidence supports any of the answers traditionally given to these questions. Those, including the authors of this book, who take seriously some versions of the slippery-slope argument should admit that the argument needs a premise on the order of a precautionary principle, such as "better safe than sorry." The likelihood of the projected moral erosion is not something we can assess by good evidence. Arguments on every side are speculative and analogical, and different assessors of the same evidence reach different conclusions. Also an intractable controversy likely will persist over what counts as good and sufficient evidence. Certainly, if legalization were to bring about unwarranted, involuntary deaths, reduce the quality of palliative care, result in deep-seated and widespread mistrust of physicians, and the like, then we would agree that these consequences would support arguments against legalizing physician assistance in hastening death. This is an important reason why the Oregon law is not merely a powerful symbol of change, but the basis on which further change may occur. How Oregon's procedural safeguards work, or fail to work, will be carefully watched in upcoming years by legislators everywhere in the United States and beyond. That state's experience is likely to shape the next steps taken in other states. Failure of the ODWDA would be a major setback for proponents of the right to die by use of prescribed drugs.

None of the abuses some predicted have materialized in Oregon.[62] The Oregon statute's restrictions have been neither loosened nor broadened. There is no evidence that any patient has died other than in accordance with his or her own wishes. The number of patients seeking prescriptions under the statute has been both low and stable (at around sixty per year), and hastened death has not been used primarily by individuals who might be thought vulnerable to intimidation or abuse. Those choosing assisted death had, on average, a higher level of education and better medical coverage than terminally ill Oregonians who did not seek assistance in dying. Women, people with disabilities, and members of disadvantaged racial minorities have not sought assistance in dying in disproportionate numbers. The overwhelming number of persons requesting assistance in dying are white, and the gender of the requesters reflects the general population. Meanwhile, reports indicate that the quality of palliative care has improved in Oregon. Perhaps most significantly, about one-third of the patients requesting assistance in dying ultimately decide not to use the prescribed drug.[63] Under the statute, mentally competent, terminally ill patients remain in control of decision making about their lives.

Oregon's experiment in physician-assisted suicide is instructive and reassuring in many respects, but questions inevitably arise about its generalizability as a model for the whole United States and for other countries, just as they arise about other national experiments—for example, in the Netherlands, with either physician-assisted suicide, or active euthanasia, or both. Although we cannot here resolve all of the many *public policy* issues about evidence, social attitudes, and legitimate practices, we can go to the heart of the *moral* issues about whether some acts of assisting another in dying are morally justified.

Valid Requests for Aid-in-Dying

At least since the passage of legislation in Oregon, the frontier of the social and legal acceptance of expanded rights to control one's death has shifted from *refusal* of treatment to *request* for aid-in-dying.[64] Assuming that the principles of respect for autonomy and nonmaleficence justify forgoing treatment, the same form of justification might extend to physicians prescribing barbiturates or providing other forms of help requested by seriously ill patients. This strategy rests on the premise that professional ethics and law need reforming because of the apparent inconsistency between (1) the strong rights of autonomy that allow persons in grim circumstances to refuse treatment so as to bring about their deaths and (2) the apparent denial of a similar autonomy right to arrange for death by mutual agreement between patient and physician under equally grim circumstances. The argument for reform is particularly compelling when a condition overwhelmingly burdens a patient, pain management fails to adequately comfort the patient, and only a physician can and is willing to bring relief. At present, medicine and law are in the awkward position of having to say to such patients, "If you were on life-sustaining treatment, you would have a right to withdraw the treatment and then we could let you die. But since you are not, we can only allow you to refuse nutrition and hydration or give you palliative care until you die a natural death, however painful, undignified, and costly." This seems tantamount to condemning the patient to live a life or to suffer a gradual end to life that he or she does not want.

Clearly the two types of authorization—refusal of treatment and request for aid-in-dying—are not perfectly analogous. A health professional is obligated to honor an autonomous refusal of a life-prolonging technology, but he or she is not obligated under ordinary circumstances to honor an autonomous request for aid-in-dying. However, the issue is not whether physicians are *obligated* to lend assistance in dying, but whether valid requests render it *permissible* for a physician (or some other person) to lend aid-in-dying. *Refusals* in medical settings have a moral force not found in requests, but requests do not lack all power to confer on another a right to act in response.

A physician's precise responsibilities to a patient may depend on the nature of the request made as well as on the nature of the pre-established patient–physician relationship. In some cases of physician compliance with requests, the patient and the physician pursue the patient's best interest under an agreement that the physician will not abandon the patient and will undertake what they jointly determine to serve the patient's best interests. In some cases, patients in a close relationship with a physician *both* refuse a medical technology *and* request a hastened death to lessen pain or suffering. Refusal and request may be parts of a single plan. If the physician accepts the plan, some form of assistance grows out of the pre-established relationship.

From this perspective, a valid request for aid-in-dying frees a responder of moral culpability for the death, just as a valid refusal precludes culpability. We can conceive of no moral grounds for restricting the liberty of a competent individual to make such a request for aid-in-dying. The only moral questions concern whether physicians are obligated not to implement such requests under conditions such as a seriously depressed state of mind that does not render a patient incompetent. We believe that physicians sometimes have sufficient moral reason to refuse to comply with such a request, but also that they sometimes have sufficient reason to comply.

These arguments suggest that causing a person's death is morally wrong, when it is wrong, because an unauthorized intervention thwarts or sets back a person's interests. It is an unjustified act when it deprives the person who dies of opportunities and goods.[65] However, if a person freely authorizes death and makes an autonomous judgment that cessation of pain and suffering through death constitutes a personal benefit rather than a setback to his or her interests, then active aid-in-dying at the person's request involves neither harming nor wronging. To the contrary, not to help such persons in their dying will frustrate their plans and cause them a loss, thereby harming them. It can also bring them indignity and despair. From this perspective, causing death is not always an evil act.

Assisting an autonomous person at his or her request to bring about death is, from this perspective, a way of showing respect for the person's autonomous choices. Similarly, denying the person access to other individuals who are willing and qualified to comply with the request shows a fundamental disrespect for the person's autonomy.

Unjustified Physician Assistance in Dying

The fact that the autonomous requests of patients for aid-in-dying should be respected in some circumstances does not entail that *all* cases of physician-assisted death by request are justifiable. Jack Kevorkian's practices provide an important historical example of the kind of *unjustified* physician-assisted suicide that society should discourage and even prohibit. In his first case of assisting in suicide, Janet Adkins, an Oregon grandmother with Alzheimer's disease, had reached a decision that she wanted to take her life rather than lose her cognitive capacities, which she was convinced were slowly deteriorating. After Adkins read about Kevorkian's machine in news reports, she communicated with him by phone and then flew from Oregon to Michigan to meet with him. Following brief discussions over a weekend, she and Kevorkian drove to a park in northern Oakland County. He inserted a tube in her arm and started saline flow. His machine was constructed so that Adkins could then press a button to inject other drugs, eventuating in potassium chloride, which would physically cause her death. She then pressed the button.[66]

This case raises several concerns. Janet Adkins was in the fairly early stages of Alzheimer's and was not yet debilitated. At fifty-four years of age, she was still capable of enjoying a full schedule of activities with her husband and playing tennis with her son, and she might have been able to live a meaningful life for several more years. A slight possibility existed that the Alzheimer's diagnosis was incorrect, and she might have been more psychologically depressed than Kevorkian appreciated. She had limited contact with him before they collaborated in her death, and he did not administer examinations to confirm either her diagnosis or her level of competence to commit suicide. He also lacked the professional expertise to evaluate her. The glare of media attention also raises the question whether Kevorkian acted imprudently to generate publicity for his social goals and for his forthcoming book.

Lawyers, physicians, and writers in bioethics have almost universally condemned Kevorkian's actions. The case raises all the fears present in the arguments mentioned previously about physician-assisted dying: abuse, lack of social control, absence of accountability, and unverifiable circumstances of a patient's death. Although Kevorkian's approach to assisted suicide is regrettable, his "patients" raise profoundly distressing questions about the lack of a support system in health care for handling their problems. Having thought for over a year about her future, Janet Adkins decided that the suffering of continued existence exceeded its benefits. Her family supported her decision. She faced a bleak future from the perspective of a person who had lived an unusually vigorous life, both physically and mentally. She believed that her brain would slowly deteriorate, with progressive and devastating cognitive loss and confusion, fading memory, immense frustration, and loss of all capacity to take care of herself. She also believed that the full burden of responsibility for her care would fall on her family. From her perspective what Kevorkian offered was preferable to what other physicians had offered her, which was a refusal to help her die.

Current social institutions, including the health care system, do not have adequate resources to help many patients in a similar condition who have reached a similar conclusion about their fates. Some dying persons face inadequate counseling, emotional support, and pain control. To them, their condition is intolerable, and no avenue of hope exists. They would rather kill themselves or be killed than face what they understand to be a bleak future without relief. To judge Kevorkian harshly is appropriate, but to say that his "patients" act immorally by arranging for death at their own hand or with a physician's assistance is, for the reasons just mentioned, an overly harsh and unwarranted judgment.

Justified Physician Assistance in Dying

Balancing the errors of the Kevorkian strategy are cases of *justified* assisted suicide. Consider the actions of physician Timothy Quill in prescribing the barbiturates desired by a forty-five-year-old patient who had refused a risky, painful, and often unsuccessful treatment for leukemia. The woman had been his patient for many years, and members of her family had, as a group, come to this decision with his counsel. The patient was competent and had already discussed and rejected all reasonable alternatives for the relief of suffering. This case satisfied most of the conditions that we consider sufficient for justified assisted suicide. These conditions include:

1. A voluntary request by a competent patient
2. An ongoing patient–physician relationship
3. Mutual and informed decision making by patient and physician
4. A supportive yet critical and probing environment of decision making
5. A considered rejection of alternatives
6. Structured consultation with other parties in medicine
7. A patient's expression of a durable preference for death
8. Unacceptable suffering by the patient
9. Use of a means that is as painless and comfortable as possible

Even though Quill's actions satisfied these conditions, some people found his involvement as a physician unsettling and unjustified. Several critics invoked the slippery-slope argument, because acts like Quill's, if legalized, can potentially affect many patients, especially the elderly. Others were troubled by the fact that Quill potentially violated a New York State law against assisted suicide. Furthermore, to reduce the risks of criminal liability, Quill lied to the medical examiner by informing him that a hospice patient had died of acute leukemia.[67]

Despite these problems, we do not oppose Quill's act, his patient's decision, or their relationship. Suffering and loss of cognitive capacity can ravage and dehumanize patients so severely that death is in their best interests. In these tragic situations—or in anticipation of them, as in this case—physicians like Quill do not act wrongly in assisting competent patients, at their request, to bring about their deaths. Public policy issues regarding how to avoid abuses and discourage unjustified acts should be a central part of our discussion about forms of appropriate physician assistance, but these issues do not affect the moral justifiability of the physician's act itself.

We maintain that physician assistance in hastening death is best viewed as part of a continuum of medical care. A physician who encounters a sick patient should initially seek, if possible, to rid the patient's body of its ills. Restoration of health is a morally mandatory goal if a reasonable prospect of success exists and the patient supports the means necessary to this end. However, to stop at this point and confine the practice of medicine to measures designed to cure diseases or heal injuries is an unduly narrow way of thinking about what the physician has to offer the patient. The value of physicians is broader. When, in the patient's eyes, the burdens of continued attempts to cure outweigh their probable benefits, the caring physician, in consultation with the patient, should redirect the course of treatment so that its primary focus is the relief of pain and suffering. For many patients, palliative care with aggressive use of analgesics will prove sufficient to accomplish this goal. For other patients, relief of intolerable distress or suffering will come only with death, which some patients will seek to hasten.[68]

Under a broader view, a physician who assists a patient in hastening his or her death is not providing a "service" that could be provided, as easily and competently, by a layperson. Discerning physicians use the full extent of their professional training and experience when they assess the patient's condition and determine whether the patient is terminally ill. They assess the prospects for effective palliative care for the patient through a meaningful dialogue. They determine whether the patient is competent to make a decision regarding the course of treatment, and they consult with other physicians to confirm the accuracy of the diagnosis, the alternatives, and the competence of the patient. These activities all require a physician's experience, knowledge, and skills.

A favorable response by a physician to a request for assistance in facilitating death by *hastening* it through fatal medication is not relevantly different from a favorable response to requests for assistance in facilitating death by *easing* it through removal of life-prolonging technology or use of coma-inducing medications. The two acts of physician assistance are morally equivalent as long as there are no other differences in the cases. That is, if the disease is relevantly similar, the request by the patient is relevantly similar, and the desperateness of the patient's circumstance is relevantly similar, then responding to a request to provide the means to hasten death seems morally equivalent to responding to a request to ease death by withdrawing treatment, sedating to coma, and the like.

We should be able to devise social policies and laws that maintain a bright line between justified and unjustified physician assistance in dying. In view of our earlier comments on wedge or slippery-slope arguments, the implementation and impact of such policies and laws need careful and ongoing monitoring, as occurs in Oregon, to ensure that they are acceptable. We also note an important practical and semantic point that arises from the discussion about the Oregon law: The person whose death is brought about makes the final decision and performs the final act. This explains the common label "physician-assisted suicide," which the Oregon law avoids and for which we have generally substituted neutral language.

To make our overall position on the legitimacy of physician-assisted dying clear, principles of respect for autonomy and beneficence—as well as justice—and virtues of care and compassion all offer strong reasons for recognizing the legitimacy of physician-assisted death. Major opposition stems from interpretations of the principle of nonmaleficence and its specifications in various distinctions and rules. We have argued on conceptual and normative grounds that many of those distinctions and rules break down on closer examination. We need richer ways to characterize when treatment is obligatory, optional, and wrong, which we have sought to provide. In arguing for changes in laws and policies to allow physician-assisted dying in carefully circumscribed contexts, we do not believe that these changes will address all of the important issues. They mainly address last-resort situations, which can often be avoided by better social policies and practices, including improved palliative care, which of course we strongly recommend.

In presenting a case involving the disconnection of a ventilator maintaining the life of a patient with Amytrophic Lateral Sclerosis (ALS, or Lou Gehrig's disease) at an international conference on "Ethical Issues in Disability and Rehabilitation," some clinical speakers framed it as an "end-of-life case," in which the "patient" decided to discontinue the ventilator. They were surprised when the audience, many of whom had disabilities and had themselves experienced long-term ventilator use, disputed this classification and argued instead that this was a "disability" case in which the clinicians should have provided better care, fuller information, and more options to the "consumer," particularly to help him overcome his felt isolation after the recent death of his spouse: "What to the clinicians was a textbook case of 'end-of-life' decision making was, for their audience, a story in which a life was ended as a result of failures of information and assistance by the presenters themselves."[69]

We clearly need further improvements and extensions of various modes of support for people who suffer from a variety of serious medical problems. Control of pain and suffering is now a moral imperative. However, significant progress will not obviate all last-resort situations, in which individuals desire and need control over their dying in ways that have often been denied them.

PROTECTING INCOMPETENT PATIENTS

In Chapter 4 we developed standards of surrogate decision making for incompetent patients. We now consult those standards in considering *who* should decide for the incompetent patient. Determining the best system for protecting such patients from negligence and harm is the central problem.[70] Most of us think first of families as the proper decision makers because they generally have the deepest interest in protecting their incompetent members. However, we also need a system that will shield incompetent individuals from family members who care little or are caught in conflicts of interest, while also protecting residents of nursing homes, psychiatric hospitals, and facilities for the disabled and mentally handicapped who rarely, if ever, see a family member. The appropriate roles of families, courts, guardians, conservators, hospital committees, and health professionals all merit consideration.

Advance Directives

In an increasingly popular procedure rooted as much in respect for autonomy as in obligations of nonmaleficence, a person, while competent, either writes a directive for health care professionals or selects a surrogate to make decisions about life-sustaining treatments during periods of incompetence.[71] Two types of *advance directive* aim at governing future decision making: (1) *living wills,* substantive directives regarding medical procedures in specific circumstances, and (2) *durable power of attorney* (DPA) for health care, or proxy directives. A DPA is a legal document in which one person assigns another person authority to perform specified actions on behalf of the signer. The power is "durable" because, unlike the usual power of attorney, it continues in effect when the signer becomes incompetent.

Early legislative action on this topic focused on the agent's decisions through living wills in the form of advance directives to physicians that specify the treatment a person welcomes or declines in foreseeable circumstances. However, individuals have difficulty making decisions and specifying guidelines that adequately anticipate the full range of medical situations that might occur. As a result, designating surrogate decision makers has become common. Living wills and DPAs protect the patient against what the patient regards as harmful outcomes and also may reduce stress for families and health professionals who fear making the wrong decision. However, these documents also generate practical and moral problems.[72]

First, relatively few persons compose them, and when they do, they often fail to leave sufficiently explicit instructions.[73] Second, a designated decision maker might be unavailable when needed, might be incompetent to make good decisions for the patient, or might have a conflict of interest, for example, because of a prospective inheritance or an improved position in a family-owned business. Third, some patients who change their preferences about treatment fail to change their directives, and a few, when legally incompetent, protest a surrogate's decision. Fourth, laws often severely restrict the use of advance directives. For example, advance directives have legal effect in some locations if and only if the patient is terminally ill and death is imminent. Decisions must be made, however, in some cases in which death is not imminent or the patient does not have a medical condition appropriately described as a terminal illness. Fifth, living wills provide no basis for health professionals to overturn a patient's instructions; yet prior decisions could turn out not to be in the patient's best medical interest, although the patient could not have reasonably anticipated the precise circumstance while competent. Surrogate decision makers also make decisions with which physicians sharply disagree, in some cases asking the physician to act against his or her conscience. Sixth, some patients do not have an adequate understanding of the range of decisions a health professional or a surrogate might have to make and, even with an adequate understanding, cannot foresee clinical situations and possible future experiences.

Vague language often permeates living wills, thus necessitating inference and discretion. Nonetheless, the advance directive is a promising and valid way for competent persons to exercise their autonomy.[74] From the perspective of biomedical ethics, adequate methods of implementation that follow the outlines of the procedures for informed consent discussed in Chapter 4 can overcome these primarily practical problems.

Surrogate Decision Making without Advance Directives

When an incompetent patient has not left an advance directive, who should make the decision, and with whom should the decision maker consult?

Qualifications of surrogate decision makers. We propose the following list of qualifications for decision makers for incompetent patients (including newborns):

1. Ability to make reasoned judgments (competence)
2. Adequate knowledge and information
3. Emotional stability
4. A commitment to the incompetent patient's interests, free of conflicts of interest and free of controlling influence by those who might not act in the patient's best interests

The first three conditions follow from the discussion of informed consent in Chapter 4. The only potentially controversial condition is the fourth. Here we endorse a criterion of *partiality*—acting as an advocate in the incompetent patient's best interests—rather than *impartiality,* which requires neutrality in consideration of the interests of the various affected parties.

Four classes of decision makers have been proposed and used in cases of withholding and terminating treatment for incompetent patients: families, physicians and other health care professionals, institutional committees, and courts. (If a court-appointed guardian exists, that person will act as the primary responsible party.) The following analysis is meant to provide a defensible structure of decision-making authority that places the caring family as the presumptive authority when the patient cannot make the decision and has not previously designated a decision maker.

The role of the family. Wide agreement exists that the patient's closest family member is the first choice as a surrogate. There is evidence that many patients strongly prefer family members in interaction with physicians as the decision-making authorities about their medical fate.[75] The family's role should be primary because of its presumed identification with the patient's interests, depth of concern about the patient, and intimate knowledge of his or her wishes, as well as its traditional role in society. Unfortunately, the term *family* is imprecise, especially if it includes the extended family. The reasons that support assigning presumptive priority to the patient's closest family member also support assigning relative priority to other family members. However, even the patient's closest family member(s) sometimes make unacceptable decisions, and the authority of the family is not final or ultimate.[76] The closest family member can have a conflict of interest, can be poorly informed, or can be too distant personally and even estranged from the patient.[77]

Consider an illustrative case: Mr. Lazarus was a fifty-seven-year-old male patient who was brought into the hospital after suffering a heart attack while playing touch football. Lazarus had five children and a loving wife. Lazarus lapsed into a coma and became ventilator-dependent. After twenty-four hours Mrs. Lazarus asked that the ventilator be withdrawn and dialysis stopped so that he could be allowed to die. The attending was very uncomfortable with this request because he thought that Mr. Lazarus had a good chance of full recovery. Mrs. Lazarus insisted that treatment be withdrawn, and she produced a DPA for health care that designated her as the surrogate. Mrs. Lazarus became angry when the health care team expressed reluctance to withdraw care, and she threatened to sue the hospital if her decision was not honored. An ethics consult was called because the attending and staff remained unwilling to carry out her wishes. The ethics consultant carefully read the DPA, only to discover that Mr. Lazarus had designated his wife as surrogate only if he was deemed to be in a PVS. Furthermore, Mr. Lazarus had stipulated on the DPA that if he was not in a PVS, he wanted "everything done." Mr. Lazarus awoke after three days and immediately revoked his DPA when told of his wife's demand.[78]

Health care professionals should seek to disqualify any decision makers who are significantly incompetent or ignorant, are acting in bad faith, or have a conflict of interest. Serious conflicts of interest in the family may be more common than either physicians or the courts have generally appreciated.

The role of health care professionals. Physicians and other health care professionals can help the family become more adequate decision makers and can safeguard the patient's interests and preferences (where known) by monitoring the quality of surrogate decision making. Often, for example, the physician will best serve both the family and the patient by helping surrogates see that rapid functional decline has set in and the time has came to shift from life-prolonging measures to palliative care centered on increased comfort and reduction of the burdens of treatments.[79] Such guidance can be wrenchingly difficult and emotionally challenging for the physician.

In the comparatively rare situation in which physicians contest a surrogate's decision and disagreements persist, physicians should seek help from an independent source of review, such as a hospital ethics committee or the judicial system. In the event that a surrogate, a member of the health care team, or an independent reviewer asks a caregiver to perform an act that the caregiver regards as contraindicated, futile, or unconscionable, the caregiver is not obligated to perform the act but may still be obligated to help the surrogate or patient make other arrangements for care.

Institutional ethics committees. Surrogate decision makers sometimes refuse treatments that would serve the interests of those they should protect, and physicians sometimes too readily acquiesce in their preferences. In other cases, surrogates need help in reaching difficult decisions. The involved parties then may need a mechanism or procedure to help make a decision or to break a private circle of refusal and acquiescence. A similar need exists for assistance in decisions regarding residents of nursing homes and hospices, psychiatric hospitals, and many residential facilities in which families often play only a small role, if any.

These hospital ethics committees now differ widely in their composition and function. Many create or recommend explicit policies to govern actions such as withholding and withdrawing treatment, and many serve educational functions in the hospital. Controversy centers on additional functions, such as whether committees should make, facilitate, or monitor decisions about patients in particular cases. The decisions of committees on occasion need to be reviewed or criticized, perhaps by an auditor or impartial party.

Nonetheless, the benefits of good committee review generally outweigh its risks. These committees help resolve disagreements, generate reasoned options, and help the parties conform to institutional guidelines and governmental regulations. A major justification for committee review is that open discussion and debate foster better thinking than can be expected of parties with narrower perspectives. These committees have a particularly robust role to play in circumstances in which physicians acquiesce too readily to parental, familial, or guardian choices that prove contrary to a patient's best interests.

The judicial system. Courts are sometimes unduly intrusive as final decision makers, but in many cases they are the last and the fairest recourse. When good reasons exist to appoint guardians or to disqualify the family or health care professionals to protect an incompetent patient's interests, the courts may legitimately be involved. The courts also sometimes need to intervene in nontreatment decisions for incompetent patients in mental institutions, nursing homes, and the like. If no family members are available or willing to be involved, and if the patient is confined to a state mental institution or is in a nursing home, it may be appropriate to establish safeguards beyond the health care team and the institutional ethics committee.[80]

CONCLUSION

We have concentrated in this chapter on the principle of nonmaleficence and its implications for refusals of treatment and requests for assistance in dying when death is a high probability or certainty. From the principle that we should avoid causing harm to persons, there is no direct step to the conclusion that a *positive obligation* exists to provide benefits such as health care and various forms of assistance. We have not entered this territory in a chapter on nonmaleficence, because obligations to provide positive benefits are the territory of beneficence and justice, which need to be distinguished as separate principles of biomedical ethics. We treat them in Chapters 6 and 7.

NOTES

1. W. H. S. Jones, *Hippocrates,* vol. I (Cambridge, MA: Harvard University Press, 1923), p. 165. See also Albert R. Jonsen, "Do No Harm: Axiom of Medical Ethics," in *Philosophical and Medical Ethics: Its Nature and Significance,* ed. Stuart F. Spicker and H. Tristram Engelhardt, Jr. (Dordrecht, Netherlands: D. Reidel, 1977), pp. 27–41. On the connection of "Do No Harm" to nonmaleficence and beneficence, see Virginia A. Sharpe, "Why 'Do No Harm'?" *Theoretical Medicine* 18 (1997): 197–215.

2. W. D. Ross, *The Right and the Good* (Oxford: Clarendon, 1930), pp. 21–26; and John Rawls, *A Theory of Justice* (Cambridge, MA: Harvard University Press, 1971; rev. ed., 1999), p. 114 (1999: p. 98).

3. William Frankena, *Ethics,* 2nd ed. (Englewood Cliffs, NJ: Prentice Hall, 1973), p. 47.

4. On the priority of avoiding harm, see criticisms by N. Ann Davis, "The Priority of Avoiding Harm," in *Killing and Letting Die,* 2nd ed., ed. Bonnie Steinbock and Alastair Norcross (New York: Fordham University Press, 1994), pp. 298–354.

5. *McFall v. Shimp, no.* 78-1771 in Equity (C. P. Allegheny County, PA, July 26, 1978); Barbara J. Culliton, "Court Upholds Refusal to Be Medical Good Samaritan," *Science* 201 (August 18, 1978): 596–97; Mark F. Anderson, "Encouraging Bone Marrow Transplants from Unrelated Donors," *University of Pittsburgh Law Review* 54 (1993): 477ff.

6. Alan Meisel and Loren H. Roth, "Must a Man Be His Cousin's Keeper?" *Hastings Center Report* 8 (October 1978): 5–6.

7. Joel Feinberg, *Harm to Others,* vol. I of *The Moral Limits of the Criminal Law* (New York: Oxford University Press, 1984), esp. pp. 32–36.

8. On the roles of harm and nonmaleficence in bioethics, see Bettina Schöne-Seifert, "Harm," in *Encyclopedia of Bioethics,* rev. ed., ed. Warren Reich (New York: Simon & Schuster Macmillan, 1995): 1021–26.

9. On rules of nonmaleficence, see Bernard Gert, *Morality: A New Justification of Morality* (New York: Oxford University Press, 1988), chaps. 6–7.

10. H. L. A. Hart, *Punishment and Responsibility* (Oxford: Clarendon, 1968), esp. pp. 136–57; Joel Feinberg, *Doing and Deserving* (Princeton, NJ: Princeton University Press, 1970), esp. pp. 187–221; and Eric D'Arcy, *Human Acts: An Essay in Their Moral Evaluation* (Oxford: Clarendon, 1963), esp. p. 121.

11. On medical negligence, physician-caused harm, and their connection to medical ethics, see Virginia A. Sharpe and Alan I. Faden, *Medical Harm: Historical, Conceptual, and Ethical Dimensions of Iatrogenic Illness* (New York: Cambridge University Press, 1998). On the legal model and the professions, see Martin Curd and Larry May, *Professional Responsibility for Harmful Actions* (Dubuque, IA: Kendall/Hunt, 1984).

12. As Quoted in Angela Roddy Holder, *Medical Malpractice Law* (New York: Wiley, 1975), p. 42.

13. This case was presented to one of the authors during a consultation. On some of the intuitions at work in this and similar cases, see Anna Maria Cugliari and Tracy E. Miller, "Moral and Religious Objections by Hospitals to Withholding and Withdrawing Life-Sustaining Treatment," *Journal of Community Health* 19 (1994): 87–100.

14. For defenses of the distinction along these or similar lines, see Daniel P. Sulmasy and Jeremy Sugarman, "Are Withholding and Withdrawing Therapy Always Morally Equivalent?" *Journal of Medical Ethics* 20 (1994): 218–22 (commented on by John Harris, pp. 223–24); and Kenneth V. Iserson, "Withholding and Withdrawing Medical Treatment: An Emergency Medicine Perspective," *Annals of Emergency Medicine* 28 (1996): 51–54.

15. *In the matter of Spring,* Mass. 405 N.E. 2d 115 (1980), at 488–89.

16. Lewis Cohen, Michael Germain, and David Poppel, "Practical Considerations in Dialysis Withdrawal," *Journal of the American Medical Association* 289 (2003): 2113–19.

17. Robert Stinson and Peggy Stinson, *The Long Dying of Baby Andrew* (Boston: Little, Brown, 1983), p. 355.

18. Susanna E. Bedell and Thomas L. Delbanco, "Choices about Cardiopulmonary Resuscitation in the Hospital: When Do Physicians Talk with Patients?," *New England Journal of Medicine* 310 (April 26, 1984): 1089–93; and Marcia Angell, "Respecting the Autonomy of Competent Patients," *New England Journal of Medicine* 310 (April 26, 1984): 1115–16.

19. This case has been adapted with permission from a case presented by Dr. Martin P. Albert of Charlottesville, VA. On problems in nursing homes, see Alan Meisel, "Barriers to Forgoing Nutrition and Hydration in Nursing Homes," *American Journal of Law and Medicine* 21 (1995): 335–82; Elizabeth H. Bradley, Vasum Peiris, and Terrie Wetle, "Discussions about End-of-Life Care in Nursing Homes," *Journal of the American Geriatrics Society* 46 (1998): 1235–41.

20. *In the matter of Quinlan,* 70 N.J. 10, 355 A.2d 647, cert. denied, 429 U.S. 922 (1976). The New Jersey Supreme Court ruled that the Quinlans could disconnect the mechanical ventilator so that the patient could "die with dignity."

21. *In re Conroy,* 98 N.J. 321, 486 A.2d 1209 (1985).

22. *Brophy v. New England Sinai Hospital, Inc.,* 398 Mass. 417, 497 N.E. 2d 626 (1986).

23. These issues were first raised in 1982, in *Barber v. Superior Court,* 147 Cal. App. 3d 1006, 195 Cal. Rptr. 484 (1983). By 1988, many courts accepted this trend as determinative. For the massive court literature, see Alan Meisel, *The Right to Die,* 2nd ed. (New York: Wiley, 1995), and Meisel, "The 'Right to Die': A Case Study in American Lawmaking," *European Journal of Health Law* 3 (1996): 49–74.

In *Cruzan v. Director, Missouri Dep't of Health,* 497 U.S. 261 (1990), the U.S. Supreme Court concluded that a competent person has a constitutionally protected right to refuse lifesaving hydration and nutrition. Its dicta reflected no distinction between medical and sustenance treatments.

24. See Joanne Lynn and James F. Childress, "Must Patients Always Be Given Food and Water?" *Hastings Center Report* 13 (October 1983): 17–21; and Joanne Lynn, ed., *By No Extraordinary Means* (Bloomington, IN: Indiana University Press, 1986).

25. Daniel Callahan, "On Feeding the Dying," *Hastings Center Report* 13 (October 1983): 22; Paolo Cattorini and Massimo Reichlin, "Persistent Vegetative State: A Presumption to Treat," *Theoretical Medicine* 18 (1997): 263–81.

26. Mark Siegler and Alan J. Weisbard, "Against the Emerging Stream: Should Fluids and Nutritional Support Be Discontinued?" *Archives of Internal Medicine* 145 (January 1985): 129–32; Gillian M. Craig, "On Withholding Nutrition and Hydration in the Terminally Ill: Has Palliative Medicine Gone Too Far?" *Journal of Medical Ethics* 20 (1994): 139–43.

27. Robert M. McCann, William J. Hall, and Ann Marie Groth-Juncker, "Comfort Care for Terminally Ill Patients: The Appropriate Use of Nutrition and Hydration," *Journal of the American Medical Association* 272 (October 26, 1994): 1263–66; Ronald Cranford, "Neurologic Syndromes and Prolonged Survival: When Can Artificial Nutrition and Hydration Be Foregone?" *Law, Medicine, and Health Care* 19 (1991): 13–22, esp. 18–19.

28. The RDE has rough precedents that predate the writings of St. Thomas Aquinas (e.g., in St. Augustine and Abelard). However, the history primarily flows from Aquinas. See Anthony Kenny, "The History of Intention in Ethics," *Anatomy of the Soul* (Oxford: Basil Blackwell, 1973), Appendix; Joseph T. Mangan, S.J., "An Historical Analysis of the Principle of Double Effect," *Theological Studies* 10 (1949): 41–61; and T. A. Cavanaugh, *Double-Effect Reasoning: Doing Good and Avoiding Evil* (New York: Oxford University Press, 2006), chap. 1.

29. Joseph Boyle reduces the RDE to two conditions: intention and proportionality. "Who Is Entitled to Double Effect?" *Journal of Medicine and Philosophy* 16 (1991): 475–94, and "Toward Understanding the Principle of Double Effect," *Ethics* 90 (1980): 527–38. For criticisms of intention-weighted views, see Sophie Botros, "An Error about the Doctrine of Double Effect," *Philosophy* 74 (1999): 71–83; and Timothy E. Quill, Rebecca Dresser, and Dan Brock, "The Rule of Double Effect—A Critique of Its Role in End-of-Life Decision Making," *New England Journal of Medicine* 337 (1997): 1768–71. For representative philosophical positions, see P. A. Woodward, ed., *The Doctrine of Double Effect: Philosophers Debate a Controversial Moral Principle* (Notre Dame, IN: Notre Dame University Press, 2001).

30. See David Granfield, *The Abortion Decision* (Garden City, NY: Image Books, 1971), which defends the RDE, and Susan Nicholson, *Abortion and the Roman Catholic Church* (Knoxville, TN: Religious Ethics, 1978). See the criticisms of the RDE in Donald Marquis, "Four Versions of Double Effect," *Journal of Medicine and Philosophy* 16 (1991): 515–44, reprinted in *The Doctrine of Double Effect,* ed. Woodward, pp. 156–85; and the defense in Daniel Sulmasy and Edmund Pellegrino, "The Rule of Double Effect," *Archives of Internal Medicine* 159 (1999): 545–50.

31. See Michael Bratman, *Intention, Plans, and Practical Reason* (Cambridge, MA: Harvard University Press, 1987).

32. Alvin I. Goldman, *A Theory of Human Action* (Englewood Cliffs, NJ: Prentice Hall, 1970), pp. 49–85.

33. Hector-Neri Castañeda, "Intensionality and Identity in Human Action and Philosophical Method," *Nous* 13 (1979): 235–60, esp. 255.

34. Our analysis here draws from Ruth R. Faden and Tom L. Beauchamp, *A History and Theory of Informed Consent* (New York: Oxford University Press, 1986), chap. 7.

35. We follow John Searle in thinking that we cannot reliably distinguish, in many situations, among acts, effects, consequences, and events. Searle, "The Intentionality of Intention and Action," *Cognitive Science* 4 (1980): 65.

36. This interpretation of double effect is defended by Boyle, "Who Is Entitled to Double Effect?"

37. For this debate, see Joseph Boyle, "Medical Ethics and Double Effect: The Case of Terminal Sedation," *Theoretical Medicine* 25 (2004): 51–60; Alison McIntyre, "The Double Life of Double Effect," *Theoretical Medicine* 25 (2004): 61–74; Sulmasy and Pellegrino, "The Rule of Double Effect"; Lynn A. Jansen and Daniel Sulmasy, "Sedation, Alimentation, Hydration, and Equivocation: Careful Conversation about Care at the End of Life," *Annals of Internal Medicine* 136 (June 4, 2002): 845–49; and Johannes J. M. van Delden, "Terminal Sedation: Source of a Restless Debate," *Journal of Medical Ethics* 33 (2007): 187–88.

38. See Quill, Dresser, and Brock, "The Rule of Double Effect"; and McIntyre, "The Double Life of Double Effect."

39. On futility, see Baruch A. Brody and Amir Halevy, "Is Futility a Futile Concept?" *Journal of Medicine and Philosophy* 20 (1995): 123–44; R. Lofmark and T. Nilstun, "Conditions and Consequences of Medical Futility," *Journal of Medical Ethics* 28 (2002): 115–19; Loretta M. Kopelman, "Conceptual and Moral Disputes about Futile and Useful Treatments," *Journal of Medicine and Philosophy* 20 (1995): 109–21; and Steven H. Miles, "Medical Futility," in *Health Care Ethics: Critical Issues,* ed. John F. Monagle and David C. Thomasma (Gaithersburg, MD: Aspen, 1994): 233–40.

40. Susan B. Rubin, *When Doctors Say No: The Battleground of Medical Futility* (Bloomington, IN: Indiana University Press, 1998); Lawrence J. Schneiderman, Nancy Jecker, and Albert R. Jonsen, "Medical Futility: Response to Critiques," *Annals of Internal Medicine* 125 (1996): 669–74; Lawrence J. Schneiderman and Nancy S. Jecker, *Wrong Medicine: Doctors, Patients, and Futile Treatment* (Baltimore, MD: The Johns Hopkins University Press, 1995).

41. For constructive proposals that take account of legitimate disagreement, see Robert Truog, "Progress in the Futility Debate," *Journal of Clinical Ethics* 6 (1995): 128–32; Rosemarie Tong, "Towards a Just, Courageous, and Honest Resolution of the Futility Debate," *Journal of Medicine and Philosophy* 20 (1995): 165–89; and Baruch A. Brody and Amir Halevy, "The Houston Process-Based Approach to Medical Futility," *Bioethics Forum* 14 (1998): 10–18.

42. *Superintendent of Belchertown State School v. Saikewicz,* Mass., 370 N.E. 2d 417 (1977), at 428.

43. Ramsey, *Ethics at the Edges of Life* (New Haven, CT: Yale University Press, 1978), p. 155.

44. See President's Commission, *Deciding to Forego Life-Sustaining Treatment,* chap. 5, and the articles on "The Persistent Problem of PVS," *Hastings Center Report* 18 (February–March 1988): 26–47.

45. Ramsey, *Ethics at the Edges of Life,* p. 172.

46. President's Commission, *Deciding to Forego Life-Sustaining Treatment.*

47. See Frank A. Chervenak and Laurence B. McCullough, "Nonaggressive Obstetric Management," *Journal of the American Medical Association* 261 (June 16, 1989): 3439–40; and their "The Fetus as Patient: Implications for Directive versus Nondirective Counseling for Fetal Benefit," *Fetal Diagnosis and Therapy* 6 (1991): 93–100.

48. Albert R. Jonsen and Michael J. Garland, "A Moral Policy for Life/Death Decisions in the Intensive Care Nursery," in *Ethics of Newborn Intensive Care,* ed. Jonsen and Garland (Berkeley, CA: University of California, Institute of Governmental Studies, 1976), p. 148. A report from the Nuffield Council on Bioethics uses the concept of "intolerability" to describe situations where life-sustaining treatment

would not be in the baby's "best interests" because of the burdens imposed by "irremediable suffering." *Critical Care Decisions in Fetal and Neonatal Medicine: Ethical Issues* (London: Nuffield Council on Bioethics, 2006).

49. See Steinbock and Norcross, *Killing and Letting Die,* 2nd ed.; Tom L. Beauchamp, ed., *Intending Death* (Upper Saddle River, NJ: Prentice Hall, 1996); Jeff McMahan, "Killing, Letting Die, and Withdrawing Aid," *Ethics* 103 (1993): 250–79; David Orentlicher, "The Alleged Distinction between Euthanasia and the Withdrawal of Life-Sustaining Treatment: Conceptually Incoherent and Impossible to Maintain," *University of Illinois Law Review* (1998): 837–59; and James Rachels, "Killing, Letting Die, and the Value of Life," in his *Can Ethics Provide Answers? And Other Essays in Moral Philosophy* (Lanham, MD: Rowman & Littlefield, 1997), pp. 69–79.

50. *Assisted suicide* is the term often used to describe this practice. Although we sometimes use this term, we also use broader language, such as "physician-assisted dying," or "physician-arranged dying," not because of a desire to find euphemisms but because the broader language often provides a more accurate description. Although the term *suicide* has the small advantage of indicating that the one whose death is brought about performs the final act, other conditions such as prescribing and transporting fatal substances may be as causally relevant as the "final act" itself.

51. The Supreme Court utilized and endorsed the distinction between "killing" and "letting die" in *Vacco v. Quill,* 521 U.S. 793, at 800–07 (1997).

52. Howard Brody, "Messenger Case: Lessons and Reflections," *Ethics-In-Formation* 5 (1995): 8–9; John Roberts, "Doctor Charged for Switching off His Baby's Ventilator," *British Medical Journal* 309 (August 13, 1994): 430. In February 1995, a jury in a lower court cleared Dr. Messenger of manslaughter charges brought in 1994.

53. Cf. James Rachels, "Active and Passive Euthanasia," *New England Journal of Medicine* 292 (January 9, 1975): 78–80; Rachels, "Killing, Letting Die, and the Value of Life," pp. 69–79; Roy W. Perrett, "Killing, Letting Die and the Bare Difference Argument," *Bioethics* 10 (1996): 131–39; and Dan W. Brock, "Voluntary Active Euthanasia," *Hastings Center Report* 22 (March–April 1992): 10–22.

54. In both *Quinlan* and *Conroy,* the New Jersey Supreme Court held that the respirator was only delaying the patient's inevitable death, which would be a "natural death" if the life-support apparatus were removed. For moral accounts that rely on this traditional medical and legal model to defend the killing–letting die distinction, see Kevin P. Quinn, "Assisted Suicide and Equal Protection: In Defense of the Distinction between Killing and Letting Die," *Issues in Law and Medicine* 13 (1997): 145–71; and Daniel Callahan, *The Troubled Dream of Life* (New York: Simon & Schuster, 1993), chap. 2.

55. In saying that the patient "needs" the respirator, we are indicating that it is not medically futile, and thus does not satisfy the other criterion that by itself would justify withdrawal. We do not here address the question whether it is justifiable to stop patient-desired medical procedures on other grounds, such as rationing or triage based on probability of successful outcomes. See our discussion of rationing in Chapter 7.

56. See Joseph J. Fins, *A Palliative Ethic of Care: Clinical Wisdom at Life's End* (Sudbury, MA: Jones & Bartlett, 2006); and Joanne Lynn et al., *Improving Care for the End of Life: A Sourcebook for Health Care Managers and Clinicians* (New York: Oxford University Press, 2007).

57. Oregon Death with Dignity Act, Ore. Rev. Stat. § 127.800 *et seq.* This Act explicitly rejects the language of "physician-assisted suicide." It prefers the language of a right patients have to make a "request for medication to end one's life in a humane and dignified manner."

58. See Lawrence O. Gostin, "Deciding Life and Death in the Courtroom: From Quinlan to Cruzan, Glucksberg, and Vacco—A Brief History and Analysis of Constitutional Protection of the 'Right to Die,'" *Journal of the American Medical Association* 278 (November 12, 1997): 1523–28.

59. For fuller discussions, see Douglas Walton, *Slippery Slope Arguments* (Oxford: Clarendon, 1992); Govert den Hartogh, "The Slippery Slope Argument," in *A Companion to Bioethics,* ed. Helga Kuhse and Peter Singer (Malden, MA: Blackwell, 1998): 280–90; Christopher James Ryan, "Pulling up the Runaway: The Effect of New Evidence on Euthanasia's Slippery Slope," *Journal of Medical Ethics* 24 (1998): 341–44; Bernard Williams, "Which Slopes Are Slippery?" in *Moral Dilemmas in Modern Medicine,* ed. Michael Lockwood (Oxford: Oxford University Press, 1985), pp. 126–37; and James Rachels, *The End of Life: Euthanasia and Morality* (Oxford: Oxford University Press, 1986), chap. 10.

60. See Timothy E. Quill and Christine K. Cassel, "Nonabandonment: A Central Obligation for Physicians," in *Physician-Assisted Dying: The Case for Palliative Care and Patient Choice,* ed. Quill and Margaret P. Battin (Baltimore, MD: Johns Hopkins University Press, 2004), chap. 2.

61. See Franklin G. Miller, Howard Brody, and Timothy E. Quill, "Can Physician-Assisted Suicide Be Regulated Effectively?" *Journal of Law, Medicine and Ethics* 24 (1996): 225–32.

62. See, for example, Timothy E. Quill, "Legal Regulation of Physician-Assisted Death—The Latest Report Cards," *New England Journal of Medicine* 356 (May 10, 2007): 1911–13; Susan Okie, "Physician-Assisted Suicide—Oregon and Beyond," *New England Journal of Medicine* 352 (April 21, 2005): 1627–30; Linda Ganzini et al., "Oregon Physicians' Attitudes about and Experiences with End-of-Life Care Since Passage of the Oregon Death with Dignity Act," *Journal of the American Medical Association* 285 (2001): 2365–66; Katrina Hedberg et al., "Five Years of Legal Physician-Assisted Suicide in Oregon," *New England Journal of Medicine* 348 (March 6, 2003): 961–64.

63. The information in this paragraph appears in Oregon Department of Human Services, *Seventh Annual Report on Oregon's Death with Dignity Act* (2005). A similar pattern appears in the *Eighth Annual Report on Oregon's Death with Dignity Act* (2006).

64. On the nature and importance of the distinction, see Bernard Gert, James L. Bernat, and R. Peter Mogielnicki, "Distinguishing Between Patients' Refusals and Requests," *Hastings Center Report* 24 (July–August 1994): 13–15; Leigh C. Bishop et al., "Refusals Involving Requests" [Letters and Responses], *Hastings Center Report* 25 (July–August 1995): 4; and Diane E. Meier et al., "On the Frequency of Requests for Physician Assisted Suicide in American Medicine," *New England Journal of Medicine* 338 (April 23, 1998): 1193–1201.

65. Cf. Allen Buchanan, "Intending Death: The Structure of the Problem and Proposed Solutions," in *Intending Death,* esp. 34–38; Frances M. Kamm, "Physician-Assisted Suicide, the Doctrine of Double Effect, and the Ground of Value," *Ethics* 109 (1999): 586–605; and Matthew Hanser, "Why Are Killing and Letting Die Wrong?" *Philosophy and Public Affairs* 24 (1995): 175–201.

66. See *New York Times,* June 6, 1990, pp. A1, B6, June 7, 1990, pp. A1, D22; June 9, 1990, p. A6; June 12, 1990, p. C3; *Newsweek,* June 18, 1990, p. 46. For Kevorkian's description, see his *Prescription: Medicide* (Buffalo, NY: Prometheus Books, 1991), pp. 221–31.

67. See Timothy E. Quill, "Death and Dignity: A Case of Individualized Decision Making," *New England Journal of Medicine* 324 (March 7, 1991): 691–94, reprinted with additional analysis in Quill, *Death and Dignity* (New York: Norton, 1993).

68. Again, under the ODWDA, many patients never ingest the drug provided via the physician's prescription. Fear of pain and the loss of bodily functions and autonomy is one of the principal causes of distress for many. Knowledge that one can readily escape these dreaded conditions if they become intolerable may, by itself, provide sufficient comfort.

69. J. K. Kaufert and T. Koch, "Disability or End-of-Life: Competing Narratives in Bioethics," *Theoretical Medicine* 24 (2003): 459–69. See also Kristi L. Kirschner, Carol J. Gill, and Christine K. Cassel, "Physician-Assisted Death in the Context of Disability," in *Physician-Assisted Suicide,* ed. Robert F. Weir (Bloomington and Indianapolis, IN: Indiana University Press, 1997), pp. 155–66.

70. For an examination of current U.S. law, see Norman L. Cantor, *Making Medical Decisions for the Profoundly Mentally Disabled* (Cambridge, MA: The MIT Press, 2005).

71. See Hans-Martin Sass, Robert M. Veatch, and Rihito Kimura, eds., *Advance Directives and Surrogate Decision Making in Health Care: United States, Germany, and Japan* (Baltimore: Johns Hopkins University Press, 1998); and Nancy M. P. King, *Making Sense of Advance Directives* (Dordrecht, Netherlands: Kluwer Academic, 1991; rev. ed. 1996).

72. For accounts of problems and promise in advance directives, see Norman L. Cantor, "Making Advance Directives Meaningful," *Psychology, Public Policy, and Law* 4 (1998): 629–52; Dan Brock, "Trumping Advance Directives," *Hastings Center Report* 21 (September–October 1991): S5–S6; The President's Council on Bioethics, *Taking Care: Ethical Caregiving in Our Aging Society* (Washington, DC: The President's Council on Bioethics, 2005), chap. 2; and Alasdair R. MacLean, "Advance Directives, Future Selves and Decision-Making," *Medical Law Review* 14 (2006): 291–320.

73. See E. R. Gamble et al., "Knowledge, Attitudes, and Behavior of Elderly Persons Regarding Living Wills," *Archives of Internal Medicine* 151 (February 1991): 277–80.

74. See the empirical study by Donald Patrick et al., "Validation of Preferences for Life-Sustaining Treatment: Implications for Advance Care Planning," *Annals of Internal Medicine* 127 (1997): 509–17.

75. Su Hyun Kim and Diane Kjervik, "Deferred Decision Making: Patient's Reliance on Family and Physicians for CPR Decisions in Critical Care," *Nursing Ethics* 12 (2005): 493–506.

76. See Judith Areen, "The Legal Status of Consent Obtained from Families of Adult Patients to Withhold or Withdraw Treatment," *Journal of the American Medical Association* 258 (July 10, 1987): 229–35; and John W. Warren et al., "Informed Consent by Proxy: An Issue in Research with Elderly Patients," *New England Journal of Medicine* 315 (October, 1986): 1124–28.

77. See Nancy Rhoden, "Litigating Life and Death," *Harvard Law Review* 102 (1988): 437; and Patricia King, "The Authority of Families to Make Medical Decisions for Incompetent Patients after the Cruzan Decision," *Law, Medicine & Health Care* 19 (1991): 76–79.

78. As reported in Mark P. Aulisio, "Standards for Ethical Decision Making at the End of Life," in *Advance Directives and Surrogate Decision Making in Illinois,* ed. Thomas May and Paul Tudico (Springfield, IL: Human Services Press, 1999), pp. 25–26.

79. See David E. Weissman, "Decision Making at a Time of Crisis Near the End of Life," *Journal of the American Medical Association* 292 (2004): 1738–43.

80. For analysis of the role of courts and the connection to valid consent, see M. Stratling, V. E. Scharf, and P. Schmucker, "Mental Competence and Surrogate Decision-Making Towards the End of Life," *Medicine, Health Care and Philosophy* 7 (2004): 209–15.

6
Beneficence

Morality requires not only that we treat persons autonomously and refrain from harming them, but also that we contribute to their welfare. These beneficial actions fall under the heading of "beneficence." Principles of beneficence potentially demand much more than the principle of nonmaleficence, because agents must take positive steps to help others, not merely refrain from harmful acts.

This chapter presents two principles of beneficence: positive beneficence and utility. *Positive beneficence* requires agents to provide benefits to others. *Utility* requires that agents balance benefits, risks, and costs to produce the best overall results. We also treat the virtue of benevolence, various forms of care, and nonobligatory ideals of beneficence. Building on these distinctions, we discuss the conflicts between beneficence and respect for autonomy that occur in paternalistic refusals to accept a patient's wishes or in public policies designed to protect or improve individuals' health. The remainder of the chapter focuses on balancing benefits, risks, and costs through analytical methods designed to implement the principle of utility in health policy and clinical care. We conclude that these analytical methods have a useful, although limited, role as aids in decision making

THE CONCEPT OF BENEFICENCE

In ordinary English, the term *beneficence* connotes acts of mercy, kindness, and charity. Forms of beneficence also typically include altruism, love, and humanity. We use *beneficence* to cover beneficent action more broadly, so that it includes all forms of action intended to benefit other persons. *Benevolence* refers to the *character trait* or *virtue* of being disposed to act for the benefit of others. *Principle of beneficence* refers to a statement of moral *obligation* to act for the benefit of others. Many acts of beneficence are not obligatory, but some forms of beneficence, in our analysis, are obligatory.

Beneficence and benevolence have played central roles in certain ethical theories. Utilitarianism, for example, is systematically arranged on a principle of beneficence (the principle of utility). During the Scottish Enlightenment, major figures such as Francis Hutcheson and David Hume made benevolence the centerpiece of their common-morality theories. These theories all closely associate beneficence with the goal of morality itself. We agree that obligations to confer benefits, to prevent and remove harms, and to weigh an action's possible goods against its costs and possible harms are central to the moral life. However, principles of beneficence are not broad enough, in our account, to determine or justify all other principles.

The principle of utility is thus not identical, in our analysis, to the classic utilitarian principle of utility. Our principle should be viewed neither as the sole principle of ethics nor as one that justifies or overrides all other principles. It is one among a number of prima facie principles, and it does not determine the overall balance of moral obligations. Although utilitarians allow society's interests to override individual interests and rights, the principle of utility that we defend can be legitimately constrained by the various other principles in our framework.

OBLIGATORY BENEFICENCE AND IDEAL BENEFICENCE

Some deny that morality includes any form of positive obligations. They hold that beneficence is purely a virtuous ideal or an act of charity, and thus that persons are not morally deficient if they fail to act beneficently. These views rightly point to a need to clarify and specify beneficence, stating the points at which beneficence is optional rather than obligatory. An instructive and classic example of this problem is found in the New Testament parable of the Good Samaritan, which illustrates several problems in interpreting beneficence. In this parable, robbers beat and abandon a "half-dead" man traveling from Jerusalem to Jericho. After two travelers pass by the injured man without rendering help, a Samaritan sees him, has compassion, binds up his wounds, and brings him to an inn to take care of him. In having compassion and showing mercy, the Good Samaritan expressed an attitude of *caring for* the injured man and also *took care* of him. Both the Samaritan's motives and his actions were beneficent. Common interpretations of the parable suggest that positive beneficence is more an *ideal* than an *obligation,* because the Samaritan's act seems to exceed ordinary morality. Nonetheless, it is not clear that beneficence itself is reducible to the category of the morally ideal.

Virtually everyone agrees that the common morality does not contain a principle of beneficence that requires severe sacrifice and extreme altruism—for example, putting one's life in grave danger to provide medical care or giving both of one's kidneys for transplantation. Everyone agrees that only *ideals* of beneficence incorporate such extreme generosity. Likewise, we are not morally required to benefit persons on all occasions, even if we are in a position to do so. For example, we are not morally required to perform all possible acts of generosity or charity that would benefit others. Much beneficent conduct therefore does constitute ideal, rather than obligatory, conduct, and the line between an obligation and a moral ideal is often unclear in the case of beneficence. (See our discussion of ideals in Chapter 2.) Nonetheless, the principle of positive beneficence supports an array of moral rules of obligation. Examples of these rules, in their most general forms, include:

1. Protect and defend the rights of others.
2. Prevent harm from occurring to others.
3. Remove conditions that will cause harm to others.
4. Help persons with disabilities.
5. Rescue persons in danger.

Distinguishing Rules of Beneficence from Rules of Nonmaleficence

Rules of beneficence differ in several ways from those of nonmaleficence, which were treated in the previous chapter. There we argued that rules of nonmaleficence (1) are negative prohibitions of action, (2) must be followed impartially, and (3) provide moral reasons for legal prohibitions of certain forms of conduct. By contrast, rules of beneficence (1) present positive requirements of action, (2) need not always be followed impartially, and (3) generally do not provide reasons for legal punishment when agents fail to abide by them.

The second condition is impartial adherence. We are morally prohibited from causing harm to anyone. However, we are morally permitted to help or benefit those with whom we have special relationships, and we often are not required to help or benefit those with whom we have no such special relationship. In certain contexts, morality thus allows us to practice our beneficence with partiality in regard to those with whom we have special relationships. We are obligated to act nonmaleficently toward all persons at all times, but it is generally not possible to act beneficently toward all persons. Accordingly, failing to act nonmaleficently toward a party is (prima facie) immoral, but failing to act beneficently toward a party is very often not immoral. Nonetheless, we are obligated to follow impartially *some* rules of beneficence, such as those requiring efforts to rescue strangers when the rescue efforts pose little risk.

General and Specific Beneficence

A distinction between *specific* and *general* beneficence can eliminate some of the confusion that surrounds the distinction between *obligatory* beneficence and *nonobligatory* moral ideals. Specific beneficence is directed at specific parties, such as children, friends, and patients, whereas general beneficence is directed beyond these special relationships to all persons.

Virtually everyone agrees that all persons are obligated to act, in certain circumstances, in the interests of their children, friends, and other special parties, but the idea of a general obligation of beneficence is more controversial. W. D. Ross suggests that obligations of general beneficence "rest on the mere fact that there are other beings in the world whose condition we can make better."[1] Such an unqualified form of general beneficence obligates us to benefit persons whom we do not know and with whose views we are not ourselves sympathetic. Obligations of beneficence, so understood, are potentially very demanding. Shelly Kagan, for example, argues that we should recognize no limits, in principle, to the sacrifice that morality can demand of us in promoting the overall good.[2]

The thesis that we have the same impartial obligation to persons we do not know as we have to our own families is both overly romantic and impractical. It is also perilous because this standard may divert attention from our obligations to those to whom we are close or indebted, and to whom our responsibilities are clear rather than clouded. The more widely we generalize obligations of beneficence, the less likely we will be to meet our primary responsibilities. For this reason, among others, the common morality recognizes significant limits to the demands of beneficence.[3]

Some writers try to set limits to our obligations by distinguishing between the removal of harm, the prevention of harm, and the promotion of benefit (see Chapter 5). For instance, in developing a principle of "the obligation to assist," Peter Singer distinguishes preventing evil from promoting good, and contends that "if it is in our power to prevent something bad from happening, without thereby sacrificing anything of comparable moral importance, we ought, morally, to do it."[4] Singer's criterion of comparable importance sets a limit on sacrifice: We ought to donate time and resources until we reach a level at which, by giving more, we would sacrifice something of comparable moral importance. For example, at this point we might cause as much suffering to ourselves as we would relieve through our gift. While Singer leaves it an open question what counts as morally important, his argument clearly implies that morality sometimes requires us to make large sacrifices to rescue needy persons around the world.[5] This account is too demanding, as judged by common-morality standards. The requirement that persons seriously disrupt their life plans in order to benefit the sick, undereducated, or starving exceeds the limits built into common-morality obligations. Standards in the common morality assume that the level of cost, risk, or sacrifice that Singer proposes as morally obligatory surpasses moral obligation—it is a commendable moral ideal, but not an obligation.

Singer would resist such claims about his theory. He would argue that there is no clear justification for the claim that common-morality obligations do not contain a very demanding principle of beneficence. He thinks that the common morality endorses a harm prevention principle. Singer would explain the almost universal lack of concern for poverty relief as a failure to draw the correct implications from the moral principle(s) of beneficence that all moral persons accept. We respond, constructively, to this line of argument in the next section, where we treat obligations of rescue. The claim that Singer-type beneficence makes excessively strong demands is best tested in rescue cases. We there offer a five-condition analysis of beneficence that we judge more satisfactory than Singer's principle(s).[6]

Later Singer attempted to take account of objections that his principle sets "too high a standard." Without giving up his strong principle of beneficence, he suggested that it might be morally wise and most productive to *publicly advocate* a lower standard or weakened principle. In this respect, he allows that his principle may need a more guarded formulation in order to motivate those who would follow it. To the question, "What level of assistance should we [publicly] advocate?," he offered this answer:

> Any figure will be arbitrary, but there may be something to be said for a round percentage of one's income like, say, 10 per cent—more than a token donation, yet not so high as to be beyond all but saints. . . . No figure should be advocated as a rigid minimum or maximum; . . . [but by] any reasonable ethical standards this is the minimum we ought to do, and we do wrong if we do less.[7]

This is a more realistic assessment of obligations of beneficence, but we are skeptical of a percentage of income as a determination of one's obligation, especially in light of vast differences in income and wealth and also in light of conditions we identify later. It is even more unlikely that "any reasonable ethical standard" sets such a figure as 10% as the minimum. Nonetheless, Singer's revised thesis rightly attempts to set clear limits on the scope of the obligation of beneficence—limits that reduce required costs and impacts on the agent's life plans and that make meeting one's obligations a realistic possibility.

Singer defended his lines of argument about beneficence, including the public advocacy thesis, in his 2007 Uehiro Lectures.[8] Here a difference of emphasis is evident. Singer is often concerned with which social conditions will motivate people to give, rather than attempting to determine precisely what our obligations of beneficence are. Singer responds to some critics[9] by conceding that perhaps the limit of what we should publicly advocate as a level of giving is no more than a person's "fair share" of what is needed to relieve poverty and other problems. Unless we draw the line at this point, we might not be able to motivate people to give at all. A fair share is a lower threshold of obligations than his earlier formulations suggested (e.g., 10%), but far more realistic. Attention to *motivation* to give provides an illuminating approach to the nature and limits of beneficence. However, *obligation* and *motivation* should not be collapsed into one another. It may prove difficult in many circumstances of obligation to motivate people to discharge their obligations, as Singer well appreciates.

The Obligation to Rescue

Some circumstances eliminate discretionary choice regarding beneficiaries of our beneficence; these circumstances render *specific* actions obligatory. Consider the stock example of a passerby who observes someone drowning, but stands in no special moral relationship with the drowning person. The obligation of beneficence is not strong enough, in our view, to require a passerby who is a very poor swimmer to risk his or her life by trying to swim a hundred yards to rescue someone drowning in deep water. Nonetheless, there is still a critical moral relationship between the victim and the passerby, because the passerby is well-placed at that moment to help the victim. As such, a specific obligation of beneficent action does arise in this circumstance. If the passerby does nothing (e.g., fails to alert a nearby lifeguard or fails to call out for help), the failure is morally culpable.

Apart from very close moral relationships, such as contracts or the ties of family or friendship, we suggest that a person X has a determinate obligation of beneficence toward a person Y if and only if each of the following conditions is satisfied (assuming that X is aware of the relevant facts):[10]

1. Y is at risk of significant loss of or damage to life or health or some other major interest.
2. X's action is necessary (singly or in concert with others) to prevent this loss or damage.
3. X's action (singly or in concert with others) has a very high probability of preventing it.[11]
4. X's action would not present very significant risks, costs, or burdens to X.[12]
5. The benefit that Y can be expected to gain outweighs any harms, costs, or burdens that X is likely to incur.

Although it is difficult to specify in the abstract "very significant risks, costs, or burdens," the implication of the fourth condition is clear: Even if X's action would probably save Y's life and would meet all of the conditions except the fourth, the action would still not be *obligatory* on grounds of beneficence.

We now test these theses about the demands of beneficence with two cases. The first is a borderline case of specific obligatory beneficence, involving rescue, whereas the second presents a clear-cut case of specific obligatory beneficence. In the first case, originally introduced in Chapter 5, Robert McFall was diagnosed as having aplastic anemia, which is often fatal, but his physician believed that a bone marrow transplant from a genetically compatible donor could increase his chances of surviving. David Shimp, McFall's cousin, was the only relative willing to undergo the first test, which established tissue compatibility. However, Shimp then refused to undergo the second test for genetic compatibility. When McFall sued to force his cousin to undergo the second test and to donate bone marrow if he turned out to be compatible, the judge ruled that the *law* did not allow him to force Shimp to engage in such acts of positive beneficence, but the judge added that Shimp's refusal was *"morally* indefensible."

Conditions 1 and 2 given earlier were met for an obligation of specific beneficence in this case, but condition 3 was not clearly satisfied. McFall's chance of surviving one year (at the time) would have only increased from 25% to between 40% and 60%. These contingencies make it difficult to determine whether principles of beneficence demanded a particular course of action. Although most medical commentators agreed that the risks to the donor were minimal, Shimp was especially concerned about what we call condition 4. Bone marrow transplants, he was told, require 100 to 150 punctures of the pelvic bone. These punctures can be painlessly performed under anesthesia, and the major risk is a one-in-10,000 chance of death from anesthesia. Shimp, however, believed that the risks were greater ("What if I become a cripple?" he asked) and that they outweighed the probability and magnitude of benefit to McFall. This case, then, is a borderline case of obligatory specific beneficence.

In the *Tarasoff* case (the first case in Chapter 1), a therapist, on learning of his patient's intention to kill an identified woman, notified the police but not the intended victim, because of constraints of confidentiality. Suppose we modify the actual circumstances in this case to create the following hypothetical situation: A psychiatrist has informed his patient that he does not believe in keeping information confidential. The patient agrees to treatment under these conditions and subsequently reveals a serious intention to kill an identified woman. The psychiatrist may now either remain aloof or take measures to protect the woman (by notifying her or the police). What does morality—and specifically beneficence—demand of the psychiatrist in this case?

Only a remarkably narrow account of moral obligation would assert that the psychiatrist is under no obligation whatever to protect the woman by contacting her or the police. The psychiatrist is not at risk and, moreover, will suffer virtually no inconvenience or interference with his life plans. If morality does not demand this much beneficence, it is hard to see how morality imposes any positive obligations at all. Even if a competing obligation exists, such as protection of confidentiality, requirements of beneficence will in some cases override it. Sometimes, for example, health care professionals have a moral obligation to warn spouses or lovers of HIV-infected patients who refuse to disclose their status and who refuse to engage in safer sex practices (see Chapter 8).

What, now, is the morally relevant difference between these rescue cases involving individuals and those discussed in the previous section involving global poverty and public health? We suggested that rescuing a drowning person involves a special obligation not present with global poverty, because the rescuer is "well-placed at that moment to help the victim." But we are all placed well enough to help people in poverty by giving modest sums of money, as we can easily do so at little risk to ourselves and with a high probability of some degree of success.

One possible response is that in the drowning case there is a specific individual toward whom we have an obligation, whereas in the poverty cases we seem to have vast obligations toward entire populations of people, only a very few of whom we can hope to help through a gift. Perhaps we are obligated only when there are specific individuals whom we can help, not when there is a whole group and we can only help some of the members.

However, this line of argument has implausible implications, particularly when the size of groups is smaller in scale. Suppose an epidemic breaks out in a reasonably small community, calling for immediate quarantine, and hundreds of persons who are not infected cannot return to their homes where there are infected persons. But they are also not allowed to leave the city limits, and all hotel rooms are filled. Authorities project that you could prevent the deaths of approximately twenty noninfected persons by offering them your house to stay in. Conditions would become unsanitary if more than twenty persons were housed in one home, but there are enough homes to house every stranded person if each house in the community takes twenty persons. It seems very implausible to say that no person in any household is morally obligated to open their houses to these people for the weeks needed to control the epidemic, even though no one person has an obligation to any one of the stranded people as specific individuals. The hypothesis might be offered that this obligation arises only because they are all members of the community, but even this principle is implausible because it would arbitrarily exclude visitors who got caught. Accordingly, it does seem that we have obligations beyond those to specific individuals. Any other conclusion is morally unacceptable, and likely would be judged unacceptable across cultures that share the common morality.

In light of these considerations, common-morality beneficence requires people who are well off to provide at least some level of aid to people in extreme poverty. From this perspective Singer's weaker principles become very plausible, as we hinted earlier they might. However, we do not think that the duty to rescue, as we have now developed it, plausibly supports Singer's strong principle of beneficence. We return to this issue, focusing on global poverty and public health, in the chapter on justice (Chapter 7, pp. 264–66, during a discussion of cosmopolitan ethical theories). We also return, in Chapter 9, to the importance of *practicability* in a normative theory (pp. 22, 77–8). We do not believe that Singer's strong principle can be made practicable, whereas the weaker principles can.

To conclude, it is doubtful that ethical theory or practical deliberation can set precise, determinate conditions of obligations of beneficence. Any attempt to do so will almost certainly be a revisionary line in the sense that it will draw a sharper boundary for our obligations than exists in the common morality. Although beneficence is unclear at its heart, it should not be concluded that we can never fix or specify obligations of beneficence with any clarity.

Role Obligations and Special Relations

Obligations of specific beneficence usually rest on special moral relations (e.g., in families and friendships) or on special commitments, such as explicit promises and acceptance of roles with accompanying responsibilities. These special moral relationships and role relationships may not appear to generate the problems about specifying the limits of obligatory beneficent risk-taking and cost-bearing that we have encountered thus far. However, there are related limits. For instance, how far are parents obligated to go in providing expensive care for their severely ill children?[13] Are physicians and other health care professionals obligated to accept extraordinary risks while caring for abusive or contagious patients?

At this stage in the discussion, we note only that there is an implicit assumption of beneficence in all medical and health care professions and their institutional contexts: Promoting the welfare of patients—not merely avoiding harm—embodies medicine's goal, rationale, and justification. Preventive medicine and public health interventions have also long embraced concerted social actions of beneficence, such as vaccination programs and health education, as obligatory, not merely optional.

A Reciprocity-Based Justification of Obligations of Beneficence

Several justifications can be proposed for obligations of general and specific beneficence. One is a reciprocity-based account, which is particularly well-suited to biomedical ethics.

David Hume argued that the obligation to benefit others arises from social interactions: "All our obligations to do good to society seem to imply something reciprocal. I receive the benefits of society, and therefore ought to promote its interests."[14] Reciprocity is the act or practice of making an appropriate and often proportional return—for example, returning benefit with proportional benefit, harm with proportional criminal sentencing, and friendly actions with gratitude. Hume's reciprocity account rightly maintains that we incur obligations to help or benefit others at least in part because we have received, will receive, or stand to receive beneficial assistance from them.

Reciprocity is a pervasive feature of social life, although not so pervasive that we can reduce all of the moral life to obligations of reciprocity. Nonetheless, many obligations of beneficence to society (as distinct from those to identified individuals) typically derive from some form of reciprocity. It is implausible to maintain that we are largely free of, or can free ourselves from, a broad range of indebtedness to our parents, to researchers in medicine and public health, to educators, and to social institutions such as schools. The claim that we make our way independent of our benefactors is as unrealistic as the idea that we can always act autonomously without affecting others.[15]

Codes of medical ethics have sometimes inappropriately viewed physicians as independent, self-sufficient philanthropists whose beneficence is analogous to generous acts of giving. The Hippocratic oath states that physicians' obligations to patients represent philanthropic service, whereas obligations to their teachers represent debts incurred in the course of becoming physicians. However, today many physicians and health care professionals owe a large debt to society (e.g., for education and privileges) and to their patients, past and present (e.g., for research and "practice"). Because of this indebtedness, the medical profession's role of beneficent care of patients is misconstrued if modeled primarily on philanthropy, altruism, and personal commitment. This care is rooted in a reciprocity of giving after having received.[16]

Obligations of specific beneficence, by contrast, typically derive from special moral relationships with persons, frequently through institutional roles and contractual arrangements. These obligations arise from implicit and explicit commitments, such as promises and roles, as well as from the acceptance of specific benefits. Both our "station and its duties" and our promises impose obligations. When a patient contracts with a physician for services, the latter assumes a role-specific obligation of beneficent treatment that would not be present apart from the relationship. Although physicians in private practice typically have no legal obligation to see patients in emergencies or to help those injured in an automobile accident, moral obligations of beneficence do, on occasion, require such acts. The obligation to render assistance in extraordinary circumstances, such as an automobile accident, is not limited to physicians or to health care professionals. Anyone who falls under our five-condition analysis of the specific obligation of beneficence has an obligation to provide such assistance, as he or she is able.

Of course, physicians are typically able to lend more assistance in a medical emergency than other citizens, and we can therefore ask whether the physician has a specific obligation of assistance unique to persons with such skills and training. Here we encounter a gray area between a role-specific obligation and a non-role-specific obligation. The physician at the scene of an accident is obligated to do more than the lawyer or student to aid the injured, to the degree there is a need for medical skills. Yet a physician-stranger is not morally required to assume the same level of commitment and risk that a prior contractual relationship with a patient or hospital would morally require.

PATERNALISM: CONFLICTS BETWEEN BENEFICENCE AND AUTONOMY

The idea that beneficence expresses the primary obligation in health care is ancient. Throughout the history of health care, the professional's obligations and virtues have generally been interpreted as commitments of beneficence. We find perhaps the most celebrated expression in the Hippocratic work *Epidemics*: "As to disease, make a habit of two things—*to help, or at least to do no harm.*"[17] Traditionally, physicians relied almost exclusively on their own judgments about their patients' needs for information and treatment. However, over the last few decades, medicine has increasingly confronted assertions of patients' rights to make independent judgments. As assertions of autonomy rights increased, the problem of paternalism loomed larger.

Disputes about the Primacy of Beneficence

Whether respect for the autonomy of patients should have priority over professional beneficence directed at those patients is a central problem in biomedical ethics. The principle of respect for autonomy has grounded several rights for patients, including rights to receive information, to consent to and refuse procedures, and to have confidentiality and privacy maintained. Others ground such obligations on the health care professional's primary obligation of beneficence, which is to act for the patient's medical benefit.

Proponents of the autonomy model and proponents of the beneficence model—as we refer to these two contrasting paradigms—sometimes fail to carefully distinguish between the principles of beneficence and respect for autonomy. For example, beneficence could be construed to *incorporate* the patient's autonomous choices in the sense that the patient's preferences help to determine what counts as a medical benefit. Along these lines, two defenders of the beneficence model, Edmund Pellegrino and David Thomasma, argue that "the best interests of the patients are intimately linked with their preferences," from which "are derived our primary duties toward them."[18] This formulation of the beneficence model simply restates the autonomy model. If the patient's preferences alone determine the content of the physician's obligation to act beneficently, respect for autonomy rather than pure medical beneficence has triumphed, and the problem of paternalism evaporates.

However, we argued earlier that beneficence provides the primary goal and rationale of medicine and health care and that it can directly conflict with respect for autonomy. This creates a serious and pervasive problem of paternalism. We now begin to address it by considering critical conceptual issues.

The Nature of Paternalism

What is paternalism? The *Oxford English Dictionary* (*OED*) dates the term *paternalism* to the 1880s, giving its root meaning as "the principle and practice of paternal administration; government as by a father; the claim or attempt to supply the needs or to regulate the life of a nation or community in the same way a father does those of his children." The analogy with the father presupposes two features of the paternal role: that the father acts beneficently (i.e., in accordance with his conception of the interests of his children) and that he makes all or at least some of the decisions relating to his children's welfare, rather than letting them make those decisions. In health care relationships, the analogy is this: A professional has superior training, knowledge, and insight and is thus in an authoritative position to determine the patient's best interests. From this perspective, a health care professional is like a loving parent with dependent and often ignorant and fearful children.

Paternalistic acts often use such forms of influence as deception, lying, manipulation of information, or nondisclosure of information, as well as coercion and force. However, they may simply involve a refusal to carry out the other's wishes. According to some definitions in the literature, paternalistic actions by definition restrict *autonomous* choices, and thus restricting nonautonomous conduct is not paternalistic. Although one author of this text prefers this conception,[19] we here accept and build on the broader definition suggested by the *OED*: intentional nonacquiescence or intervention in another person's preferences, desires, or actions with the intention of either preventing or reducing harm to or benefiting the person. Even if a person's desires, intentional actions, and the like are *not substantially autonomous,* overriding them can still be paternalistic under this definition.[20] For example, if a man ignorant of his fragile, life-threatening condition and sick with a raging fever attempts to leave a hospital, it is paternalistic to detain him, even if his attempt to leave does not derive from a substantially autonomous choice.

Accordingly, we define "paternalism" as *the intentional overriding of one person's preferences or actions by another person, where the person who overrides justifies this action by appeal to the goal of benefiting or of preventing or mitigating harm to the person whose preferences or actions are overridden.* This definition is normatively neutral—it does not presume that paternalism is either justified or unjustified. Although the definition assumes an act of beneficence analogous to parental beneficence, it does not prejudge whether the beneficent act is justified, obligatory, misplaced, and so forth.

Problems of Medical Paternalism

Throughout the history of medical ethics both the principles of nonmaleficence and beneficence have been invoked as a basis for paternalistic actions toward patients. For example, physicians have traditionally held that disclosing certain kinds of information can cause harm to patients under their care and that medical ethics obligates them not to cause such harm. Consider a typical case: A man brings his father, who is in his late sixties, to his physician because he suspects that his father's problems in interpreting and responding to daily events may indicate Alzheimer's disease. The man also makes an "impassioned plea" that the physician not tell his father if the tests suggest Alzheimer's. Tests subsequently indicate that the father probably does have the disease. The physician now faces a dilemma, because of the conflict between demands of respect for autonomy (assuming that the father has substantial autonomy and is competent at least some of the time) and demands of beneficence. The physician first considers the now widely recognized obligation to inform patients of a diagnosis of cancer. This obligation typically presupposes accuracy in the diagnosis, a relatively clear course of the disease, and a competent patient—none of which is clearly present in this case. The physician also notes that disclosure of Alzheimer's disease adversely affects patients' coping mechanisms, and thus could harm the patient, particularly by causing further decline, depression, agitation, and paranoia.[21] (See also our discussion of veracity in Chapter 8.)

Some patients—for example, those who are depressed or addicted to potentially harmful drugs—are unlikely to reach adequately reasoned decisions, at least not likely under certain conditions or mental states. Other patients who are competent and deliberative may make poor choices, judged by the courses of action that their physicians recommend. When patients of either type choose harmful courses of action, some health care professionals respect autonomy (in the case of stated preferences that are autonomous) by not interfering beyond attempts at persuasion, whereas others act beneficently by attempting to protect patients against the potentially harmful consequences of their own stated preferences. Discussions of medical paternalism focus on how to specify these principles, which principle to follow under which conditions, and how to intervene in the decisions and affairs of such patients when intervention is warranted.

Insofar as depression, drug addiction, and the like substantially interfere with the exercise of a patient's autonomy, beneficent acts to protect the patient and promote his or her interests represent soft paternalism. Here there is generally no troublesome conflict between autonomy and beneficence because of the absence of substantial autonomy. Because the beneficiary lacks substantial autonomy, the intervention is much easier to justify than it would be if a comparable preference or action were substantially autonomous. However, in contrast to much of the literature on paternalism, we also argue that beneficence sometimes provides grounds for justifiably restricting substantially autonomous actions.

Soft and Hard Paternalism

We have already suggested an important distinction between soft and hard paternalism.[22] In soft paternalism, an agent intervenes in the life of another person on grounds of beneficence or nonmaleficence with the goal of preventing substantially *nonvoluntary* conduct. Substantially nonvoluntary actions include cases such as poorly informed consent or refusal, severe depression that precludes rational deliberation, and addiction that prevents free choice and action. Hard paternalism, by contrast, involves interventions intended to prevent or mitigate harm to or to benefit a person, despite the fact that the person's risky choices and actions are informed, voluntary, and autonomous. The hard paternalist will restrict forms of information available to the person or will otherwise override the person's informed and voluntary choices. The intended beneficiary's choices need not be *fully* informed or voluntary, but for the interventions to qualify as hard paternalism, these choices must be *substantially* autonomous.

Soft paternalistic actions are morally complicated only because of the difficulty of determining whether a person's actions are substantially nonautonomous and of determining appropriate means of action. That we should protect persons from harm caused to them by conditions beyond their control is not a controversial premise. Hence, soft paternalism does not involve a real conflict between the principles of respect for autonomy and beneficence. Refraining from soft paternalism is not an example of respect for autonomy because soft paternalism only tries to prevent the harmful consequences of a patient's actions that the patient did not autonomously choose.

This conclusion is not inconsistent with our earlier definition of paternalism as involving an intentional overriding of one person's known preferences or actions by another person. Some behaviors that express preferences are not autonomous. For example, some patients on medication or recovering from surgery insist that they do not want a certain physician to touch or examine them. They may be experiencing temporary hallucinations around the time of the statement. A day later they have no idea why they stated this preference. A person's preferences can be motivated by many states and desires. Whether one should call such a (nonautonomous) expression a preference or an action is an important question, but not one that we need to pursue now that we have clarified our meaning. This analysis also explains why we will be concerned largely, almost exclusively, with the justification of hard paternalism

Debates about paternalism appear in health policy as well as in clinical ethics. "Neopaternalists" have argued for government policies intended to protect or benefit individuals through shaping or steering their choices without, in fact, altogether disallowing or coercing those choices.[23] In clinical care, similar arguments have supported the physician's manipulation of some patients to select proper goals of care.[24]

Soft paternalists recommend policies and actions that pursue the values that they believe the intended beneficiary holds but cannot realize because of limited capacities, commitment, or limited self-control.[25] Here, the individual's own stated preferences, choices, and actions are deemed unreasonable in light of his or her own standards. By contrast, in hard paternalism the intended beneficiary does not accept the values used to define his or her own best interests. Hard paternalism reflects the benefactor's conception of best interests and may ban, prescribe, or regulate conduct in ways that manipulate individuals' actions to secure the benefactor's intended result. These interventions usually involve clear trade-offs, as in "sin taxes" directed at harmful conduct such as smoking cigarettes. Soft paternalism, by contrast, reflects the intended beneficiary's own conception of his or her best interests, even if the intended beneficiary fails to fully understand or recognize those interests or to fully pursue them because of inadequate voluntariness, commitment, or self-control.

This conception has problems. It is reasonable to assume that our knowledge of what an informed and competent person chooses to do is the *best evidence* we have of what his or her values are. For example, if a very religious man fails to follow the dietary restrictions of his religion, although he is strongly committed to all aspects of the religion, his departures from dietary laws may be the best evidence we have of his true values. If so, then it would be morally unjustified for a religious leader or the man's family to be soft paternalists while basing their best-interest judgments on the patient's own values. Because it seems correct—short of counterevidence in particular cases—that competent informed choice is the best evidence of a person's values, a justified soft paternalism must have adequate evidence that this assumption is misguided in a particular case.

Some proponents of soft paternalism reach the conclusion that the position is compatible with, not contrary to, liberty. Some even use the paradoxical label "libertarian paternalism." Drawing on psychology and behavioral economics, Cass Sunstein and Richard Thaler defend this position: "The idea of libertarian paternalism might seem to be an oxymoron, but it is both possible and desirable for private and public institutions to influence behavior while also respecting freedom of choice."[26] This form of paternalism focuses on two limitations on the intended beneficiary's preferences, choices, and actions that can serve to justify interventions to benefit him or her. The limitations are sometimes labeled "bounded rationality" and "bounded self-control" (in contrast to the economic model of unbounded rationality and self-control). For instance, if the available evidence were to establish that smokers discount the risks of smoking because of an "optimism bias," among other factors, "it is hardly obvious," Christine Jolls and Sunstein argue, "that government would violate their autonomy by giving a more accurate sense of those risks, even if the best way of giving that accurate sense were through concrete accounts of suffering."[27]

If this account truly is soft paternalism (which is unclear), it is not because these authors eschew overriding autonomy and prefer behavioral inducements. Rather, it must be based on the claim that people's limited rationality is itself a limitation on their capacity to act autonomously and that therefore we are justified in arranging their choice situation in a way that likely will correct their cognitive biases. However, if the position is that we should use our knowledge of cognitive biases not only to correct for failures of rationality, but to manipulate people into doing what is good for them, then this position looks more like *hard* paternalism, depending on the nature of the manipulation.

Although we agree that paternalism—be it soft or hard—is sometimes justified in health care and in health-related public policies, there are good reasons for caution even about some forms of soft paternalism.[28] One supposed advantage of the theory may actually be an ethical disadvantage. This paternalism reflects many values that individuals would recognize or realize themselves if they did not encounter internal limits of rationality and control. The means employed, whether by health care professionals or the government, *shape and steer* persons without *thwarting* their free choice. As a result, these prima facie appealing paternalistic policies and practices may face little opposition and may even be implemented without the transparency and publicity needed for public assessment. Hence soft paternalistic governmental policies or health care practices may be susceptible to abuse if they lack public scrutiny.

Soft paternalistic policies sometimes work by stigmatizing certain conduct. Stigmatization can change behavior, but with psychosocial costs. Proponents insist that they target *acts,* not *persons.* However, in practice, it is easy to slide from stigmatizing conduct to stigmatizing people who engage in that conduct. For example, in the United States stigmatization of smoking and smokers has played an increasingly explicit role in private and public efforts to curtail smoking.[29] The slide from stigmatization of acts (smoking) to stigmatization of people (smokers) who engage in those acts can lead to hostility and antipathy for population subgroups.[30] Because smoking is now more common among lower socioeconomic groups in the United States, stigmatization is directed at socially vulnerable members of society—a matter of moral concern from the standpoint of both beneficence and justice.[31]

Acceptance of soft paternalistic interventions also runs the risk of preparing the way for hard paternalistic interventions.[32] Some paternalistic policies appear to be based entirely on the value of the predicted outcomes for the beneficiary, without consideration of whether a person's autonomy is diminished. This looks to be hard paternalism. However, when the theory is based on evidence that certain people cannot make rational decisions, the appeal is to limited autonomy, which looks to be soft paternalism. Justifications based on evidence of limited agency are more attractive than those based on good outcomes that take no account of autonomy. However, because good outcomes (beneficence) justify the positions taken in both soft and hard cases, it is easy to slide from the soft to the hard side.

Soft paternalistic interventions often succeed, in part, by increasing support for the social values and norms that warrant the use of those interventions to control situations of limited rationality and limited self-control. The campaign against cigarette smoking is again an instructive example because there was a social movement from disclosure of information, to sharp warnings, to soft paternalistic public measures to reduce addiction-controlled unhealthy behavior, to hard paternalistic measures such as increasing taxation of cigarettes.[33] In this example, paternalism remains beneficent, but increasingly loses touch with, and may even violate, respect for autonomy.

The Justification of Paternalism and Antipaternalism

Three general positions dominate the literature on the justification of paternalism: (1) antipaternalism, (2) paternalism that appeals to the principle of respect for autonomy as expressed in some form of consent, and (3) paternalism that appeals to principles of beneficence. All three positions agree that some acts of soft paternalism are justified, such as preventing a man under the influence of a hallucinogenic drug from killing himself. Even antipaternalists do not object to such interventions because substantially autonomous actions are not at stake.

Antipaternalism. Antipaternalists may oppose hard paternalistic interventions for various reasons. The serious adverse consequences of giving (hard) paternalistic authority to the state or to physicians or any other group provide one basis for the rejection of hard paternalism, but another and more influential basis is that rightful authority resides in the individual. The argument for this conclusion rests on the analysis of autonomy rights discussed in Chapter 4: Hard paternalistic interventions display disrespect toward autonomous agents and fail to treat them as moral equals, treating them instead as less-than-independent determiners of their own good. If others impose their conception of the good on us, they deny us the respect they owe us, even if they have a better conception of our needs than we do and are acting to benefit us.[34]

Antipaternalists hold that paternalistic standards are too broad and would authorize and institutionalize too much intervention if made the basis of policy. Hence, paternalism allows an unacceptable latitude of judgment in contexts involving potential abuses of power. For example, suppose a sixty-five-year-old man who has donated a kidney to one of his sons now volunteers to donate his second kidney when another son needs a transplant, an act most would think not in his best interests even though he contends that he could survive on dialysis. Are we to commend him, ignore him, or deny his request? Hard paternalism suggests that it would be permissible and perhaps obligatory to restrain him as well as to refuse to carry out his request. If so, antipaternalists argue, the state is permitted, in principle, to restrain its morally heroic citizens if they act in a manner "harmful" to themselves.

A medical example with an extensive antipaternalistic literature is the involuntary hospitalization of persons who have neither been harmed by others nor actually harmed themselves, but who are thought to be at risk of such harm. In this case, a double paternalism is common—a paternalistic justification for both therapy and commitment. Antipaternalists would regard the intervention as justified by the intent to benefit, emphasizing that, in such a case, beneficence does not conflict with respect for autonomy because the intended beneficiary lacks substantial autonomy.

Paternalism justified by consent. Some theories appeal to *consent* to justify paternalistic interventions—be it rational consent, subsequent consent, hypothetical consent, or some other type of consent. As Gerald Dworkin puts it, "The basic notion of consent is important and seems to me the only acceptable way to try to delimit an area of justified paternalism." Paternalism, he says, is a "social insurance policy" to which fully rational persons would subscribe in order to protect themselves.[35] Such persons would know, for example, that they might be tempted at times to make decisions that are far-reaching, potentially dangerous, and irreversible. At other times, they might suffer irresistible psychological or social pressures to take actions that are unreasonably risky. In still other cases, persons might not sufficiently understand the dangers of their actions, such as medical facts about the effects of smoking, although they might believe they have a sufficient understanding. Those who use consent as a justification conclude that we would consent to a limited authorization for others to control our actions if our autonomy becomes defective or we are unable to make the prudent decision that we otherwise would make.[36]

A theory that appeals to rational consent to justify paternalistic interventions has attractive features, particularly its attempt to harmonize principles of beneficence and respect for autonomy. However, this approach does not incorporate an individual's actual *consent,* and thus is not truly consent-based. It is best to keep autonomy-based justifications at arm's length from paternalism. Beneficence alone justifies truly paternalistic actions, just as it justifies parental actions that override children's preferences.[37] We do not control children because we believe that they will subsequently consent to or would rationally approve our interventions. We control them because we believe they will have better, or at least less dangerous, lives.

Paternalism justified by prospective benefit. Accordingly, the most plausible justification of paternalistic actions places benefit on a scale with autonomy interests and balances both: As a person's interests in autonomy increase and the benefits for that person decrease, the justification of paternalistic action becomes less plausible; conversely, as the benefits for a person increase and that person's autonomy interests decrease, the justification of paternalistic action becomes more plausible. Thus, preventing minor harms or providing minor benefits while deeply disrespecting autonomy lacks plausible justification, but actions that prevent major harms or provide major benefits while only trivially disrespecting autonomy have a plausible paternalistic rationale. Indeed, as we now argue, even hard paternalistic actions can sometimes be justified.

Justified hard paternalism. Two cases can provide starting points for reflection on the conditions of justified hard paternalism. In the first, a physician obtains the results of a myelogram (a graph of the spinal region) following examination of a patient. Although the test yields inconclusive results and needs to be repeated, it also suggests a serious pathology. When the patient asks about the test results, the physician decides on grounds of beneficence to withhold potentially negative information, knowing that, on disclosure, the patient will be distressed and anxious. Based on her experience with other patients and her ten-year knowledge of this particular patient, the physician is confident that the information would not affect the patient's decision to consent to another myelogram. Her sole motivation in withholding the information is to spare the patient the emotional distress of thinking through a painful decision prematurely and perhaps unnecessarily. However, the physician intends to be completely truthful with the patient about the results of the second test and intends to disclose the information well before the patient will need to decide about surgery. This physician's act of temporary nondisclosure is morally justified, although beneficence has (temporarily) received priority over respect for autonomy. (See also our discussion of the disclosure of "bad news" in Chapter 8.)

A commonplace example of justified hard paternalism appears in the following case:

> After receiving his preoperative medicine, C, a 23-year-old male athlete scheduled for a hernia repair, states that he does not want the side rails up. C is of clear mind and understands why the rule is required, however, C does not feel the rule should apply to him because he is not the least bit drowsy from the preoperative medication and he has no intention of falling out of bed. After considerable discussion between the nurse and patient, the nurse responsible for C's care puts the side rails up. Her justification is as follows: C is not drowsy because he has just received the preoperative medication, and its effects have not occurred. Furthermore, if he follows the typical pattern of patients receiving this medication in this dosage, he will become drowsy very quickly. A drowsy patient is at risk for a fall. Since there is no family at the hospital to remain with the patient, and since the nurses on the unit are exceptionally busy, no one can constantly stay with C to monitor his level of alertness. Under these circumstances the patient must be protected from the potential harm of a fall, despite the fact that he does not want this protection.... The nurse restricted this autonomous patient's liberty based on...protection of the patient from potential harm...and *not* as a hedge against liability or for protection from criticism.[38]

Such minor hard paternalistic actions are common in hospitals, and, in our view, warranted.

To consolidate the discussion thus far, hard paternalism is justified in health care only if the following conditions are satisfied:

1. A patient is at risk of a significant, preventable harm.
2. The paternalistic action will probably prevent the harm.
3. The projected benefits to the patient of the paternalistic action outweigh its risks to the patient.
4. There is no reasonable alternative to the limitation of autonomy.
5. The least autonomy-restrictive alternative that will secure the benefits and reduce the risks is adopted.

We could add a sixth condition requiring that a paternalistic action not damage *substantial* autonomy interests, such as would be present if a Jehovah's Witness refuses a blood transfusion because of a deeply held conviction. To intervene forcefully by providing the transfusion would substantially infringe the patient's autonomy and thus could not be justified under this additional condition. However, some cases of justified hard paternalism may cross the line of minimal infringement. In general, as the risk to a patient's welfare increases or the likelihood of an irreversible harm increases, the likelihood of a justified paternalistic intervention correspondingly increases.[39]

The following case plausibly supports hard paternalistic intervention, even though it involves more than minimal infringement of respect for autonomy: A psychiatrist is treating a patient who is not insane, but who acts in what appear to be bizarre ways. He is acting conscientiously on his unique religious views. He asks a psychiatrist a question about his condition, a question that has a definite answer but which, if answered, would lead him to engage in seriously self-maiming behavior such as plucking out his right eye to fulfill what he believes to be his religion's demands. Many, including the present authors, would maintain that the doctor acts paternalistically, and justifiably, by concealing information from this patient, even though he is rational and otherwise informed. Because the infringement of the principle of respect for autonomy is *more than minimal* in this case (the religious views being central to the patient's life plan), a sixth condition requiring no substantial infringement of autonomy cannot be a necessary condition for *all* cases of justified hard paternalism.

Problems of Suicide Intervention

The state, religious institutions, and health care professionals have all traditionally assumed some jurisdiction to intervene in suicide attempts. Those who intervene do not always justify their actions on paternalistic grounds, but paternalism, in both soft and hard forms, has been the primary justification.

Thousands of certified suicides occur in the United States each year, and many other suicides are classified as accidental deaths because too little is known about the decedents' intentions. Several conceptual questions about the term *suicide* make it difficult to classify acts as suicides.[40] For example, when

Barney Clark became the first human to receive an artificial heart, one report indicated that he was given a key that he could use to turn off the compressor if he decided he wanted to die. As Dr. Willem Kolff noted, if the patient "suffers and feels it isn't worth it any more, he has a key that he can apply.... I think it is entirely legitimate that this man whose life has been extended should have the right to cut it off if he doesn't want it, if [his] life ceases to be enjoyable."[41] Would Clark's use of the key to turn off the artificial heart have been an act of suicide? If he had refused to accept the artificial heart in the first place, few would have labeled his act a suicide. His overall condition was extremely poor, the artificial heart was experimental, and no suicidal intention was evident. If, on the other hand, Clark had intentionally shot himself with a pistol while on the artificial heart, his act would have been classified as suicide. If Clark had used the key to turn off his artificial heart, controversy would have erupted about whether to characterize his act as forgoing life-sustaining treatment, withdrawing from an experiment, suicide, or all of the above.

Pursuit of these conceptual problems about the vagueness of *suicide* would divert us from our main topic. Our concern is paternalistic intervention in cases that are generally agreed to be acts of attempted suicide. The primary moral issue is the following: If suicide is a protected moral right, then the state, health professionals, and others have no legitimate grounds for intervention in autonomous suicide attempts. No one doubts that we should intervene to prevent suicide by nonautonomous persons, and few wish to return to the days when suicide was a criminal act. But if we accept an autonomy right to commit suicide, then we could not legitimately attempt to prevent the autonomous but imprudent individual from committing suicide.

A clear and relevant example of attempted suicide appears in the following case, involving John K., a thirty-two-year-old lawyer. Two neurologists independently confirmed that his facial twitching, which had been evident for three months, was an early sign of Huntington's disease, a neurological disorder that progressively worsens, leads to irreversible dementia, and is uniformly fatal in approximately ten years. His mother suffered a horrible death from the same disease, and John K. had often said that he would prefer to die than to suffer the way his mother had suffered. Over several years he had been anxious, had drunk heavily, and had sought psychiatric help for intermittent depression. Following this diagnosis, he told his psychiatrist about his situation and asked for help in committing suicide. After the psychiatrist refused to help, John K. attempted to take his own life by ingesting his antidepressant medication, leaving a note of explanation to his wife and child.[42]

Several interventions occurred or were possible in this case. First, the psychiatrist refused to assist John K.'s suicide and would have sought involuntary commitment had John K. not insisted that he did not plan to kill himself anytime soon. The psychiatrist appears to have thought that he could provide appropriate psychotherapy over time. Second, John K.'s wife found him unconscious and rushed him to the emergency room. Third, the emergency room staff decided to treat him despite the suicide note. The question is which, if any, of these possible or actual interventions was justifiable?

A widely accepted account of our obligations relies on John Stuart Mill's strategy of *temporary* intervention. On this account, intervention is justified to ascertain whether a person is acting autonomously; further intervention is unjustified once it is clear that the person's actions are substantially autonomous. Glanville Williams used this strategy in a classic statement of the position:

> If one suddenly comes upon another person attempting suicide, the natural and humane thing to do is to try to stop him, for the purpose of ascertaining the cause of his distress and attempting to remedy it, or else of attempting moral dissuasion if it seems that the act of suicide shows lack of consideration for others, or else again from the purpose of trying to persuade him to accept psychiatric help if this seems to be called for....But nothing longer than a temporary restraint could be defended. I would gravely doubt whether a suicide attempt should be a factor leading to a diagnosis of psychosis or to compulsory admissions to a hospital. Psychiatrists are too ready to assume that an attempt to commit suicide is the act of mentally sick persons.[43]

This antipaternalist stance is vulnerable to criticism on two grounds. First, failure to intervene with strong efforts symbolically communicates to potentially suicidal persons a lack of communal concern and diminishes our sense of communal responsibility. Second, many persons who commit or attempt to commit suicide are mentally ill, clinically depressed, or destabilized by a crisis and are, therefore, not acting autonomously. From a clinical perspective, many suicidal persons are beset with ambivalence or are under the influence of drugs, alcohol, or intense pressure. Many mental health professionals believe that suicides almost always result from maladaptive attitudes or illnesses needing therapeutic attention and social support.

In a typical circumstance, from this perspective, the suicidal person plans how to end life while simultaneously holding fantasies about how rescue will occur, not only rescue from death but from the negative circumstances prompting the suicide. If the suicide springs from clinical depression or constitutes a call for help, a failure to intervene seems to show disrespect for the person's deepest autonomous wishes, including his or her hopes for the future. Surface intentions do not always capture deeper desires or inclinations, and, in a matter as serious as suicide, deeper motives should be heavily weighted in justifying intervention.

Another worry is that revised suicide laws would foster insensitive attitudes on the part of health care professionals, especially in a medical system organized around cost control. Some institutions devoted to caring for the ill and elderly, such as the modern nursing home, frequently communicate a message of indifference to forms of suffering that lead patients to end their lives. These institutions contrast sharply with the ethos of a hospice, which provides a supportive community. Hospices are but one of many examples of social institutions that recognize but counterbalance rights of autonomy, independence, and self-reliance with appropriate communal care and support.

However, caution is needed in calls for communal beneficence, which may express itself paternalistically through forceful interventions. Although suicide has been decriminalized, a suicide attempt, irrespective of motive, almost universally provides a legal basis for public officers to intervene, as well as grounds for involuntary hospitalization.[44] Often the burden of proof is appropriately placed on those who claim that the patient's judgment is not autonomous or is imprudent.

For example, Ida Rollin, seventy-four years old, suffered from ovarian cancer. Her physicians told her that she had only a few months to live and that her dying would be painful and upsetting. Rollin indicated to her daughter that she wanted to end her life and requested assistance. The daughter secured some pills and conveyed a doctor's instructions about how they should be taken. When the daughter expressed reservations about these plans, her husband reminded her that they "weren't driving, she [Ida Rollin] was," and that they were only "navigators."[45]

This metaphor-laden reference to rightful authority is a reminder that those who propose suicide intervention to prevent such persons from control over their lives require a moral justification that fits the context. Occasions arise in health care (and elsewhere) when it is appropriate to step aside and allow a person to bring life to an end, and perhaps even to assist in facilitating the death, just as occasions exist when it is appropriate to intervene. (See Chapter 5 on physician-assisted forms of ending life.)

Denying Requests for Nonbeneficial Procedures

Patients and surrogates sometimes request medical procedures that the clinician is convinced will not be beneficial. Sometimes denials of such requests are paternalistic.

Passive paternalism. Discussion of medical paternalism typically focuses on paternalistic interventions when the patient prefers nonintervention. A comparatively neglected form of paternalism, which might be called *passive paternalism,* appears in the professional's refusal, for reasons of patient-centered beneficence, to execute a patient's positive preferences for an intervention.[46] The following is a case of passive paternalism: Elizabeth Stanley, a sexually active twenty-six-year-old intern, requests a tubal ligation, insisting that she has thought about this request for months, dislikes available contraceptives, does not want children, and understands that tubal ligation is irreversible. When the gynecologist suggests that she might someday want to get married and have children, she responds that she would either find a husband who did not want children or adopt children. She thinks that she will not change her mind and wants the tubal ligation to make it impossible for her to reconsider. She has scheduled vacation time from work in two weeks and wants the surgery then.[47]

If a physician refuses to perform the tubal ligation on grounds of the patient's benefit, the decision is paternalistic. However, if the physician refuses purely on grounds of conscience ("I won't do such procedures as a matter of personal moral policy"), it may not be a paternalistic decision. Passive paternalism is usually easier to justify than active paternalism, because physicians do not have a moral obligation to carry out their patients' desires when they are incompatible with acceptable standards of medical practice or are against the physicians' conscience. If a physician believes that providing a requested "treatment," such as a worthless drug for cancer, is not in any patient's best interests, he or she is not compelled to violate his or her professional or personal conscience by providing it, even when the patient is substantially autonomous. (See our discussion of conscientious refusals in Chapter 2.)

Medical futility. Passive paternalism is central to debates about medical futility, a topic we introduced in Chapter 5. Consider the classic case of eighty-five-year-old Helga Wanglie, who was maintained on a respirator in a persistent vegetative state. The hospital sought to stop the respirator on grounds that it was "nonbeneficial," in that it could not heal her lungs, palliate her suffering, or enable her to experience the benefits of life. The surrogate decision makers—her husband, a son, and a daughter—wanted life support continued on grounds that Mrs. Wanglie would not be better off dead, that a miracle could occur, that physicians should not play God, and that efforts to remove her life support indicated "moral decay in our civilization."[48]

If life support for such patients is futile, denying patients' or surrogates' requests for treatment is warranted. In these circumstances "clinically nonbeneficial interventions" is preferable to the term *futility*.[49] Typically a claim of futility is not that an intervention will harm the patient (in violation of the principle of nonmaleficence), but that it will not produce the benefit the patient or the surrogate seeks. A justified claim of futility cancels a professional's obligation to provide a medical procedure. However, it is not clear that the language of futility illuminates the range of ethical issues in passive paternalism, in part because of its variable and vague uses (which we discussed in Chapter 5). Furthermore, in the relevant cases, physicians' decisions often involve balancing the probable benefits and burdens to patients, a judgment that goes beyond judgments of medical futility.

Like passive paternalism, conceptions of medical futility are often presented as independent of considerations of financial costs, even though the need to control the costs of health care has fueled much of the interest in medical futility. We next examine ways to balance benefits, costs, and risks to determine how they should and should not play a role in judgments about acceptable care and the distribution of care.

BALANCING BENEFITS, COSTS, AND RISKS

Thus far, we have concentrated on the role of the principle of beneficence in clinical medicine and health care with some attention to beneficent policies. We now turn to the examination and evaluation of beneficent health policies through tools that analyze and assess appropriate benefits relative to costs and risks. These tools often are morally unobjectionable and may even be morally required to illuminate trade-offs and to enhance our ability to make reasoned assessments of health-related policies to maximize beneficent outcomes. Nonetheless, moral problems do surround the use of these tools.

Physicians routinely base judgments about the most suitable medical treatments on the balance of probable benefits and harms for patients. This criterion is also used in judgments about the ethical acceptability of research involving human subjects; these judgments consider whether the probable overall benefits—usually *for society*—outweigh the risks *to subjects.* In submitting a research protocol involving human subjects to an institutional review board (IRB) for approval, an investigator is expected to array the risks to subjects and probable benefits to both subjects and society, and then to explain why the probable benefits outweigh the risks. When IRBs array risks and benefits, determine their respective weights, and reach decisions, they typically use *informal* techniques such as expert judgments based on reliable data and analogical reasoning based on precedents. However, we focus in this section on techniques that employ *formal, quantitative* analysis of costs, risks, and benefits. These methods have been at the center of recent controversies over appropriate health policies.

The Nature of Costs, Risks, and Benefits

Costs include the resources required to bring about a benefit, as well as the negative effects of pursuing and realizing that benefit. They represent sacrifices made in the attempt to reach some important objective. We concentrate on costs expressed in monetary terms—the primary interpretation of costs in cost–benefit and cost-effectiveness analysis. The term *risk,* by contrast, refers to a possible future harm, where harm is defined as a setback to interests, particularly in life, health, and welfare. Expressions such as *minimal risk, reasonable risk,* and *high risk* usually refer to the chance of a harm's occurrence—its *probability*— but sometimes they also refer to the severity of the harm if it occurs—its *magnitude.*

Statements of risk are *descriptive* inasmuch as they state the probability that harmful events will occur. These statements of risk are also *evaluative* inasmuch as they attach a value to the occurrence or prevention of these events. No statement of risk occurs without a prior negative evaluation of some condition. At its core, a circumstance of risk involves a possible occurrence of something that has been evaluated as harmful and an uncertainty about its actual occurrence that can be expressed in terms of its probability. Several types of risks exist, including physical, psychological, financial, and legal risks, among others. The term *benefit* sometimes refers to cost avoidance and risk reduction, but, more commonly in biomedicine, it refers to something of positive value, such as life or health. Unlike *risk, benefit* is not a probabilistic term. *Probable benefit* is the proper contrast to risk, and benefits are comparable to harms rather than to risks of harm. Thus, we can best conceive risk–benefit relations in terms of a ratio between the probability and magnitude of an anticipated benefit and the probability and magnitude of an anticipated harm.

Cost–Effectiveness and Cost–Benefit Analyses

Cost-effectiveness analysis (CEA) and cost–benefit analysis (CBA) are widely used but controversial tools of formal analysis underlying public policies regarding health, safety, and medical technologies. Some policies are directed at burgeoning demands for expensive medical care and the need to contain the costs of health care. CEA and CBA appear precise and helpful because they present trade-offs in quantified terms.[50]

Defenders of these techniques praise them as ways of reducing intuitive weighing of options and avoiding subjective and political decisions. However, critics claim that these methods of analysis are not sufficiently comprehensive, that they fail to include all relevant values and options, that they frequently conflict with principles of justice, and that they are often themselves subjective and biased. Critics also charge that these techniques concentrate decision-making authority in the hands of narrow, technical professionals (e.g., health economists) who often fail to understand moral, social, legal, and political constraints that legitimately limit use of these methods.

CEA and CBA use different terms to state the value of outcomes. CBA measures both the benefits and the costs in monetary terms, whereas CEA measures the benefits in nonmonetary terms, such as years of life, quality-adjusted life-years, or cases of disease. CEA offers a bottom line such as "cost per year of life saved," whereas CBA offers a bottom line of a benefit–cost ratio stated in monetary figures that express the common measurement. Although CBA often begins by measuring different quantitative units (such as number of accidents, statistical deaths, and number of persons treated), it attempts to convert these seemingly incommensurable units of measurement into a common figure.

Because it uses the common metric of money, CBA in theory permits a comparison of programs that save lives with, for example, programs that reduce disability or accomplish other goals, such as public education. By contrast, CEA does not permit an evaluation of the inherent worth of programs or a comparative evaluation of programs with different aims. CEA functions best to compare and evaluate different programs sharing an identical aim, such as saving years of life.

Many CEAs involve comparing alternative courses of action that have similar health benefits to determine which is the most cost-effective. A simple and now classic example is the use of the guaiac test, an inexpensive test for detecting minute amounts of blood in the stool. Such blood may result from several problems, including hemorrhoids, benign intestinal polyps, or colonic cancer. A guaiac test cannot identify the cause of the bleeding, but if there is a positive stool guaiac and no other obvious cause for the bleeding, physicians undertake other tests. In the mid-1970s, the American Cancer Society proposed using six sequential stool guaiac tests to screen for colorectal cancers. Two analysts prepared a careful CEA of the six stool guaiac tests. They assumed that the initial test costs four dollars, that each additional test costs one dollar, and that each successive test detects many fewer cases of cancer. They then determined that the marginal cost per case of *detected* cancer increased dramatically: $1,175 for one test; $5,492 for two tests; $49,150 for three tests; $469,534 for four tests; $4.7 million for five tests; and $47 million for the full six-test screen.[51]

Such findings do not dictate a conclusion, but the analysis provides relevant data for a society needing to allocate resources, for insurance companies and hospitals setting policies, for physicians making recommendations to patients, and for patients considering diagnostic procedures. This analysis is a CEA rather than a CBA, because it does not attempt to convert the benefit of detection of colorectal cancer into a measure, such as dollars, that can then be compared with the costs. It also does not include other effects that may be hard to measure, such as the reassurance given to patients.

Conceptual confusion surrounds CEA. In some cases, when two programs are compared, the cost savings of one may be sufficient to view it as more cost-effective than the other. Yet some analysts contend that we should not confuse CEA with either reduced costs or increased effectiveness alone, because it often depends on both together. A program may be more cost-effective than another even if it (1) *costs more,* because it may increase medical effectiveness, or (2) leads to an overall *decrease in medical effectiveness,* because it may greatly reduce the costs. Also, no form of analysis has the moral power to dictate the use of a particular medical procedure simply because that procedure has the lowest cost-effectiveness ratio (e.g., because it provides the greatest benefit for each dollar). To assign priority to the alternative with the lowest cost-effectiveness ratio is to view medical diagnosis and therapy in unjustifiably narrow terms.

Risk Assessment and Values in Conflict

Risk assessment is another important analytic technique. It involves the analysis and evaluation of probabilities of negative outcomes, especially harms. Risk *identification* involves locating some hazard. Risk *estimation* determines the probability and magnitude of harms from that hazard. Risk *evaluation* determines the acceptability of the identified and estimated risks, often in relation to other objectives. Evaluation of risk in relation to probable benefits is often labeled *risk–benefit analysis* (RBA), which may be formulated in terms of a ratio of expected benefits to risks and may lead to a judgment about the acceptability of the risk under assessment. Risk identification, estimation, and evaluation are all stages in risk assessment. The next stage in the process is risk *management*—the set of individual, institutional, or policy responses to the analysis and assessment of risk, including decisions to reduce or control risks. For example, risk management in hospitals includes setting policies to reduce the risk of medical malpractice suits.

This section focuses on risk assessment, which frequently informs technology assessment, environmental impact statements, and public policies protecting health and safety. The following schema of magnitude and probability of harm is useful for understanding risk assessment:

		Magnitude of Harm	
		Major	*Minor*
	High	1	2
Probability of Harm			
	Low	3	4

As category 4 suggests, a question exists about whether some risks are so insignificant, in terms of either probability or magnitude of harm or both, as not to merit attention. So-called *de minimis* risks are acceptable risks because they can be interpreted as effectively zero. For example, according to the U.S. Food and Drug Administration (FDA), a risk of less than one cancer per million persons exposed is *de minimis*. However, the quantitative threshold or cutoff point used in a *de minimis* approach is problematic. For instance, an annual risk of one cancer per million persons for the U.S. population would produce the same number of fatalities (i.e., 275) as a risk of one per one hundred in a town with a population of 27,500. In focusing on the annual risk of cancer or death to one individual per million, the *de minimis* approach may neglect the cumulative, overall level of risk created for individuals over their lifetimes by the addition of several one-per-million risks.[52]

Risk assessment also focuses on the acceptability of risks relative to the benefits sought. With the possible exception of *de minimis* risks, most risks will be considered acceptable or unacceptable in relation to the probable benefits of the actions that carry those risks—for example, the benefits of radiation or a surgical procedure in health care, or the benefits of nuclear power or toxic chemicals in the workplace.[53]

Risk–benefit analyses in the regulation of drugs and medical devices. Some of the conceptual, normative, and empirical issues in risk assessment and, specifically, in RBA are evident in the FDA's regulation of drugs and medical devices.

The FDA requires three phases of human trials of drugs. Each stage involves RBA to determine whether to proceed to the next stage and whether to approve a drug for wider use. Patients, physicians, and other health care professionals have often criticized the process of drug approval in the United States because of the length of time required for approval. Critics contend that the standard of evidence for a favorable risk–benefit ratio is too high and thus severely limits patients' access to promising new drugs, often in times of dire need created by serious, even fatal, medical conditions. Other critics charge that the process is not rigorous enough in view of the problems that sometimes appear after drug approval.[54]

In the absence of satisfactory alternatives, many patients and their families have been keenly interested in gaining access to promising drugs that are in clinical trials but not yet approved. Societal perceptions of clinical research have shifted significantly. In the 1970s and early 1980s, the major concern was to protect individuals from burdens and risks associated with research. Beginning in the 1980s, the emphasis shifted to increasing access to clinical trials. Particularly in response to the AIDS epidemic and the demands of AIDS activists, the FDA developed mechanisms to provide expanded access to experimental drugs, especially for patients with seriously debilitating or life-threatening conditions and with no satisfactory alternative treatments.[55] Accordingly, the agency authorized procedures for compassionate treatment uses of unapproved experimental drugs on patients with an illness that is serious or poses an imminent threat to life and that lacks a satisfactory therapeutic alternative. Other FDA initiatives included a "fast track" of expedited approval and a "parallel track." The fast track allows patients with "seriously debilitating" or "life-threatening" conditions to accept greater risks in taking new drugs in the absence of acceptable alternatives. This approach was used in the approval of zidovudine (AZT) to treat AIDS. The parallel track, by contrast, allows limited access to experimental AIDS drugs that, according to early studies, are reasonably safe and promising (although clinical investigations continue).

A tension often exists between the need for scientific evidence about risks and benefits to protect patients, and patients' strong desires for access to certain drugs for specific conditions. In deciding a lawsuit filed by the Abigail Alliance, a patient-advocacy group, two members of a three-judge panel of the U.S. Court of Appeals for the D.C. Circuit ruled in 2006 that terminally ill patients have a constitutional right to access to "potentially life-saving medication to which those in Phase II clinical trials have access." Moreover, "barring a terminally ill patient from the use of a potentially life-saving treatment impinges on [the] right of self-preservation."[56] Counterarguments stressed that the FDA already has expanded access programs, that it is examining further extensions of these programs, and that early and wide access may limit researchers' and the FDA's efforts to complete important clinical trials to establish a firmer RBA of treatments. These counterarguments note that drug companies would have fewer incentives to conduct clinical trials, and that allowing companies to promote drugs without sufficient evidence of efficacy could lead to fraudulent exploitation of sick and desperate patients.[57] In an eight-to-two decision overturning the panel's ruling, the full court of appeals rejected arguments that terminally ill patients have a constitutional right of access to drugs that are still being tested.[58]

Clearly, a prudent RBA and assessment is needed. It is ethically difficult to oppose expanded access to experimental drugs for patients with serious, life-threatening medical conditions, where no effective alternative treatments are available. However, the latitude patients have in balancing risks and benefits of new drugs for themselves should not become so great as to subvert the FDA's regulation of new drugs to protect the public.

An example from medical devices presents another classic case of difficult RBAs and assessments undertaken by the FDA in its regulatory decisions. For more than thirty years, thousands of women used silicone-gel breast implants to augment their breast sizes, to reshape their breasts, or to reconstruct their breasts following mastectomies for cancer or other surgery. These implants were already on the market when legislation in 1976 required that manufacturers provide data about safety and efficacy for certain medical devices. As a result, implant manufacturers were not required to provide these data unless questions arose. The health and safety concerns that emerged centered on the implants' longevity, rate of rupture, and link with various diseases.

Defenders of complete prohibition contended that no woman should be allowed to take a risk of unknown but potentially serious magnitude because her consent could not be informed. FDA Commissioner David Kessler and others defended a restrictive policy, which was implemented in 1992. Kessler argued that for "patients with cancer and others with a need for breast reconstruction," a favorable risk–benefit ratio could exist in carefully controlled circumstances.[59] He sharply distinguished candidates for reconstruction following surgery from candidates for *augmentation* and held that a favorable risk–benefit ratio existed only for candidates for *reconstruction.*

Because candidates for augmentation still had breast tissue, they were con-sidered to be at "higher risk" from these implants. In the presence of an implant, the argument went, mammography might not detect breast cancer, and the use of mammography could create a risk of radiation exposure in healthy young women with breast tissue who have silent ruptures of the gel implant without symptoms. Kessler wrote: "In our opinion the risk–benefit ratio does not at this time favor the unrestricted use of silicone breast implants in healthy women."

Although Kessler denied that this decision involved "any judgment about values," critics charged that it was, in fact, based on contested values and was inappropriately paternalistic. There is evidence that the FDA gave massive weight to unknown risks largely because it discounted the self-perceived benefits of breast implants for women, except in cases of reconstruction. The agency then held these implants to a high standard of safety, instead of allowing women to decide for themselves whether to accept the risks for their own subjective benefits—a clear act of hard paternalism.[60]

If the evidence had indicated high risk relative to benefit, as well as unreasonable risk-taking by women, a different conclusion might have been sustained, but evidence available at the time and since points in the other direction. The FDA policy was unjustifiably paternalistic, noticeably so when compared to the less restrictive public decisions reached in European countries.[61] A more defensible, nonpaternalistic policy would have permitted the continued use of silicone-gel breast implants, regardless of the users' biological conditions and aims, while requiring adequate disclosure of information about risks. Raising the level of disclosure standards, as the FDA has done in some cases, would have been more appropriate than restraining choice. In 2006, as a result of new data from manufacturers and assessments by its advisory committees, the FDA approved the marketing of silicone-gel breast implants to women of all ages for breast reconstruction and to women twenty-two years and older for breast augmentation, but the companies involved must monitor patients for ten years postimplant.[62]

We reach two general conclusions from this discussion. First, it is morally legitimate and often obligatory for society to act beneficently through the government and its agencies to protect citizens from medical drugs and devices that are harmful or that have not been established to be safe and efficacious. Hence, the FDA plays an important role. Our conclusion that the FDA should not have severely restricted or prohibited the use of silicone-gel breast implants should not be interpreted as an argument against its indispensable role. Second, RBAs are not value-free. Values are evident in the FDA's programs of expanded access to drugs, in its limits on those programs, and in many of its other decisions such as the one on silicone-gel breast implants.

Risk perception. An individual's perception of risks may differ from an expert's assessment. Variations may reflect not only different goals and "risk budgets," but also different qualitative assessments of particular risks, including whether the risks in question are voluntary, controllable, highly salient, novel, or dreaded.[63] Public and professional responses to accidental exposure to the blood of HIV-infected patients early in the HIV/AIDS epidemic provide an instructive case. Such exposure produced greater fear than did accidental exposure to the blood of patients with hepatitis B several years ago, before a vaccine became available, even though statistically both exposures carried an approximately equal overall risk of death. The probability of HIV infection was lower (apparently less than 1%), but death from the infection appeared close to a certainty over time, despite improved treatments. The probability of infection by the hepatitis B virus was higher, at approximately 25%, but, conservatively estimated, the death rate was only 5%. According to one study, the fear of certain death for someone infected with HIV appeared to account for the greater fear of HIV infection through accidental exposure.[64]

Differences in risk perception suggest some limits of attempts to use quantitative statements of probability and magnitude in reaching conclusions about the acceptability of risk. The public's informed but subjective perception of a harm needs to be considered and given substantial weight when formulating public policy, but the weight will vary with each case. However, the public sometimes holds factually mistaken views about risks that experts can identify. Some of the mistaken public views can and should be corrected through public policies.[65]

Precaution: Principle or Process?

Suppose that a new technology or a novel activity appears to pose a threat or create a hazard, thus evoking public fear. Suppose, further, that scientists lack evidence to determine the magnitude of the possible negative outcome or the probabilities of its occurrence, perhaps because of uncertain cause–effect relations. The risks cannot be quantified and an appropriate benefit–risk–cost analysis is not possible. At most, beneficence can be implemented only through *precautionary* measures. But which actions, if any, are justifiable in the face of uncertain risks?

Several common maxims come to mind: Better safe than sorry; look before you leap; an ounce of prevention is worth a pound of cure; and so forth. As rough guides for decision making, these maxims are unobjectionable and have sometimes been incorporated into a "precautionary principle." The precautionary principle has been implemented in international treaties as well as in laws and regulations in several countries to protect the environment and public health.[66] However, it is difficult to talk about *the* precautionary principle because there are so many different versions, with different advantages and problems. One assessment reports that there are as many as nineteen different formulations.[67]

A general and universal precautionary principle may be incoherent. There are different threats, hazards, and uncertain risks; and efforts to avoid any single one must attend to the others. The failure to develop some technologies may create risks just as much as the failure to stop development of those technologies. The principle, in its strong versions, could be a recipe for paralysis, giving almost no guidance at all. The principle, in context, may focus on only one set of risks, ignoring those from the other side.[68]

However, properly formulated, some precautionary measures are justified. Depending on what is valued and what is at risk, it may be ethically justifiable and even obligatory to take steps, in the absence of conclusive scientific evidence, to avoid a hazard where the harm would be both serious and irreversible. Hence, unsurprisingly, not all critics wholly reject the precautionary principle. Some accept a "modest version," which might be called an "anti-catastrophe principle."[69]

Triggering conditions for the principle's application include plausible evidence of possible harm where it is not possible to adequately characterize and quantify risk because of scientific uncertainty and ignorance. The precautionary process should not be viewed as an alternative to risk analysis and scientific research. Rather, the precautionary process should be viewed as a way to supplement risk appraisals when the available scientific evidence does not permit firm characterizations of the probability or magnitude of plausible risks.

Measures commonly associated with the precautionary principle include transparency, involvement of the public, and consultation with experts about possible responses to threats marked by uncertainty or ignorance about probabilities and magnitudes. Transparent policies, including public communication of risks, sometimes heighten fears, but such risks are acceptable because of the importance of developing risk-avoidance policies that are generally consistent with the society's basic values and the public's reflective preferences.

Perils created by some versions of the precautionary principle include distortion through speculative and theoretical threats and risks that divert attention away from real, albeit less dramatic, threats. The acceptance or rejection of any precautionary approach will depend on a careful weighing of social, cultural, and psychological perspectives.[70] However, we should not oversimplify contrasts by suggesting, for instance, that Europe is more precautionary than the United States. Even though precautionary principles appear to have more traction in laws, regulations, and discourse in Europe than in the United States, both adopt a variety of precautionary measures, often in response to different perceived threats or hazards.

In conclusion, a general precautionary principle does not help us interpret and implement principles of beneficence directed at the prevention of harm. However, this conclusion does not minimize the value of precaution or of societal and governmental interventions in certain cases on grounds of beneficence even in the absence of conclusive scientific evidence.

THE VALUE AND QUALITY OF LIFE

We turn, finally, to controversies regarding how to place a value on life, which have centered on CBAs. We also examine controversies over the value of quality-adjusted life-years (QALYs), which have centered on CEAs.

Valuing Lives

One method assigns an economic value to human life. As analysts note, a society may spend amount x to save a life in one setting (e.g., by reducing the risk of death from causes such as cancer and mining accidents), but only spend amount y to save a life in another setting. One objective in determining the value of a life is to develop consistency across practices and policies.

Analysts have developed several methods to determine the value of human life. These include discounted future earnings (DFE) and willingness to pay (WTP). According to DFE, we can determine the monetary value of lives by considering what people at risk of some disease or accident could be expected to earn if they survived. Although this approach can help measure the costs of diseases, accidents, and death, it reduces people's value to their potential economic value and gives priority to those who would be expected to have greater future earnings, such as young, adult white men and people with wealth.

WTP considers how much individuals would be willing to pay to reduce the risks of death, either through their revealed preferences (i.e., decisions people actually make in their lives) or through their expressed preferences (i.e., what people say in response to hypothetical questions). For revealed preferences to be meaningful, individuals would have to understand the risks in their lives and voluntarily assume those risks—assumptions that may not be met in decisions many people make. Also, individuals' answers to hypothetical questions may not accurately indicate how much they would be willing to spend on actual programs to reduce their (and others') risk of death.

Although we rarely put an explicit *monetary* value on human life, this is precisely what proponents of CBA urge. Qualitative factors, such as how deaths occur, are often more important to us than purely economic factors. In addition, beneficence may be expressed in policies, such as rescuing trapped coal miners, that symbolize society's benevolence and affirm the value of the victims, even though these policies would often not be supported by a CBA focused on the economic value of life determined by either DFE or WTP.

In our judgment, data gained from CBA and other analytic techniques are relevant to the formulation of public policies and can provide very valuable insights. However, they provide only *one* set of indicators of appropriate social beneficence. It is often not necessary to put a specific economic value on human life to evaluate possible risk-reduction policies and to compare their costs.

Evaluation may reasonably focus on the life-years saved, without attempting to convert them into monetary terms. In health care, CBA has, quite appropriately, diminished in importance by comparison to CEA, which often promotes the goal of maximizing QALYs, a topic to which we now turn.[71]

Valuing Quality-Adjusted Life-Years

Quality of life and QALYs. In health policy and health care, quality of life can be as important as saving lives and years of life. Improving the quality of a patient's life is especially important in chronic and rehabilitative care. Many individuals, when contemplating different treatments for a particular condition, are willing to trade some life-years for improved quality of life during their remaining life-years. Hence, researchers and policymakers have sought measures, called health-adjusted life-years (HALYs), that combine longevity with health status. QALYs are the most widely used type of HALY.[72]

An influential premise underlying use of QALYs is that, "if an extra year of healthy (i.e., good quality) life-expectancy is worth one, then an extra year of unhealthy (i.e., poor quality) life-expectancy must be worth less than one (for why otherwise do people seek to be healthy?)."[73] On this scale, the value of the condition of death is zero. Various states of illness or disability better than death but short of full health receive a value between zero and one. The value of particular health outcomes depends on the increase in the utility of the health state and the number of years it lasts.[74]

QALYs bring length of life and quality of life into a single framework of evaluation.[75] They can be used to monitor the effects of treatments on patients in clinical practice or in clinical trials, to determine what to recommend to patients, and to provide information to patients about the effects of different treatments. In some contexts, it may be sufficient to consider only the net effectiveness of different treatments measured by their QALYs. However, in the allocation of health care resources, the costs relative to the QALYs provided by different treatments must often be examined.

British health economist Alan Williams used QALYs to examine the cost-effectiveness of coronary artery bypass grafting. In his well-known analysis, bypass grafting compares favorably with pacemakers for heart block. It is superior to heart transplantation and the treatment of end-stage renal failure, but less cost-effective than hip replacement. He also found that bypass grafting for severe angina and extensive coronary artery disease is more cost-effective than for less severe cases. The rate of survival can be misleading for coronary artery bypass grafting and many other therapeutic procedures that have a major impact on quality of life. Ultimately, Williams recommended that resources "be redeployed at the margin to procedures for which the benefits to patients are high in relation to the costs."[76]

How to determine quality of life is a difficult question. Analysts often start with rough measures, such as physical mobility, freedom from pain and distress, and the capacity to perform the activities of daily life and to engage in social interactions. Quality-of-life discussions thus appear theoretically attractive as one way to provide information about the ingredients of a good life, but this notion is so amorphous and variable as to be virtually unusable in actual health policy and health care.

Despite such practical problems, some instruments can and should be developed and refined to present meaningful and accurate measures of health-related quality of life. This goal is worthwhile because, without such instruments, we are likely to operate with implicit and unexamined views about trade-offs between quantity and quality of life in relation to cost.

Ethical assumptions of QALYs. Many ethical assumptions are involved in QALY-based CEA. Utilitarianism is CEA's philosophical parent, and some of its problems carry over to its offspring, even though there are important differences.[77] Implicit in QALY-based CEA is the idea that health maximization is the only relevant objective of health services. But some nonhealth benefits or utilities of health services also contribute to quality of life. As our discussion of silicone-gel breast implants noted, conditions such as asymmetrical breasts may affect a person's subjective estimate of quality of life and may constitute a source of distress. The problem is that QALY-based CEA attaches utility only to selected outcomes while neglecting values such as how care is provided (e.g., whether it is personal care) and how it is distributed (e.g., whether universal access is provided).[78]

Related questions arise about whether the use of QALYs in CEA is adequately egalitarian. Proponents of QALY-based CEA hold that each healthy life-year is equally valuable for everyone. A QALY is a QALY, regardless of who possesses it.[79] However, QALY-based CEA may discriminate against older people, because (conditions being equal) saving the life of a younger person is likely to produce more QALYs than saving the life of an older person.[80]

QALY-based CEA also does not attend adequately to some aspects of justice. It does not consider how life-years are distributed among patients, and it may not entail efforts to reduce the number of individual victims in its attempts to increase the number of life-years. From this standpoint, no difference exists between saving one person who can be expected to have forty QALYs and saving two people who can be expected to have twenty QALYs each. In principle, CEA will give priority to saving one person with forty expected QALYs over saving two persons with only nineteen expected QALYs each. Hence, QALY-based CEA favors life-years over individual lives, and the number of life-years over the number of individual lives, while failing to recognize societal and professional obligations of beneficence that require rescuing endangered individual lives.[81]

A tension also thus exists between QALY-based CEA and the duty to rescue, even though both are ultimately grounded on considerations of beneficence. This tension appeared in an effort by the Oregon Health Services Commission to develop a prioritized list of health services so that the State of Oregon could expand its Medicaid coverage to all of its poor citizens. In commenting on a draft priority list that ranked some life-saving procedures below some routine procedures, David Hadorn noted that, "The cost-effectiveness analysis approach used to create the initial list conflicted directly with the powerful 'Rule of Rescue'—people's perceived duty to save endangered life whenever possible."[82] He is right. QALY-based CEA's methodological assignment of priority to life-years over individual lives implies that beneficence-based rescue (especially life-saving) is less significant than cost utility, that the distribution of life-years is unimportant, that saving more lives is less important than maximizing the number of life-years, and that quality of life is more important than quantity of life. These priorities raise serious moral questions that must be addressed independently of methodological questions about QALY-based CEA. (We return to the Oregon prioritized list in Chapter 7.)

CONCLUSION

Our conclusions in this chapter build on conclusions reached in previous chapters. We have distinguished between two principles of beneficence and have defended a version of paternalism that justifies a very restricted range of both soft and hard paternalistic actions. However, we acknowledged that, in addition to its disrespect for personal autonomy, a policy or rule permitting a hard paternalism in professional practice is generally not worth the risk of abuse that it invites. We also argued that even some forms of soft paternalism are ethically problematic. Finally, we examined formal techniques of analysis—CEA, CBA, and RBA—and concluded that they can be morally unobjectionable ways to implement the principle of utility, but that principles such as respect for autonomy and justice help set limits on the uses of these techniques. The next chapter develops principles of justice that began to surface in the final parts of this chapter.

NOTES

1. W. D. Ross, *The Right and the Good* (Oxford: Clarendon, 1930), p. 21.

2. Shelly Kagan, *The Limits of Morality* (Oxford: Clarendon, 1989), pp. 1–2, 402–03.

3. One limit is that agents often have discretion about when, where, how, and toward whom to act beneficently. John Stuart Mill argued that we are obligated to practice beneficence, "but not towards any definite person, nor at any prescribed time." Mill, *Utilitarianism,* in vol. 10 of the *Collected Works of John Stuart Mill* (Toronto: University of Toronto, 1969), chap. 5.

4. Peter Singer, "Famine, Affluence, and Morality," *Philosophy and Public Affairs* 1 (1972): 229–43.

5. Singer formulated a weak version of the obligation to assist in this article, but he endorsed only the strong version. The weak version says that we must help until the point at which we would have to sacrifice something of *moral significance,* by contrast to *comparable moral significance.* He does not say what counts as morally significant, leaving it a matter to be decided by moral theory.

6. Arguably, we present a *weakened* version of Singer's ideal principles, but we do not pursue this interpretive question here.

7. Peter Singer, *Practical Ethics,* 2nd ed. (Cambridge: Cambridge University Press, 1993), p. 246.

8. Singer, "Global Poverty," Lectures 1–3, Oxford Uehiro Centre for Practical Ethics, Uehiro Lectures 2007 (forthcoming as a book, 2009), http://www.practicalethics.ox.ac.uk/Events/ Uehiro%20Lectures/nuehirolectures.htm.

9. In particular to Liam B. Murphy, "The Demands of Beneficence," *Philosophy and Public Affairs* 22 (1993): 267–92.

10. Our formulations are indebted to Eric D'Arcy, *Human Acts: An Essay in Their Moral Evaluation* (Oxford: Clarendon, 1963), pp. 56–57. We have added the fourth condition and altered others. We also profited from Joel Feinberg, *Harm to Others,* vol. I of *The Moral Limits of the Criminal Law* (New York: Oxford University Press, 1984), chap. 4.

11. This third condition will need a finer-grained analysis to avoid some problems of what is required if there is a small (but not insignificant) probability of saving millions of lives at minimal cost to a person. It is not plausible to hold that a person has *no obligation* to so act. Condition 3 here could be refined to show that there must be some appropriate proportionality between probability of success, the value of outcome to be achieved, and the sacrifice that the agent would incur. Perhaps the formulation should be: a high ratio of probable benefit relative to the sacrifice made.

12. This condition may seem to imply that if various beneficent actions would carry a very demanding financial cost, one is not obligated to rescue—again a counterintuitive implication for some rescue cases. This problem needs more attention than we can provide here.

13. See Arthur L. Caplan, Robert H. Blank, and Janna C. Merrick, eds., *Compelled Compassion: Government Intervention in the Treatment of Critically Ill Newborns* (Totowa, NJ: Humana, 1992); and John D. Lantos and William A. Meadows, *Neonatal Bioethics: The Moral Challenges of Medical Innovation* (Baltimore: Johns Hopkins University Press, 2006).

14. David Hume, "Of Suicide," in *Essays Moral, Political, and Literary,* ed. Eugene Miller (Indianapolis, IN: Liberty Classics, 1985), pp. 577–89.

15. See David A. J. Richards, *A Theory of Reasons for Action* (Oxford: Clarendon, 1971), p. 186; Lawrence Becker, *Reciprocity* (Chicago: University of Chicago Press, 1990); Aristotle, *Nicomachean Ethics,* bks. 8–9.

16. See William F. May, "Code and Covenant or Philanthropy and Contract?" in *Ethics in Medicine,* ed. S. Reiser, A. Dyck, and W. Curran (Cambridge, MA: MIT Press, 1977), pp. 65–76. See also May, *The Healer's Covenant: Images of the Healer in Medical Ethics,* 2nd ed. (Louisville, KY: Westminster-John Knox Press, 2000).

17. *Epidemics,* 1:11, in *Hippocrates,* vol. I, ed. W.H.S. Jones (Cambridge, MA: Harvard University Press, 1923), p. 165.

18. Edmund Pellegrino and David Thomasma, *For the Patient's Good: The Restoration of Beneficence in Health Care* (New York: Oxford University Press, 1988), p. 29.

19. See Tom L. Beauchamp and Laurence B. McCullough, *Medical Ethics: The Moral Responsibilities of Physicians* (Englewood Cliffs, NJ: Prentice Hall, 1984), p. 84.

20. See Donald VanDeVeer, *Paternalistic Intervention: The Moral Bounds on Benevolence* (Princeton, NJ: Princeton University Press, 1986), pp. 16–40; John Kleinig, *Paternalism* (Totowa, NJ: Rowman & Allanheld, 1983), pp. 6–14.

21. This case has been formulated on the basis of and incorporates language from Margaret A. Drickamer and Mark S. Lachs, "Should Patients with Alzheimer's Be Told Their Diagnosis?" *New England Journal of Medicine* 326 (April 2, 1992): 947–51.

22. First introduced as the distinction between strong and weak paternalism by Joel Feinberg, "Legal Paternalism," *Canadian Journal of Philosophy* 1 (1971): 105–24, esp. 113, 116. See, further, Feinberg, *Harm to Self,* vol. III of *The Moral Limits of the Criminal Law* (New York: Oxford University Press, 1986), esp. pp. 12ff. In the latter (p. 14), Feinberg argued that it may be "severely misleading to think of [soft paternalism] as any kind of [real] paternalism."

23. See Cass R. Sunstein and Richard H. Thaler, "Libertarian Paternalism Is Not an Oxymoron," *University of Chicago Law Review* 70 (Fall 2003): 1159–202.

24. Erich H. Loewy, "In Defense of Paternalism," *Theoretical Medicine and Bioethics* 26 (2005): 445–68.

25. James F. Childress, *Who Should Decide? Paternalism in Health Care* (New York: Oxford University Press, 1982), p. 18. Contrast Thaddeus Mason Pope's use of the terms soft and hard paternalism, "Counting the Dragon's Teeth and Claws: The Definition of Hard Paternalism," *Georgia State University Law Review* 20 (2004): 660–722.

26. Sunstein and Thaler, "Libertarian Paternalism Is Not an Oxymoron," p. 1159. See also Richard H. Thaler and Cass R. Sunstein, "Libertarian Paternalism," *American Economics Review* 93 (2003): 175–79. Contrast Gregory Mitchell, "Review Essay: Libertarian Paternalism Is an Oxymoron," *Northwestern University Law Review* 99 (Spring 2005): 1245–77.

27. Jolls and Sunstein, "Debiasing through Law," *The Journal of Legal Studies* 33 (January 2006): 232.

28. See Edward L. Glaeser, "Symposium: Homo Economicus, Homo Myopicus, and the Law and Economics of Consumer Choice: Paternalism and Autonomy," *University of Chicago Law Review* 73 (Winter 2006): 133–57.

29. Ronald Bayer and Jennifer Stuber, "Tobacco Control, Stigma, and Public Health: Rethinking the Relations," *American Journal of Public Health* 96 (January 2006): 47–50.

30. Glaeser, "Symposium: Homo Economicus, Homo Myopicus . . . ," pp. 152–53.

31. Bayer and Stuber, "Tobacco Control, Stigma, and Public Health: Rethinking the Relations," p. 49.

32. Cf. Glaeser, "Symposium: Homo Economicus, Homo Myopicus. . . . ," pp. 153–54.

33. W. Kip Vicusi, "The New Cigarette Paternalism," *Regulation* (Winter 2002–2003): 58–64.

34. For interpretations of (hard) paternalism as insult, disrespect, and treatment of individuals as unequals, see Ronald Dworkin, *Taking Rights Seriously* (Cambridge, MA: Harvard University Press, 1978), pp. 262–63; and Childress, *Who Should Decide?,* chap. 3.

35. Gerald Dworkin, "Paternalism," *The Monist* 56 (January 1972): 65.

36. See Dworkin, "Paternalism"; and John Rawls, *A Theory of Justice* (Cambridge, MA: Harvard University Press, 1971; rev. ed., 1999), pp. 209, 248–49 (1999: pp. 183–84, 218–20).

37. Dworkin himself says, "The reasons which support paternalism are those which support any altruistic action—the welfare of another person." "Paternalism," in *Encyclopedia of Ethics,* ed. Lawrence Becker (New York: Garland, 1992), p. 940. For a variety of consent and nonconsent defenses of paternalism, see Kleinig, *Paternalism,* pp. 38–73; VanDeVeer, *Paternalistic Intervention, passim;* and see Kultgen, *Autonomy and Intervention,* esp. chaps. 9, 11, 15.

38. Mary C. Silva, *Ethical Decision-Making in Nursing Administration* (Norwalk, CT: Appleton & Lange, 1989), p. 64. Of course, someone might interpret this case as an instance of soft paternalism because the patient does not fully understand the risks of the medication, but we here take it as an example of hard paternalism.

39. Compare Kleinig's similar conclusion, *Paternalism,* p. 76.

40. We do not here address philosophical problems surrounding the definition of suicide. See Tom L. Beauchamp, "Suicide," in *Matters of Life and Death,* 3rd ed., ed. Tom Regan (New York: Random House, 1993), esp. part I; and the articles in John Donnelly, ed., *Suicide: Right or Wrong?* (Buffalo, NY: Prometheus Books, 1991).

41. See James Rachels, "Barney Clark's Key," *Hastings Center Report* 13 (April 1983): 17–19, esp. p. 17.

42. We have adapted this case from Marc Basson, ed., *Rights and Responsibilities in Modern Medicine* (New York: Alan R. Liss, 1981), pp. 183–84.

43. Glanville Williams, "Euthanasia," *Medico-Legal Journal* 41 (1973): 27.

44. See President's Commission for the Study of Ethical Problems in Medicine and Biomedical and Behavioral Research, *Deciding to Forego Life-Sustaining Treatment,* p. 37.

45. Betty Rollin, *Last Wish* (New York: Linden Press/Simon & Schuster, 1985).

46. Childress, *Who Should Decide?,* chap. 1. See also Timothy E. Quill and Howard Brody, "Physician Recommendations and Patient Autonomy: Finding a Balance between Physician Power and Patient Choice," *Annals of Internal Medicine* 125 (1996): 763–69; Allan S. Brett and Laurence B. McCullough, "When Patients Request Specific Interventions: Defining the Limits of the Physician's Obligation," *New England Journal of Medicine* 315 (November 20, 1986): 1347–51.

47. We have adapted this case from "The Refusal to Sterilize: A Paternalistic Decision," in *Rights and Responsibilities in Modern Medicine,* ed. Basson, pp. 135–36.

48. See Steven H. Miles, "Informed Demand for Non-Beneficial Medical Treatment," *New England Journal of Medicine* 325 (August 15, 1991): 512–15; and Ronald E. Cranford, "Helga Wanglie's Ventilator," *Hastings Center Report* 21 (July–August 1991): 23–24; "Brain-Damaged Woman at Center of Lawsuit Over Life-Support Dies."

49. Catherine A. Marco and Gregory L. Larkin, "Case Studies in 'Futility'—Challenges for Academic Emergency Medicine," *Academic Emergency Medicine* 7 (2000): 1147–51.

50. Our description of these analytic techniques draws on David Eddy, "Cost-Effectiveness Analysis," *Journal of the American Medical Association* 267 (March 25, 1992): 1669–75; 267 (June 24, 1992): 3342–48; and 268 (July 1, 1992): 132–36; Marthe R. Gold, Joanna E. Siegel, Louise B. Russell, and Milton C. Weinstein, eds., *Cost-Effectiveness in Health and Medicine* (New York: Oxford University Press, 1996); and Wilhelmine Miller, Lisa A. Robinson, and Robert S. Lawrence, eds., *Valuing Health for Regulatory Effectiveness Analysis* (Washington, DC: National Academies Press, 2006).

51. On this now classic example, see Duncan Neuhauser and Ann M. Lewicki, "What Do We Gain from the Sixth Stool Guaiac?" *New England Journal of Medicine* 293 (July 31, 1975): 226–28.

See also "American Cancer Society Report on the Cancer-Related Checkup," *CA—A Cancer Journal for Clinicians* 30 (1980): 193–240, which recommended the full set of six guaiac tests.

52. See Sheila Jasanoff, "Acceptable Evidence in a Pluralistic Society," in *Acceptable Evidence: Science and Values in Risk Management,* ed. Deborah G. Mayo and Rachelle D. Hollander (New York: Oxford University Press, 1991).

53. See Richard Wilson and E. A. C. Crouch, "Risk Assessment and Comparisons: An Introduction," *Science* 236 (April 17, 1987): 267–70.

54. Curt D. Burberg, Arthur A. Levin, Peter A. Gross, et al., "The FDA and Drug Safety," *Archives of Internal Medicine* 166 (October 9, 2006): 1938–42; and Alina Baciu, Kathleen Stratton, and Sheila P. Burke, eds., *The Future of Drug Safety: Promoting and Protecting the Health of the Public* (Washington, DC: The National Academies Press, 2006).

55. On the significant role of AIDS activists, see Steven Epstein, *Impure Science: AIDS, Activism, and the Politics of Knowledge* (Berkeley, CA: University of California Press, 1996), Loretta M. Kopelman, "How AIDS Activists Are Changing Research," in *Health Care Ethics: Critical Issues,* ed. John Monagle and David C. Thomasma (Gaithersburg, MD: Aspen, 1994), pp. 199–209; Robert J. Levine, "The Impact of HIV Infection on Society's Perception of Clinical Trials," *Kennedy Institute of Ethics Journal* 4 (1994): 93–98.

56. *Abigail Alliance for Better Access to Developmental Drugs and Washington Legal Foundation v. Andrew C. von Eschenbach, M.D., In His Official Capacity as Acting Commissioner, Food and Drug Administration,* United States Court of Appeals for the District of Columbia Circuit, No. 04–5350, May 2, 2006.

57. See William Schultz, a former deputy commissioner for policy at the FDA, as quoted in Susan Okie, "Access before Approval—A Right to Take Experimental Drugs?" *New England Journal of Medicine* 355 (August 3, 2006): 437–40. See also Society for Clinical Trial Board of Directors, "The Society for Clinical Trials Opposes U.S. Legislation to Permit Marketing of Unproven Medical Therapies for Seriously Ill Patients," *Clinical Trials* 3 (2006): 154–57, for opposition to the legislation that the Abigail Alliance supports.

58. *Abigail Alliance for Better Access to Developmental Drugs and Washington Legal Foundation v. Andrew C. von Eschenbach, M.D., In His Official Capacity as Acting Commissioner, Food and Drug Administration,* United States Court of Appeals for the District of Columbia Circuit, No. 04–5350, August 7, 2007.

59. David A. Kessler, "Special Report: The Basis of the FDA's Decision on Breast Implants," *New England Journal of Medicine* 326 (June 18, 1992): 1713–15. All references to Kessler's views are to this article.

60. See Marcia Angell, "Breast Implants—Protection or Paternalism?" *New England Journal of Medicine* 326 (June 18, 1992): 1695–96. Angell's criticisms also appear in her *Science on Trial: The Clash of Medical Evidence and the Law in the Breast Implant Case* (New York: Norton, 1996); and Angell, "Evaluating the Health Risks of Breast Implants: The Interplay of Medical Science, the Law, and Public Opinion," *New England Journal of Medicine* 334 (1996): 1513–18.

61. For reviews and evaluations of the scientific data, see E. C. Janowsky, L. L. Kupper, and B. S. Hulka, "Meta-Analyses of the Relation between Silicone Breast Implants and the Risk of Connective Tissue Diseases," *New England Journal of Medicine* 342 (2000): 781–90; *Silicone Gel Breast Implants: Report of the Independent Review Group* (Cambridge, MA: Jill Rogers Associates, 1998); and S. Bondurant, V. Ernster, and R. Herdman, eds., *Safety of Silicone Breast Implants* (Washington, DC: National Academy Press, 2000). See also P. C. Gerszten, "A Formal Risk Assessment of Silicone Breast Implants," *Biomaterials* 20 (1999): 1063–69.

62. "FDA Approves Silicone Gel-Filled Breast Implants After In-Depth Evaluation," *FDA News* (November 17, 2006), http://www.fda.gov/bbs/topics/NEWS/2006/NEW01512.html

63. See Paul Slovic, "Perception of Risk," *Science* 236 (April 17, 1987): 280–85; Slovic, *The Perception of Risk* (London and Sterling, VA: Earthscan, 2000); and Richard J. Zeckhauser and W. Kip Viscusi, "Risk Within Reason," *Science* 248 (May 4, 1990): 559–64.

64. Lawrence J. Schneiderman and Robert M. Kaplan, "Fear of Dying and HIV Infection vs Hepatitis B Infection," *American Journal of Public Health* 82 (April 1992): 584–89. However, several studies have shown that nurses and surgeons *undervalue* the importance of practices of protection against blood-borne pathogens.

65. See Cass Sunstein, *Laws of Fear: Beyond the Precautionary Principle* (Cambridge: Cambridge University Press, 2005) and *Risk and Reason* (Cambridge: Cambridge University Press, 2002).

66. For defenses of the precautionary principle, see United Nations Educational, Scientific and Cultural Organization (UNESCO), The Precautionary Principle (2005), http://unesdoc.unesco. org/images/001395/139578ee.pdf; Poul Harremoes, David Gee, Malcolm MacGarvin, et al., *The Precautionary Principle in the 20th Century: Lessons from Early Warnings* (London: Earthscan, 2002); Tim O'Riordan, James Cameron, and Andrew Jordan, eds., *Reinterpreting the Precautionary Principle* (London: Earthscan, 2001); Carolyn Raffensperger and Joel Tichner, eds., *Protecting Public Health and the Environment: Implementing the Precautionary Principle* (Washington, DC: Island Press, 1999); Carl Cranor, "Toward Understanding Aspects of the Precautionary Principle," *Journal of Medicine and Philosophy* 29 (June 2004): 259–79. For critical perspectives on the precautionary principle, see Sunstein, *Laws of Fear: Beyond the Precautionary Principle*; H. Tristram Engelhardt, Jr. and Fabrice Jotterand, "The Precautionary Principle: A Dialectical Reconsideration," *Journal of Medicine and Philosophy* 29 (June 2004): 301–12; Julian Morris, ed., *Rethinking Risk and the Precautionary Principle* (Oxford: Butterworth-Heinemann, 2000); and Indur M. Goklany, *The Precautionary Principle: A Critical Appraisal of Environmental Risk Assessment* (Washington, DC: Cato Institute, 2001).

67. See P. Sandin, "Dimensions of the Precautionary Principle," *Human and Ecological Risk Assessment* 5 (1999): 889–907.

68. Sunstein, *Laws of Fear: Beyond the Precautionary Principle.* See also Engelhardt and Jotterand, "The Precautionary Principle: A Dialectical Reconsideration," and Soren Holm and John Harris, "Precautionary Principle Stifles Discovery" (correspondence), *Nature* 400 (July 1999): 398.

69. Cass Sunstein accepts the former—see his *Laws of Fear: Beyond the Precautionary Principle,* whereas Richard A. Posner accepts the latter—see his *Catastrophe: Risk and Response* (New York: Oxford University Press, 2004).

70. See several chapters in O'Riordan, Cameron, and Jordan, eds., *Reinterpreting the Precautionary Principle.*

71. For a philosophical critique of CBA, see Elizabeth Anderson, *Values in Ethics and Economics* (Cambridge, MA: Harvard University Press, 1993), esp. chap. 9. See also Peter A. Ubel, *Pricing Life: Why It's Time for Health Care Rationing* (Cambridge, MA: The MIT Press, 2000), esp. p. 68.

72. See Miller, Robinson, and Lawrence, eds., *Valuing Health for Regulatory Cost-Effectiveness Analysis.* For an examination and a call for further clarification of different types of measures, see Marthe R. Gold, David Stevenson, and Dennis G. Fryback, "HALYs and QALYs and DALYs, Oh My: Similarities and Differences in Summary Measures of Population Health," *Annual Review of Public Health* 23 (2002): 115–34. For a critical examination of DALYs, see Sudhir Anand and Kara Hanson, "Disability-Adjusted Life Years: A Critical Review," in *Public Health, Ethics, and Equity,* ed. Sudhir Anand, Fabienne Peter, and Amartya Sen (Oxford: Oxford University Press, 2004), chap. 9.

73. Alan Williams, "The Importance of Quality of Life in Policy Decisions," in *Quality of Life: Assessment and Application,* ed. Stuart R. Walker and Rachel M. Rosser (Boston: MTP Press, 1988), p. 285.

74. See Erik Nord, *Cost-Value Analysis in Health Care: Making Sense out of QALYs* (Cambridge: Cambridge University Press, 1999), passim, and Gold et al., *Cost-Effectiveness in Health and Medicine,* passim.

75. See David Eddy, "Cost-Effectiveness Analysis: Is It up to the Task?" *Journal of the American Medical Association* 267 (June 24, 1992): 3344.

76. Alan Williams, "Economics of Coronary Artery Bypass Grafting," *British Medical Journal* 291 (August 3, 1985): 326–29. See also M. C. Weinstein and W. B. Stason, "Cost-Effectiveness of Coronary Artery Bypass Surgery," *Circulation* 66, Suppl. 5, pt. 2 (1982): III, 56–66.

77. See Paul Menzel, Marthe R. Gold, Erik Nord, et al., "Toward a Broader View of Values in Cost-Effectiveness Analysis of Health," *Hastings Center Report* 29 (May–June 1999): 7–15. For a defense of the utilitarian perspective of CEA and QALYs, see John McKie, Jeff Richardson, and Helga Kuhse, *The Allocation of Health Care Resources: An Ethical Evaluation of the 'QALY' Approach* (Aldershot, England: Ashgate, 1998). See also Joshua Cohen, "Preferences, Needs and QALYs," *Journal of Medical Ethics* 22 (1996): 267–72; Dan W. Brock, "Ethical Issues in the Use of Cost Effectiveness Analysis for the Prioritisation of Health Care Resources," in *Public Health, Ethics, and Equity,* ed. Anand, Peter, and Sen, chap. 10; and Madison Powers and Ruth Faden, *Social Justice: The Moral Foundations of Public Health and Health Policy* (Oxford: Oxford University Press, 2006), chap. 6.

78. Gavin Mooney, "QALYs: Are They Enough? A Health Economist's Perspective," *Journal of Medical Ethics* 15 (1989): 148–52.

79. Alan Williams, "The Importance of Quality of Life in Policy Decisions," in *Quality of Life,* ed. Walker and Rosser, p. 286; Williams, "Economics, QALYs and Medical Ethics—A Health Economist's Perspective," *Health Care Analysis* 3 (1995): 221–26.

80. Some proposals to modify or limit QALY-based CEA by societal values would require even lower weight for the elderly, in line with dominant societal values. See, for example, Nord, *Cost-Value Analysis in Health Care*; Menzel et al., "Toward a Broader View of Values in Cost-Effectiveness Analysis of Health"; and Ubel, *Pricing Life.*

81. John Harris argues that QALYs are a "life-threatening device," because they suggest that life-years rather than individual lives are valuable. "QALYfying the Value of Life," *Journal of Medical Ethics* 13 (1987): 117. See also Peter Singer, John McKie, Helga Kuhse, and Jeff Richardson, "Double Jeopardy and the Use of QALYs in Health Care Allocation," *Journal of Medical Ethics* 21 (1995): 144–50; John Harris, "Double Jeopardy and the Veil of Ignorance—A Reply," *Journal of Medical Ethics* 21 (1995): 151–57; McKie, Kuhse, Richardson, and Singer, "Double Jeopardy, the Equal Value of Lives and the Veil of Ignorance: A Rejoinder to Harris," *Journal of Medical Ethics* 22 (1996): 204–08; Harris, "Would Aristotle Have Played Russian Roulette?" *Journal of Medical Ethics* 22 (1996): 209–15; and McKie, Kuhse, Richardson, and Singer, "Another Peep Behind the Veil," *Journal of Medical Ethics* 22 (1996): 216–21.

82. David C. Hadorn, "Setting Health Care Priorities in Oregon: Cost-Effectiveness Meets the Rule of Rescue," *Journal of the American Medical Association* 265 (May 1, 1991): 2218. See, further, Peter Ubel, D. Scanlon, and M. Kamlet, "Individual Utilities Are Inconsistent with Rationing Choices: A Partial Explanation of Why Oregon's Cost-Effectiveness List Failed," *Medical Decision Making* 16 (1996): 108–16. See also John McKie and Jeff Richardson, "The Rule of Rescue," *Social Science & Medicine* 56 (2003): 2407–19.

7

Justice

Inequalities in access to health care, in health insurance, and in health status, combined with dramatic increases in the costs of health care, have fueled debates about what social justice requires of particular societies and of the global community. But is *inequality* a problem of justice? Should all age groups have equal access to health care resources? Do all persons in all countries have an equal claim on global resources? In attempting to answer such questions, we encounter uncertainty over how to reconcile, for example, fair access to health care, the alleviation of global poverty, the freedom to choose a health plan, a free-market economy, social efficiency, and the beneficent state.

In "The Lottery in Babylon," Jorge Luis Borges depicts a society that distributes all social benefits and burdens solely on the basis of a periodic lottery.[1] Each person is assigned a social role such as slave, factory owner, priest, or executioner, purely by the lottery. This random selection system disregards achievement, training, merit, experience, contribution, need, deprivation, and effort. The ethical and political oddity of the system described in Borges's story is jolting because assigning positions in this way does not cohere with conventional standards. Borges's system appears capricious and unfair, because we expect valid principles of justice to determine how social burdens, benefits, opportunities, and positions ought to be allocated.

However, if we attempt to specify principles of justice for the many contexts in which they might be invoked, they seem as elusive as the lottery method seems capricious. The construction of a comprehensive and unified theory of justice that captures our diverse conceptions is even more elusive. Moreover, many principles of justice that have been proposed in biomedical ethics are not distinct from and independent of other principles, such as nonmaleficence and beneficence.[2]

We begin this chapter by analyzing the terms *justice* and *distributive justice*. Later we examine substantive principles of justice, problems of national and international policy, and complicated and sometimes intractable moral problems of social justice in several areas.

THE CONCEPT OF JUSTICE

The terms *fairness, desert* (what is deserved), and *entitlement* have been used by various philosophers in attempts to explicate *justice*. These accounts interpret justice as fair, equitable, and appropriate treatment in light of what is due or owed to persons. Standards of justice are needed whenever persons are due benefits or burdens because of their particular properties or circumstances, such as being productive or having been harmed by another person's acts. A holder of a valid claim based in justice has a right, and therefore is due something. An injustice involves a wrongful act or omission that denies people resources or protections to which they have a right.

The term *distributive justice* refers to fair, equitable, and appropriate distribution determined by justified norms that structure the terms of social cooperation.[3] Its scope includes policies that allot diverse benefits and burdens such as property, resources, taxation, privileges, and opportunities. *Distributive justice* refers broadly to the distribution of all rights and responsibilities in society, including civil and political rights. It is distinguished from other types of justice, including *criminal* justice, which refers to the just infliction of punishment, and *rectificatory* justice, which refers to just compensation for transactional problems such as breaches of contracts and malpractice.

A compelling example of distributive justice appears in the history of research involving human subjects. Until the 1990s, the paradigm for ethical analysis focused on the risks and burdens of research, especially nontherapeutic research, and on the need to protect potential and actual research subjects from harm, abuse, and exploitation. The regulation of research sought to protect vulnerable persons from exploitation in scientific efforts to benefit others. The dominant model in protectionist policies is research that offers no prospect of direct therapeutic benefit to the subject. The concern is about an unfair distribution of burdens. However, a paradigm shift occurred in the 1990s, in part because of the interest of patients with HIV/AIDS in gaining access to new, experimental drugs within as well as outside of clinical trials. The focus shifted to the possible benefits of clinical trials and deemphasizing their risks. As a result, justice as fair access to research (participation in research and access to the results of research) became as important as protection from exploitation.[4]

No single principle can address all problems of justice. Several principles of justice arguably merit acceptance. One principle is *formal*, the others *material*. In this chapter we discuss how to specify and balance these principles. Sometimes conditions of scarcity force a society to make "tragic choices." In these situations, principles of justice may be infringed, compromised, or sacrificed.[5]

The Formal Principle of Justice

Common to all theories of justice is a minimal requirement traditionally attrib-
uted to Aristotle: Equals must be treated equally, and unequals must be treated
unequally. This principle of formal justice (sometimes called the *principle of
formal equality*) is "formal" because it identifies no particular respects in which
equals ought to be treated equally and provides no criteria for determining
whether two or more individuals are in fact equals. It merely asserts that persons
equal in *whatever* respects are the relevant respects should be treated equally.

   This formal principle lacks all substance. That equals ought to be treated
equally provokes no debate. But how shall we express *equality,* and which
differences are relevant in comparing individuals or groups? Presumably, all
citizens should have equal political rights, equal access to public services, and
equal treatment under the law. But how far should equality extend? A typical
problem in bioethics is the following: Virtually all accounts of justice in health
care hold that delivery programs and services designed to assist persons of
a certain class, such as the poor, the elderly, or the disabled should be made
available to all members of *that class.* To deny benefits to some when others in
the same class receive benefits is unjust. But is it also unjust to deny access to
equally needy persons outside of the delineated class, such as workers with no
health insurance?

Material Principles of Justice

Principles that specify the relevant characteristics for equal treatment are called
material because they identify the substantive properties for distribution. One
such principle is the principle of need, which declares that social resources,
including health care, should be distributed according to need. To say that a
person needs something is to say that, without it, the person will be harmed, or
at least detrimentally affected. However, we are not required to distribute all
goods and services to satisfy all needs, such as needs for athletic equipment and
antilock brakes. Presumably our obligations are limited to *fundamental needs.*
To say that someone has a fundamental need is to say that the person will be
harmed or detrimentally affected in a fundamental way if the need is not fulfilled. For example, the person might be harmed through malnutrition, bodily
injury, or nondisclosure of critical information. In bioethics literature it is widely
held that health care is a special good and that needs for it are special needs for
a theory of justice.

   If we were to analyze the notion of fundamental needs, we could progressively specify and shape the material principle of need into a public policy for
purposes of distribution. For the moment, however, we are emphasizing only
the significance of the step of accepting the principle of need as a valid material

principle of justice. This principle is only one among the set of plausible material principles of justice. If, by contrast, one were to accept only a principle of free-market distribution, then one would oppose a principle of need as a basis for public policy. All public and institutional policies based on distributive justice ultimately derive from the acceptance or rejection of some material principles and some procedures for specifying, refining, or balancing them, and many disputes over the right policy of distribution spring from rival, or at least alternative, starting points using different material principles.

Each of the following principles has been proposed as a valid, general material principle of distributive justice (as have other principles).[6]

1. To each person an equal share
2. To each person according to need
3. To each person according to effort
4. To each person according to contribution
5. To each person according to merit
6. To each person according to free-market exchanges

No obvious barrier prevents acceptance of more than one of these principles, and some theories of justice accept all six as valid. A plausible moral thesis is that each of these material principles identifies a prima facie obligation whose weight cannot be assessed independently of particular goods and domains in which it is applicable. Most societies invoke several of these material principles in framing public policies, appealing to different principles in different contexts. For example, unemployment subsidies, welfare payments, and many health care programs are distributed on the basis of need (and to some extent on criteria such as previous length of employment); jobs and promotions in many sectors are awarded on the basis of demonstrated achievement and merit; the higher incomes of some persons are allowed and often encouraged on grounds of free-market wage scales, superior effort, merit, or potential social contribution; and, at least theoretically, the opportunity for a basic education is distributed to all citizens.

Conflicts among the preceding principles create a serious priority problem as well as a challenge to a moral system that aims for a coherent framework of principles. These conflicts indicate the vital need for both specification and balancing of these principles.

Relevant Properties

Material principles identify relevant properties that persons must possess to qualify for a particular distribution, but theoretical and practical difficulties confront the justification of allegedly relevant properties. Tradition, convention, and moral and legal principle can and do function in some cases to establish relevant properties. However, in many contexts it is appropriate either to institute a new policy establishing relevant properties where none previously existed or to develop a new policy that revises established criteria. For example, a country needs to establish a policy about whether nonresident aliens will be allowed on waiting lists for cadaveric organ transplantation in that country. It thus has to decide whether citizenship is a relevant property and, if so, on what basis and in what ways.

Courts sometimes mandate policies that revise entrenched notions about relevant properties. For example, the United States Supreme Court decided in the case of *Auto Workers v. Johnson Controls, Inc.*[7] that employers cannot legally adopt "fetal protection policies" that specifically exclude women of childbearing age from a hazardous workplace, because these policies discriminate illegally based on gender. Under the policy that was challenged, only fertile men could choose whether they wished to assume reproductive risks. The majority of justices held that this policy used the irrelevant property of gender even though mutagenic substances affect sperm as well as eggs.

These problems again show that abstract principles provide only rough guidelines for forming specific policies or taking concrete actions. We need further moral argument that specifies and balances principles. However, many philosophers believe that a general framework or theory of justice can provide assistance, a subject to which we turn now.

THEORIES OF JUSTICE

Theories of distributive justice attempt to connect properties of persons with morally justifiable distributions of benefits and burdens. Philosophers have proposed several theories to determine how to distribute, or, in some cases, redistribute, social burdens and goods and services, including health care.

Several types of theory have been influential: *Utilitarian* theories emphasize a mixture of criteria for the purpose of maximizing public utility; *libertarian* theories emphasize rights to social and economic liberty, invoking fair procedures rather than substantive outcomes; *communitarian* theories stress the principles and practices of justice that evolve through traditions and practices in a community; and *egalitarian* theories emphasize equal access to the goods in life that every rational person values, often invoking material criteria of need and equality. We also, in a later section, consider *cosmopolitan* theories.

We can expect these theories to succeed only partially in bringing coherence and comprehensiveness to our fragmented visions of social justice. Policies for health care access and distribution in many countries provide an example of the problems that confront these theories. Many countries seek to provide the best available health care for all citizens, while protecting public resources through cost-containment programs. They also promote the ideal of equal access to health care for everyone, including the indigent, while maintaining aspects of a competitive, free-market environment. These laudable goals of superior care, equal access, free choice, and social efficiency are extremely difficult to render coherent in a social system. Different conceptions of the just society underlie them, and pursuing one goal may undercut another.

Utilitarian Theories

Utilitarian theories, which are treated in more detail in Chapter 9, regard distributive justice as one among several problems of maximizing value. Utilitarians argue that the standard of justice depends on the principle of utility, which demands that we seek to maximize social welfare. Justice, they contend, is merely the name for the paramount and most stringent forms of obligation created by the principle of utility. Typically, utilitarian obligations of justice establish correlative rights for individuals that in this theory should be enforced by law, if necessary. These rights are strictly contingent upon social arrangements that maximize net social utility. Rights have no other basis, and disputes emerge even among utilitarians as to whether rights have a meaningful place in moral theory. However, if a system of rights is justified entirely on the grounds that its existence will maximize social utility, utilitarians cannot consistently object to rights.

Nevertheless, various moral problems surround the use of utilitarian principles to justify rights. Individual rights, such as the right to health care, have a tenuous foundation when they rest on overall utility maximization, because social utility could change at any time. Furthermore, some utilitarian approaches neglect considerations of justice governing how benefits and burdens are distributed. For example, it would be unjust for a society to maximize utility by denying access to health care for some of its sickest and most vulnerable populations, yet some utilitarian theories seem committed to such a policy.

While utilitarian moral theories present problems for theory of justice, these theories help in forming just health policies, as we often note in this chapter.

Libertarian Theories

The United States has traditionally, although not exclusively, accepted the free-market ideal that distributions of health care are best left to the marketplace, which operates on the material principle of ability to pay, either directly or indirectly through insurance. Under this conception, a just society protects rights of property and liberty, allowing persons to improve their circumstances and protect their health on their own initiative. Health care is not a right, and the ideal health care system is privatized. A libertarian interpretation of justice focuses neither on public utility nor on meeting the health needs of citizens, but on the unfettered operation of fair procedures under conditions of law and order.

One libertarian, Robert Nozick, argues for an "entitlement theory" of justice in which government action is justified if and only if it protects citizens' liberty and property rights.[8] He contends that a theory of justice should affirm individual rights rather than create patterns of economic distribution in which governments redistribute the wealth acquired by persons under the free market. Governments act coercively and unjustly when they tax the wealthy at a progressively higher rate than those who are less wealthy, and then use the proceeds to underwrite state support of the indigent through welfare payments and unemployment compensation.

Nozick proposes three principles of justice, all centered on private property rights: justice in acquisition, justice in transfer, and justice in rectification. More specifically, no pattern of just distribution exists independent of free-market procedures of acquiring property, legitimately transferring that property, and providing rectification for those whose property was illegitimately taken or who otherwise were illegitimately obstructed in the free market. Accordingly, justice consists in the operation of just procedures, not in the production of just outcomes (such as an equal distribution of health resources). There are no welfare rights, and therefore no rights or claims to health care can be based on justice.

Libertarians do not oppose utilitarian or egalitarian patterns of distribution if these patterns are freely chosen by participants. Any distribution of goods, including public health measures and health care, is just and justified if and only if individuals in the relevant group freely choose it. As a result, libertarians generally support a health care system in which health care insurance is privately and voluntarily purchased. In this system, the state does not coercively take anyone's personal property to benefit another. Investors in health care and insured persons have property rights, physicians have liberty rights, and society is not morally obligated to provide health care. Indeed, society is morally obligated to refrain from providing funds by coercive taxation and from assigning physicians by conscription.

Communitarian Theories

Communitarians react negatively to models of society (such as those developed by Mill, Rawls, and Nozick) that base human relationships on rights and contracts and that attempt to construct a single theory of justice by which to judge every society. Communitarians regard principles of justice as pluralistic, deriving from as many different conceptions of the good as there are diverse moral communities. What is owed to individuals and groups depends on these community-derived standards.[9]

Communitarians emphasize the responsibility of the community to the individual and the responsibility of the individual to the community. Some communitarians eschew the language of justice and adopt the language of solidarity, which is both a personal virtue of commitment and a principle of social morality.

For example, in the Netherlands solidarity is sometimes viewed as a collective obligation. A report of a Committee assembled under the Dutch Secretary for Public Health argued that supplying certain health services and goods is "consonant with the basic values of Dutch society." The report assigned an "absolute priority... to care for the elderly, the handicapped, and psychiatric patients."[10]

Some communitarian writers in biomedical ethics assign major roles to both personal choice and community. For example, Ezekiel Emanuel envisions small deliberative democratic communities that develop shared conceptions of the good life and justice.[11] He proposes thousands of community health programs (CHPs), each involving citizen-members who join in a federation. Justice resides in the guarantee that services will be provided to fulfill community-endorsed social goals.

Egalitarian Theories

Egalitarian theories of justice hold that persons should receive an equal distribution of certain goods such as health care, but no prominent egalitarian theory requires equal sharing of all possible social benefits. Qualified egalitarianism requires only some basic equalities among individuals and permits inequalities that benefit the least advantaged.

John Rawls's theory of justice, the most celebrated recent egalitarian theory, challenges libertarian, utilitarian, and communitarian theories. He argues that "what justifies a conception of justice is not its being true to an order antecedent and given to us, but its congruence with our deeper understanding of ourselves and our aspirations."[12] A theory of justice matches our commonly accepted judgments of fairness with our general principles. Rawls argues that impartial persons would agree on two fundamental principles of justice. The first requires that each person be permitted the maximum amount of basic liberty compatible with a similar measure of liberty for others. The second stipulates that once this equal basic liberty is assured, inequalities in social primary goods (including, for example, income, rights, and opportunities) are to be allowed only if they benefit everyone and if they are attached to positions open to all based on fair equality of opportunity. Rawls considers social institutions just if, and only if, they conform to these two basic principles.

Although Rawls never pursued the implications of his theory for health policy, others have. In an influential interpretation and extension, Norman Daniels argues for a just health care system based primarily on a Rawlsian principle of "fair equality of opportunity." Daniels argues that health care needs are special and that fair opportunity is central to any acceptable theory of justice. Social institutions affecting health care distribution thus should be arranged, as far as possible, to allow each person to achieve a fair share of the normal range of opportunities present in that society.

This theory, like Rawls's, recognizes a positive societal obligation to reduce or eliminate barriers that prevent fair equality of opportunity, an obligation that extends to programs to correct or compensate for various disadvantages. It views disease and disability as undeserved restrictions on persons' opportunities to realize basic goals. Health care, then, is needed to achieve, maintain, or restore adequate or "species-typical" levels of functioning so that individuals can realize basic goals. A health care system designed to meet these needs should attempt to prevent disease, illness, or injury from reducing the range of opportunity open to the individual. The allocation of health care resources, then, is constructed to ensure justice through fair equality of opportunity.[13]

This Rawls-inspired theory has far-reaching egalitarian implications for national health policy, and perhaps for international policy as well. On this account, each member of society, irrespective of wealth or position, would have equal access to an adequate, although not maximal, level of health care—the exact level of access being contingent on available social resources and public processes of decision making. We return to this issue in the later section "The Right to a Decent Minimum of Health Care."

Later in this chapter, we also discuss "cosmopolitan" theories, which are built on egalitarian foundations. We do not attempt to assess the relative merits of the theories. Rather, we use the theories as resources. Among the most influential elements of egalitarian thinking, especially in Rawlsian theory, is the role of the rule of fair opportunity in a theory of social justice, a topic to which we now turn.

FAIR OPPORTUNITY AND UNFAIR DISCRIMINATION

What kind of fair opportunity in life does justice require? To address this question, we consider first certain properties that have often served, unjustly, as bases of distribution. These properties include gender, race, IQ, linguistic accent, ethnicity, national origin, and social status. In anomalous contexts these properties may be relevant and acceptable. But general rules such as "To each according to gender" and "To each according to IQ" are unacceptable material principles. These properties are irrelevant, discriminatory, and based on differences for which the affected individual is not responsible.

The Fair-Opportunity Rule

The fair-opportunity rule says that no persons should receive social benefits on the basis of undeserved advantageous properties (because no persons are responsible for having these properties) and that no persons should be denied social benefits on the basis of undeserved disadvantageous properties (because they also are not responsible for these properties). Properties distributed by the lotteries of social and biological life do not provide grounds for morally accept-able discrimination between persons in social allocations if people do not have a fair chance to acquire or overcome these properties.

The attempt to supply all citizens with a basic education raises moral prob-lems analogous to those in health care. Imagine a community that offers a high-quality education to all students with basic abilities, regardless of gender or race, but does not offer a comparable educational opportunity to students with reading difficulties or mental deficiencies. This system is unjust. The students with dis-abilities lack basic skills and need special training to overcome their problems. They should receive an education suitable to their needs and opportunities, even if it costs more. The fair-opportunity rule requires that they receive the benefits needed to ameliorate the unfortunate effects of life's lottery. By analogy, persons with functional disabilities lack capacity and need health care to reach a higher level of function and have a fair chance in life. If they are responsible for their disabilities, they might not be entitled to health care services. But if they are not responsible, the fair-opportunity rule demands that they receive that which will help them reduce or overcome the unfortunate effects of life's lottery of health.

Mitigating the Negative Effects of Life's Lotteries

Numerous properties might be disadvantageous and undeserved—for example, a squeaky voice, an ugly face, inarticulate speech, an inadequate early educa-tion, malnutrition, or disease. But which undeserved properties create a right *in justice* to some form of assistance?

One hypothesis is that virtually all abilities and disabilities are functions of what Rawls calls the natural lottery and the social lottery. "Natural lottery" refers to the distribution of advantageous and disadvantageous genetic proper-ties, and "social lottery" refers to the distribution of assets or deficits through family property, school systems, government agencies, and the like. It is possible that all talents and disabilities result from heredity, natural environment, family upbringing, education, inheritance, and the like, in some combination. From this perspective, even the ability to work long hours, the ability to compete, and a warm smile are biologically, environmentally, and socially engendered. If so, talents, abilities, and successes are not to our credit, just as genetic disease is acquired through no fault of the afflicted person.

Rawls uses fair opportunity as a rule of redress. To overcome disadvantag-ing conditions (whether from biology or society) that are not deserved, the rule demands compensation for disadvantages. The full implications of this approach are uncertain, but his conclusions are challenging:

> [A free-market arrangement] permits the distribution of wealth and income
> to be determined by the natural distribution of abilities and talents. Within
> the limits allowed by the background arrangements, distributive shares

are decided by the outcome of the natural lottery; and this outcome is arbitrary from a moral perspective. There is no more reason to permit the distribution of income and wealth to be settled by the distribution of natural assets than by historical and social fortune. Furthermore, the principle of fair opportunity can be only imperfectly carried out, at least as long as the institution of the family exists. The extent to which natural capacities develop and reach fruition is affected by all kinds of social conditions and class attitudes. Even the willingness to make an effort, to try, and so to be deserving in the ordinary sense is itself dependent upon happy family and social circumstances.[14]

At a minimum, current social systems of distributing benefits and burdens would undergo massive revision if this approach were accepted. Rather than allowing broad inequalities in social distribution based on effort, contribution, and merit, justice is achieved only if radical inequalities are reduced. Inequalities are permissible only if disadvantaged persons benefited more from them than from an equal distribution of benefits.

At some point the process of reducing inequalities introduced by life's lotteries must stop, and at that point persons who are disadvantaged will lose meaningful protection by the fair-opportunity rule.[15] Libertarians rightly stress that limited resources will constrain the implementation of this rule, but they draw the line at a different place. Some disadvantages are merely *unfortunate,* they argue, whereas others are *unfair,* and therefore obligatory in justice to correct. Tristram Engelhardt has argued that society should call a halt to claims of fairness or justice precisely at the point of this distinction between the unfair and the unfortunate.[16]

However, we argue that the problems addressed in this chapter create a need for criteria other than the distinction between the unfortunate and the unfair, a criterion that may only beg the central questions of what is fair. We will see that no bright lines distinguish the unfair from the unfortunate or fair from unfair allocation schemes. Nevertheless, if one accepts the fair-opportunity rule, as we do, it will deeply affect moral reflection about health policy and other areas.

Racial, Ethnic, and Gender Disparities in Health Care

Disparities in health care based on racial and gender properties are social problems that fall under the fair-opportunity rule. Health care has often been covertly distributed on the basis of these properties, resulting in a differential impact in many countries on the health of racial and ethnic minorities as well as women.[17] Many studies in the United States indicate that blacks and women have poorer access to various forms of health care in comparison to white males. For example, gender and racial inequities in employment have an impact on job-based health insurance; and the race and gender of physicians often play a role in the quality of patient–physician interaction.[18]

In the face of apparent disparities, studies conducted in various parts of the health care system have led to efforts, partially successful but largely unsuccessful, to overcome racial and ethnic disparities.[19] One controversy centers on the rates of coronary artery bypass grafting (CABG) between white and black Medicare patients, as well as between male and female Medicare patients. Differences have been evident since the mid-1980s in many parts of the United States.[20] Differences in need cannot entirely account for the variance, and it remains unclear to what extent the rates can be explained by physician supply, poverty, awareness of health care opportunities, reluctance among blacks and women to undergo surgery, and racial prejudice. One study found that, after controlling for age, payer, and appropriateness and necessity for CABG, African American patients in New York State had significant access problems unrelated to patient refusals.[21] Disparities also appear in the management of acute myocardial infarction[22] and in the care of chronic conditions such as glucose control for patients with diabetes or cholesterol control among patients with cardiovascular disorders.[23]

A major report from the Institute of Medicine on racial and ethnic disparities in health care identifies several "unacceptable" racial and ethnic disparities across a wide range of medical conditions and health care services, leading to "worse health outcomes."[24] While insurance status, income, and level of education are important in access, the report stresses that other, independent factors are also significant. These include the broader context of historic and continuing social and economic inequality; patient-level variables such as cultural preferences and some biological differences; system-level factors, such as language barriers, time constraints in health care, geographic availability; and care process-level variables, including bias, stereotyping, and uncertainty based in part on racial and ethnic differences and on the clinician's need to make medical decisions under the pressure of time and with limited information.[25]

Renal transplantation provides another informative case study because financial barriers play a less significant role in kidney transplantation than in most other areas of health care. The federal End-Stage Renal Disease (ESRD) Program ensures coverage for kidney dialysis and transplantation for virtually everyone who needs them if their private insurance does not provide the coverage. However, concerns about costs can still be a factor because immunosuppressant medications needed for life are not covered under the ESRD program after three years. Evidence suggests that discrimination against blacks, other minorities, and women occurs leading up to and at the point of referral to transplantation centers and admission to waiting lists, where criteria may vary considerably. For instance, blacks are much less likely than whites to be referred for evaluation at transplant centers and to be placed on a waiting list or to receive a transplant.[26] Factors include minority distrust of the system (in part based on prior experience), delayed or limited access to health care, and inadequate guidance through the system by health care professionals.

Once patients are admitted to the waiting list, the criteria for selecting recipients of donated cadaveric organs are public and are, to a significant extent, represented through point systems. Disputes continue about how much weight to give to different factors in the distribution of kidneys for transplantation, with particular attention to human lymphocyte antigen (HLA) matching. The degree of HLA match between a donor and a recipient affects the long-term survival of the transplanted kidney. However, assigning priority to tissue matching—and giving less weight to time on the waiting list and other factors—has been shown to produce "disparate effects" for minorities. Most organ donors are white; certain HLA phenotypes are different in white, black, and Hispanic populations; and the identification of HLA phenotypes is less complete for blacks and Hispanics. Yet nonwhites have a higher rate of end-stage renal disease and are also disproportionately represented on dialysis rolls. Blacks on the waiting list also, on average, wait much longer than whites to receive a first kidney transplant, if they receive one at all.

In an interim report on one policy change, analysts predicted that eliminating the relevant HLA matching (HLA-B) as a priority would increase the number of kidney transplantations among nonwhites by 6.0% while reducing the number for whites by 4.0% and, at the same time, increasing the rate of graft loss by 2.0%. They conclude that, "Such a change would reduce the tension inherent in the current allocation policy by improving equity without sacrificing utility."[27] Normatively, the tension between utility and providing fair opportunity persists, and critics have challenged the use of "disparate impact tests" to shift from policies that seek to maximize the number of quality-adjusted life-years per organ to trying to increase the access of racial or ethnic groups to transplantation.[28]

The problems plaguing minority patients are similar to those facing women patients. Several years ago, the Council on Ethical and Judicial Affairs of the American Medical Association examined data that raised concerns about whether women are disadvantaged because of inadequate attention to research, diagnosis, and treatment of their health problems.[29] The Council found gender disparities, for example, in the diagnosis and treatment of cardiac disease. Biological differences do not account for these disparities. The Council notes that gender bias need not be manifest in an overt manner. Social attitudes involving stereotypes, prejudices, and gender-role attributions may be present, including the attribution of women's health complaints to emotional rather than physical causes. In the use of diagnostic and therapeutic procedures for patients with coronary heart disease, for example, evidence exists that men and women are treated differently for reasons that appear unrelated to their medical conditions.

In a review of studies of cardiovascular disease, the leading cause of women's death, women were less aggressively screened and treated for cholesterol problems than men.[30] However, in a sign of progress beginning in 2004, virtually the same percentage of women and men with Medicare received recommended care in the hospital following a heart attack.[31] In another area, HIV-infected women were less likely than HIV-infected men to be placed on highly active antiretroviral therapy and to receive medications to prevent possible opportunistic infections.[32]

In short, while some disparities in health care for women and men have declined, others persist. The best available interpretations of known causal factors suggest many violations of the fair-opportunity rule.

VULNERABILITY AND EXPLOITATION

We turn now to some quite different problems of fair opportunity. These are not problems of health care distribution, but problems about the vulnerability of human research subjects at risk of exploitation. We concentrate on the recruitment and enrollment in clinical research (primarily pharmaceutical trials) of the economically disadvantaged, who are often disadvantaged by the social lottery.

By "economically disadvantaged," we mean persons who are impoverished, may lack significant access to health care, may be homeless, may be malnourished, and so forth, and yet possess mental capacity to "volunteer" in, for example, safety and toxicity (phase I) drug studies. Thus, we are considering only persons who possess a basic competence to reason, deliberate, decide, and consent. Data indicate that somewhere between 50% and 100% of research subjects who are healthy volunteers self-report that financial need or financial reward is their primary motive for volunteering.[33] We know that such persons are involved in some research in North America, but we do not know the full extent of their involvement, just as we do not know the scope of the use of poor persons as research subjects in other parts of the world, including developing countries. [34]

Vulnerability and Vulnerable Groups

It should not be assumed that there is a straightforward connection between economically disadvantaged groups and vulnerability or between vulnerability and exploitation by researchers. The connections are subtle and the concepts complicated. The literature has sometimes viewed the class of the economically disadvantaged who are vulnerable as narrow, at other times broad. Those so classified may or may not include individuals living on the streets, low-income persons who are the sole financial support of a large family, persons desperately lacking access to health care, persons whose income falls below a certain threshold level, and so forth. Their situation of economic distress could be long-term or only temporary.

The notion of a "vulnerable group" was considered very significant in bioethics and health policy between the 1970s and the early 1990s. However, over the years it has suffered from overexpansion because so many groups have now been declared vulnerable—from the infirm elderly, to the undereducated, to those with inadequate resources, to whole countries whose members lack rights or are subject to exploitation.[35] The language of "vulnerable groups" suggests that all members of a vulnerable group—for example, all prisoners, all poor people, and all pregnant women—are by category vulnerable. The problem is that for many groups a label covering all members of the group serves to overprotect, stereotype, and even disqualify members capable of making their own decisions.[36] "Vulnerable" is an inappropriate label for any class of persons when some members of the class are not vulnerable in the relevant respects. For example, pregnant women as a class are not vulnerable, although some pregnant women are. Accordingly, we do not speak of the economically disadvantaged as a categorically vulnerable group. Instead, we speak of *vulnerabilities.* Ideally, research ethics can supply a schema of forms and conditions of vulnerability, rather than a list of vulnerable groups.[37]

The concept of vulnerability. In biomedical ethics, the notion of vulnerability often focuses on a person's susceptibility, whether as a result of internal or external factors, to inducement or coercion, on the one hand, or to harm, loss, or indignity, on the other.[38] The economically disadvantaged may be vulnerable in several ways to influences that introduce a significant risk of harm. Their situation may leave them lacking in critical resources and forms of social powers that might have been created on their behalf. Hence, they may not be able to resist or refuse acceptance of the risk involved, requiring trade-offs among their interests.[39]

Categorical exclusion of the economically disadvantaged? A tempting strategy to protect their interests is to exclude economically disadvantaged persons categorically, even if they are not categorically vulnerable. This remedy would eliminate the problem of their unjust exploitation, but it would deprive them of the freedom to choose and would often be harmful to their financial interests. Nothing about economically disadvantaged persons justifies their exclusion, as a group, from participation in research, just as it does not follow from their status as disadvantaged that they should be excluded from participation in any legal activity. To be sure, there is an increased risk of taking advantage of the economically distressed, but to exclude them categorically would be an inexcusable, paternalistic form of discrimination and deprivation of fair opportunity that may only serve to further marginalize, deprive, stigmatize, or discriminate against them.

Consider the weakly analogous case of what has long been the paradigm of competent persons who are categorically excluded from phase I clinical trials—namely, prisoners. The right to volunteer as a research subject has been denied to prisoners in most nations on grounds of the potential for manipulation or coercion in penal institutions.[40] Were this same potential to exist for economically disadvantaged persons, the same categorical exclusion might be appropriate. However, this problem needs to be examined in each context to determine if competent persons, whatever their vulnerabilities, are able to consent freely in that circumstance.

We turn now to the major moral problems about enrolling the economically disadvantaged in research: undue inducement, undue profit, and exploitation.

Undue Inducement, Undue Profit, and Exploitation

Some persons report feeling heavily pressured to enroll in clinical trials, even though their enrollment is correctly classified as voluntary.[41] These individuals are in desperate need of money. Attractive offers of money and other goods can leave a person with a sense of having no meaningful choice but to accept research participation. Such a person feels constrained by influences that many individuals easily resist.

Constraining situations. In these constraining situations—sometimes mis-leadingly termed *coercive* situations—there is no coercion, strictly speaking, because no one has intentionally issued a threat to gain compliance. (See our discussion of coercion in Chapter 4.) A person feels controlled by the constraints of a situation, such as severe illness or lack of food and shelter, rather than by the design or threat of another person. Sometimes people unintentionally make other persons feel "threatened" by their actions, and sometimes illness, power-lessness, and lack of resources are perceived as harms that a person feels com-pelled to prevent or ameliorate. These situations significantly constrain choices, even though they do not involve threats. The prospect of another night on the streets or another day without food can constrain a person to accept an offer of research participation, just as such conditions could constrain a person to accept an unpleasant or risky job that the person would otherwise not accept. A person can rightly report in both cases, "I had no choice; it was unthinkable to refuse the offer."

Undue inducement. In constraining situations, monetary payments and related offers such as shelter or food give rise to questions of *undue inducement,* on the one hand, and *undue profit,* on the other. The "Common Rule" in the United States requires investigators to "minimize the possibility of" coercion and undue inducement, but it does not define, analyze, or explain these notions.[42] The bioethics and public policy literatures also do not adequately handle issues of exploitation, undue inducement, and undue profit.

Monetary payments seem unproblematic if the payments are welcome offers that persons do not want to refuse and the risks are at the level of everyday activities.[43] But inducements become increasingly problematic as (1) risks are increased, (2) more attractive inducements are introduced, and (3) the subjects' economic disadvantage is increased. The problem of exploitation centers on whether solicited persons are situationally disadvantaged and without viable alternatives, feel forced or compelled to accept attractive offers that they otherwise would not accept, and assume increased risk in their lives. As these conditions are mitigated, the problem of exploitation diminishes and may vanish. As these conditions are increased, the problem of exploitation looms larger.

The presence of an irresistibly attractive offer is a *necessary* condition of "undue inducement," but this condition is not by itself *sufficient* to make an inducement *undue*. A situation of undue inducement must also involve a person's assumption of a sufficiently serious risk of harm that he or she would not ordinarily assume. We will not try to pinpoint a precise threshold level of risk, but it would have to be above the level of common job risks such as those of unskilled construction work. Inducements are not undue unless they are both above the level of standard risk (hence "excessive" in risk) and irresistibly attractive (hence "excessive" in payment) in light of a constraining situation. Although these offers are not coercive, because no *threat* of excessive risk or of taking money away from the person is involved, the offer can still be manipulative. Indeed, since irresistibly attractive payment is involved, these offers almost certainly should be categorized as manipulative, although not necessarily as unjustifiably manipulative (see analysis of these distinctions in Chapter 4, pp. 133–35).

Undue profit. Undue inducements should be distinguished from *undue profits,* which occur from a distributive injustice of too small a payment, rather than an irresistibly attractive, large payment. In the undue-profit situation, the subject of research receives an unfairly low payment, while the sponsor of research gets more than is justified. Often, this seems to be what critics of pharmaceutical research believe happens: Those approached are in a weak to nonexistent bargaining situation, constrained by their poverty, and are given a pitifully small amount of money and unjust share of the benefits, while companies reap unseemly profits. If this is the worry, the basic question is how to determine a nonexploitative, fair payment.

How should we handle these two moral problems of exploitation—undue inducement (unduly large and irresistible payments) and undue profit (unduly small and unfair payments)? One possible answer is that if the research involves excessive risk, it should be prohibited categorically, even if a good oversight system is in place. This answer is appealing, but we would still need to determine what constitutes excessive risk, irresistibly attractive payment, unjust underpayment, and constraining situations—all difficult and unresolved problems.

The moral dilemma can be very challenging here: To avoid undue inducement, payment schedules must be kept reasonably low, approximating an unskilled labor wage, or possibly even lower. Even at this low level, payment might still be sufficiently large to constitute an undue inducement for some research subjects. As payments are lowered to avoid undue inducement, research subjects (in some circumstances) will be recruited largely or entirely from the ranks of the economically disadvantaged. Somewhere on this continuum the amount of money paid will be so little that it is exploitative by virtue of undue profits yielded by taking advantage of a person's misfortune. If the payment scales were increased to avoid undue profit, they would at some point become high enough to attract persons from the middle class. At or around this point, the offers would be declared excessively attractive and judged undue inducements for impoverished persons interested in the payments.[44] This dilemma becomes a profound problem of potential injustice if the pool of research subjects is comprised more or less exclusively of the economically disadvantaged.

There may be situations in which payments that are too high (creating undue inducements) are, *at the same time,* payments that are too low (creating undue profits). To the desperate, $.25/hr. or $10/hr. might be irresistibly attractive, while distributively unfair. Critics charge that pharmaceutical companies routinely take advantage of such situations, but insufficient information is available at present for a definite judgment. However, from what we know, at least some contexts of research conducted in North America do not seem to involve either undue inducement or undue profit. Whatever the actual situation in North America or elsewhere, we have attempted to locate the moral problems that must be addressed and to consider possible paths to their resolution.

Finally, some brief comments are in order that should help frame discussion of these issues: An important reason for caution about prohibiting research or about encouraging pharmaceutical companies to pull out of poor communities is that payments for studies are a vital source of needed funds for the economically disadvantaged and a way to build an infrastructure and jobs in these communities.[45] One of the few readily available sources of money for some economically distressed persons are jobs such as day labor that expose them to more risk and generate less money than the payments generated by participation in phase I clinical trials.[46] To deny these persons the right to participate in clinical research on grounds of the potential exploitation already discussed can be paternalistic and demeaning, as well as economically distressing.

It is often unclear when a practice becomes a way to exploit the disadvantaged for the benefit of the privileged. This question of justice can be answered only by specifying and defending the precise conditions under which an arrangement is unfair—a task beyond the scope of this chapter. However, we ought not to assume that a fair system of incentives for research subjects cannot be constructed, including one with effective committee and regulatory oversight.

NATIONAL HEALTH POLICY AND THE RIGHT TO HEALTH CARE

Questions about who shall receive what share of a society's resources have generated many controversies about appropriate national health policies, unequal distributions of health advantages, and rationing of health-related goods and services. The primary economic barrier to health care access in many countries—most visibly the United States—is the lack of adequate insurance. Close to 50 million U.S. citizens (approximately 18% of the nonelderly population) lack health insurance of any kind.[47] Inadequate insurance affects persons who are uninsured, uninsurable, underinsured, or only occasionally insured. In many other countries the primary barriers to both health and health care are poverty and limited government resources. Problems of justice are very different in different parts of the world.

Some problems of unfairness arise in the United States because of the extraordinary reliance on employers for financing the system. Persons with medium to large size employers are not only better covered, but are also subsidized by tax breaks in the system. When employed persons who are not covered become ill, taxpayers rather than free-riding employers usually pick up the bill. The financing of health care is also regressive. Low-income families pay premiums comparable to and often higher than the premiums paid by high-income families, and many individuals who do not qualify for group coverage pay dramatically more for the same coverage than those who qualify in a group.

Despite various controversies, a social consensus appears to be emerging in the United States that all citizens should be able to secure equitable access to health care, including insurance coverage. The problem with this consensus is its content-thinness: Citizens and politicians disagree sharply on a range of solutions proffered to improve access, on the role of government in these solutions, and on methods of financing them. It is unclear whether such a fragile consensus can generate a secondary consensus about how to implement equitable access in public policy.

Arguments Supporting Rights to Health Care

Two main arguments support a moral right to government-funded health care: (1) an argument from collective social protection and (2) an argument from fair opportunity.

The first argument focuses on the similarities between health needs and other needs that government has conventionally protected. Threats to health are relevantly similar to threats presented by crime, fire, and pollution. Collective actions and resources have conventionally been used to resist such threats, and many collective schemes to protect health exist in virtually all societies, including programs of public health and environmental protection. Consistency suggests that critical health care assistance in response to threats to health should likewise be a collective responsibility. This argument by analogy makes an appeal to coherence: If the government has an obligation to provide one type of essential service, then it must have an obligation to provide another relevantly similar service.

This argument has been criticized on grounds that government responsibilities are nonobligatory and nonessential. However, this perspective is favored by few beyond those committed to libertarianism. On each of the nonlibertarian theories of justice previously explicated, the argument from other comparable government services successfully generates a public obligation to provide some level of goods and services to protect health. Relevant *dissimilarities* do exist between the individual good of health care and other public programs, including social goods such as public health. The argument from collective social protection therefore might seem to fail.

However, additional premises supporting the right to health care are found in society's right to expect a decent return on the investment it has made in physicians' education, funding for biomedical research, and funding for other parts of the medical system that pertain to health care. The return to be expected on this taxed investment is health care protection. The scope of protection extends beyond public health measures to training and research in medicine. Nevertheless, we cannot reasonably expect a direct individual return on all collective investments. Some investments seek only the discovery of cures or treatments, not the provision of cures and treatments once discovered. Even if the government funds drug research and regulates the drug industry, this activity does not justify the expectation that the government will subsidize or reimburse individuals' drug purchases. This first argument in support of a moral right to health care can secure only a decent return on our investment, not a full return or refund.

A second argument buttresses this first argument, by appeal to the fair-opportunity rule. The justice of social institutions should be judged by their tendency to counteract lack of opportunity caused by unpredictable misfortune over which the person has no meaningful control. The need for health care is greater among the seriously diseased and injured, because the costs of health care for them can be uncontrollable and overwhelming, particularly as health status worsens. Insofar as injury, disability, or disease creates profound disadvantages and reduces agents' capacity to function properly, justice requires that we use societal health care resources to counter these effects and to restore to persons a fair chance to use their capacities.[48]

The Right to a Decent Minimum of Health Care

An intractable problem about the right to health-related goods and services is how to specify the entitlements. One approach proposes a right of *equal access* to health resources. This goal might entail merely that all persons have a right not to be prevented from obtaining health care, but this right does not entail that others must provide anything in the way of goods, services, or resources. Although some libertarians favor this limited right, it is not a serious proposal from any other perspective. Any significant right of access to health care refers to a right to obtain specified goods and services to which every entitled person has an equal claim. A very demanding interpretation of this right requires that everyone have equal access to every good and service that is available to anyone. But unless the world's economic systems are radically revised, this conception of a right is utopian. Rights to health-related resources will always have limits.

The right to a *decent minimum* of health care is therefore an attractive one.[49] This moderate egalitarian point of view requires equal access only to fundamental health care and health-related resources. The first concern in this theory is that basic health care be universally accessible. To this end, the decent-minimum approach entails acceptance of a two-tiered system of health care: enforced social coverage for basic and catastrophic health needs (tier 1), together with voluntary private coverage for other health needs and desires (tier 2). At the second tier, better services, such as luxury hospital rooms and optional, cosmetic dental work, are available for purchase at personal expense. The first tier distributes health care based on need, and meets needs by universal access to basic services. This tier presumably covers at least public health protections and preventive care, primary care, acute care, and special social services for those with disabilities. In this conception, society's obligations are not limitless but fall under a general model of a safety net for everyone.

The decent minimum, so understood, offers a possible compromise among libertarians, utilitarians, communitarians, and egalitarians, because it incorporates some moral premises that each theory stresses. It guarantees basic health care for all on a premise of equal access while allowing unequal additional purchases by individual initiative, thereby mixing private and public forms of distribution. Utilitarians should find the proposal attractive because it serves to minimize public dissatisfaction, to maximize social utility, and to permit allocation decisions based on cost-effectiveness analysis. The egalitarian finds an opportunity to use an equal access principle and to see fair opportunity embedded in the distributional system. The communitarian perspective is also not neglected. A societal consensus about values, even if only rough and incomplete, is required for a practicable system. The common good is a basic point of reference for public deliberation about how to establish the decent minimum. Finally, the libertarian sees a substantial opportunity for free-market production and distribution. The two-tiered system provides indigent persons with opportunities for health care that would otherwise not be available to them, but leaves a tier for free choice and charity. In addition, various forms of competition and incentives may be used as tools to increase the system's productivity and the quality of health care.

A health care system that finds pockets of support from each of these four types of theory could also turn out to be the fairest approach to democratic reform of the system.[50] We do not now have—and are not likely ever to have—a single viable theory of social justice. Experience suggests that, while appeals to one of these accounts of justice work well in some contexts, each can fail or even yield disastrous results in others.

Although attractive theoretically, the decent-minimum proposal will be difficult to explicate and implement practically. The plan raises questions about whether society can fairly, consistently, and unambiguously devise a public policy that recognizes a right to care for primary needs without creating a right to expensive forms of treatment, such as liver transplantation, that reduce resources that could be put to use elsewhere. The model is purely programmatic until society delineates the decent minimum in operational terms.

In light of the current flux in national health systems, this task is probably the major problem confronting health policy in many, and perhaps all, countries today. (We include in its scope the problem of *setting priorities*; see the later section on this subject.) Fair public participation is indispensable in any process of setting the threshold of a decent minimum. When substantive standards are contested—for example, regarding a decent or sufficient level of health care—fair procedures will be our only recourse.

Public preferences should play a role in setting the decent minimum, as Ronald Dworkin proposes in his hypothetical test of what "ideal prudent insurers" would choose under stated conditions.[51] Dworkin rightly criticizes what he perceives to be an undue use of the "rescue principle." This principle asserts that it is intolerable when a society allows people to die who could have been saved by spending more money on health care. He argues that this principle grows out of an "insulation model" that treats health care as different from and superior to all other goods and that calls for its equal distribution even if society distributes no other goods equally. In place of this model, Dworkin proposes that we try to imagine a "prudent insurance" ideal, which envisions health care under "a free and unsubsidized market." This ideal market presupposes a fair distribution of wealth and income; full information about the benefits, costs, and risks of various medical procedures; and ignorance about the likelihood that any particular person will experience morbidity, either life-threatening or non-life-threatening, from diseases and accidents. Under these circumstances, whatever aggregate amount a well-informed community decides to spend on health care is just, as is the distribution pattern it chooses. Dworkin's strategy will be difficult to implement, but it should facilitate determination of what justice requires in the way of a decent minimum.

Forfeiting the Right to Health Care

If we assume that all citizens enjoy a right to a minimum of health care, can individuals forfeit that right even though they wish to preserve it? The question is whether a person forfeits the right to certain forms of care through actions that result in personal ill health and that generate health care needs. Examples include patients who acquired AIDS as a result of unsafe sexual activities or intravenous drug use, smokers with lung cancer, and alcoholics who develop liver disease. It is unfair, some charge, to ask individuals in an insurance scheme to pay higher premiums or taxes to support people who voluntarily engage in risky actions.[52] This conclusion does not conflict with the rule of fair opportunity, they argue, because risk-takers' voluntary actions reduced their opportunity.

However, many questions arise about how far society can fairly exclude risk-takers from coverage. First, it must be possible to identify and differentiate various causal factors in morbidity, such as natural causes, the social environment, and personal activities. Once these factors have been identified, solid evidence must establish that a particular disease or illness resulted from personal activities, rather than some other cause. Second, the personal activities in question must have been autonomous. If risks are unknown at the time of action, individuals cannot be justly held responsible for their choices.

It is virtually impossible to isolate causal factors in many cases of ill health because of complex causal links and limited knowledge. Medical needs often result from the conjunction of genetic predispositions, personal actions, effects of prior disease, and environmental and social conditions. The respective roles of these different factors are often impossible to establish, as in the example of whether a particular individual's lung cancer resulted from personal cigarette smoking, passive smoking, environmental pollution, occupational conditions, or heredity (or some combination of these causal conditions). If ill health is broadly rooted in socially induced causes such as environmental pollutants and infant feeding practices, then the class of diseases covered by the right to a decent minimum will presumably expand as evidence about the causal roles of these factors increases.

It would, nonetheless, be fair in many cases to require individuals to pay higher premiums or taxes if they accept well-documented risks that may result in costly medical attention. Risk-takers might be required to contribute more to particular pools, such as insurance plans, or to pay a tax on their risky conduct, such as an increased tax on cigarettes.

A vexing example of health policy problems has emerged for patients with alcohol-related end-stage liver failure (ESLF) who need liver transplants. Donated livers are scarce, and many patients suffering from end-stage liver failure die before they can obtain transplants. A major cause of ESLF is excessive alcohol intake that causes cirrhosis of the liver. Hence, the question arises whether patients who have alcohol-related ESLF should be excluded from waiting lists for liver transplants or should be given lower priority ratings. Arguments for their lower priority or total exclusion often appeal to the probability that they will resume a pattern of alcohol abuse and again experience ESLF, thereby wasting the transplanted liver. However, studies have demonstrated that patients with alcohol-related ESLF who receive a liver transplant and abstain from alcohol do as well as patients whose ESLF resulted from other causes (although conditions such as a smoking history complicate this generalization).[53] Thus, a good case exists for not excluding alcohol-related ESLF patients altogether, instead introducing conditions that require demonstrated and extended abstention from alcohol.

Nonetheless, Alvin Moss and Mark Siegler have proposed that patients with alcohol-related ESLF (over 50% of the patients with ESLF) automatically receive a lower priority ranking in the allocation of donated livers than patients who develop ESLF through no fault of their own.[54] Their argument appeals to fairness, fair opportunity, and utility. They argue that it is fair to hold people responsible for their decisions, and then to allocate organs with a view to utilitarian outcomes. They judge that it is "fairer to give a child dying of biliary atresia an opportunity for a first normal liver than it is to give a patient with [alcohol-related ESLF] who was born with a normal liver a second one."[55] Even if alcoholism is a chronic disease for which individuals are not responsible, Moss and Siegler contend that individuals who have this disease have the responsibility to seek and use available treatments to prevent the late-stage complications, including liver failure. Their failure to do so becomes a morally relevant consideration.

In addition, Moss and Siegler use the utilitarian argument that public support is indispensable for liver transplantation, both for securing funds and for securing organ donations. Giving patients with alcohol-related ESLF equal priority for donated livers could reduce public support for liver transplantation, and this consequence could be devastating for transplant programs. This utilitarian argument is plausible but speculative, and it is not clear that it should override other considerations of justice.

In our judgment, all patients should be evaluated on a case-by-case basis, considering medical need and probability of successful transplantation, rather than any being excluded altogether (few argue for this) or automatically receiving a lower priority.[56] An individual can then receive a lower priority rating, as warranted. Examples of conditions under which personal responsibility should affect priorities and lead to a lower rating are the following: (1) The alcoholic who fails to seek effective treatment for alcoholism and develops alcohol-related ESLF should receive a lower priority, but, unlike Moss and Siegler, we do not view a diagnosis of alcohol-related ESLF as itself categorically sufficient for a lower priority score. (2) A transplant recipient who through personal negligence does not take sufficient immunosuppressant medication, causing the transplant to fail, should be given a lower priority or be rejected for a second transplant.

The issues raised by this debate will intensify as lung transplantation becomes more common and more cigarette smokers seek transplants, often in competition with patients who have lethal genetic conditions.

GLOBAL HEALTH POLICY AND THE RIGHT TO HEALTH

The right to a decent minimum of health care is typically conceived in terms of *national* health policy, but the idea of a right to a decent minimum of health (through public health measures, sanitation, supply of clean drinking water, and the like) can and should be conceived as a matter of the global order that reaches beyond national health systems. Globalization has brought a realization that problems of protecting health and maintaining healthy conditions are international in nature and that serious attempts at their alleviation will require a justice-based restructuring of the global order. One model of international justice is found in the Commission on Human Rights of the United Nations:

> [T]he right of everyone to the enjoyment of the highest attainable stan-
> dard of physical and mental health is a human right....[F]or millions
> of people throughout the world, the full realization of th[is] right...still
> remains a distant goal and..., especially for those living in poverty, this
> goal is becoming increasingly remote....[P]hysical and mental health is
> a most important worldwide social goal, the realization of which requires
> action by many other social and economic sectors in addition to the health
> sector.[57]

Ethical and political theories that explicitly address questions of global justice are now widely referred to as "cosmopolitan theories." This approach, which has strongly influenced the authors of this volume, takes as its starting point large and usually catastrophic social conditions—in particular, famine, poverty, and epidemic disease. The theory then attempts to delineate which obligations extend across national borders to address these problems. The obligations advanced in the theory are similar to those traditionally found in moral and political theory, but globalized.

An early and profound influence on cosmopolitan thinking came from Peter Singer's work on global obligations, which we treated in Chapter 6. One reason for Singer's influence in turning philosophers' attention in a global direction was his trenchant way of pointing to the gap between fundamental principles of morality (such as those treated in our book) and the practice of those principles at the international level. Singer succeeded in convincing many philosophers that, despite the apparently overdemanding nature of his conclusions, they only show that morality demands more of us than many had thought, especially in addressing global poverty and ill health.

Singer's theory, which is grounded in utilitarian beneficence, is oriented toward the obligations of agents such as persons and governments. By contrast, the perspective of egalitarian social justice that we often take (much like Rawls) in this chapter proposes that we orient theory around the moral evaluation of *social institutions* and their responsibilities, legitimacy, and weaknesses. The focus is not on the morality of individual choices, but on the morality of the basic structure of society from within which moral choices are made. The most influential cosmopolitan theories attempt to apply Rawls's theory of justice to achieve global institutional reform (e.g., in the structure and commitments of the World Health Organization and in pharmaceutical companies).

Thomas Pogge, a prominent defender of cosmopolitan theory, argues that Rawls's thesis that the principles of justice are limited to specific nation-states unduly limits the theory of justice. A consistent moral theory will apply principles of justice everywhere. If the worst-off are the focal point of concern, as they are in Rawls's theory, we need to address the situation of the truly worst-off—the global poor. The basic structure of society lies in the scattered norms and institutions that affect almost everyone, including those found in commerce and public policy. Here there seems no good reason to distinguish sharply between citizens and foreigners. The criterion of national citizenship, from the point of view of justice, is as morally arbitrary as race, class, or gender. Applying rules of justice only within given nations also will increase disparities in wealth and well-being rather than alleviate the fundamental problem. We also will lack a coherent theory of social justice if it is restricted only to local conditions.[58]

A major problem of international health is the role that poverty plays in causing and perpetuating poor health. Here it is the right to *health,* not the right to health *care,* that is the major concern. A framework for international health policy and public health has been constructed in bioethics by Madison Powers and Ruth Faden. They start with a basic premise about justice: "Social justice is concerned with human well-being," not only health, but what they call six core dimensions of well-being: health, personal security, reasoning, respect, attachment, and self-determination. They argue that the list presents a particularly useful set of criteria for expressing the requirements of justice within public health and health policy.[59] Each of the six dimensions is an independent concern of justice, and the "job of justice" is to secure a sufficient level of each dimension for each person. The justice of societies and of the global order can be judged by how well they implement these dimensions.

The job of justice is here closely associated with what we have called beneficence—the obligation to benefit. Nonetheless, Powers and Faden see their problems as ones of egalitarian *justice,* not merely beneficence and social utility (the centerpiece of Singer's theory). The goal of their account is to reduce inequality in the face of human misery, not to use a utilitarian measuring and balancing device. Their egalitarian approach begins with the world as we encounter it—a world characterized by profound inequalities in well-being and resources. They target the inequalities that are the most unjust and the most in need of redress. Although only the first of the six dimensions of well-being in this account is health, Powers and Faden argue that the moral justification for health policies depends as much on the other five dimensions of well-being as it does on health. An absence of any of the other conditions can be seriously destructive to health. A constellation of inequalities can systemically magnify and reinforce initial conditions of ill health, creating ripple effects that attack various aspects of health. They are offering an account of interactive effects: Poor education and lack of respect, for example, can affect core forms of reasoning and health status. Social structures can compound these adverse effects. The result is a mixture of interactive and cascading effects that require urgent attention from the point of view of justice.[60]

Cosmopolitan theory captures a critical aspect of egalitarian justice. Poor health and growing inequalities are the result of many interactive effects. It would be absurd to look, in a theory of justice, only at the distribution of health care, ignoring the many causes of poor health and poor delivery of care. Deprivations of education cause deprivations of health, just as ill health can make it difficult to obtain a good education. Any one dimension of well-being can affect development of other dimensions of well-being, and all can make for poor health. In some societies, there is a constantly compounding body of deprivations. Inequalities in these circumstances are among the most urgent for a theory of justice to address, regardless of the nation in which they occur.

Inequalities are not merely a matter of bad luck or personal failings. They are often distributed by social institutions that can be structured explicitly to reduce the inequalities. If, for example, lower level public schools distribute woeful educational outcomes, which in turn contribute to poor diet and poor health, it is within our power to alter this situation. Rawls was certainly right to point to the pervasive effects of these institutions and their place in the theory of justice. Both Pogge and Powers–Faden are right in arguing that inequalities in health and well-being brought about by severe poverty have a particular moral urgency. Internationally, the world is one of radical inequalities in almost every respect, most notably in life expectancies. Somewhere around twenty million people in the developing world die each year, including several million young children, from malnutrition and diseases that can be inexpensively prevented or treated by cheap and available means. If the reach of social justice is global, this kind of inequality from disadvantaging conditions must be at the top of the conditions to be remedied.

While it remains unclear what would constitute an adequate strategy for attacking these problems, we can again hold out the model of a decent minimum—in this case a decent minimum standard of health. It would be an enormous improvement in global justice if the target were taken seriously that all persons have a fair opportunity at reasonably good health and welfare over the course of a decent life span.

ALLOCATING, SETTING PRIORITIES, AND RATIONING

Rights to health and health care encounter theoretical and practical difficulties of allocating, rationing, and setting priorities. The practical problems of justice are important and pressing, but we begin with some basic conceptual and structural matters.

Allocation

Decisions about allocation in particular cases often have far-reaching effects on other allocations. For example, the funds allocated for medical and biological research may affect the availability of training programs for physicians. Problems of allocation usually involve competition among desirable programs. We can identity four distinct, but interrelated, types of allocation. The third and fourth are of particular importance for the discussion of rationing later in this chapter.

1. *Partitioning the comprehensive social budget.* Every large political unit operates with a budget, which includes allocations for health and for other social goods, such as housing, education, culture, defense, and recreation. Health is not our only value or goal, and expenditures for other goods inevitably compete for limited resources with health-targeted expenditures. However, apart from an emergency state of affairs, if a well-off society fails to allocate sufficient funds to provide adequate public health measures and a decent minimum of health care, it has an unjust allocational system.

2. *Allocating within the health budget.* Allocation decisions must be made from within the budget portion devoted to health. We protect and promote health in many ways besides the provision of medical care. Health policies and programs for public health, disaster relief, poverty aid, occupational safety, environmental protection, injury prevention, consumer protection, and food and drug control are all parts of society's effort to protect and promote the health of not only its citizens, but often citizens of other nations. The budget for health vastly exceeds the specific portion for health care.

3. *Allocating within the health care budget.* Once society has determined its budget for sectors such as public health and health care, it still must allocate its resources within each sector by selecting certain projects and procedures for funding.[61] For example, determining which categories of injury, illness, or disease (if any) should receive a priority ranking in

the allocation of health care resources is a major aspect of allocation. Policymakers will examine various diseases in terms of their communicability, frequency, cost, associated pain and suffering, and impact on length of life and quality of life, among other factors. It might be justified, for instance, to concentrate less on fatal diseases, such as some forms of cancer, and more on widespread disabling diseases, such as arthritis.

4. *Allocating scarce treatments for patients.* Because health needs and desires are virtually limitless, every health care system faces some form of scarcity, and not everyone who needs a particular form of health care can gain access to it. At one time or the other, medical resources and supplies such as penicillin, insulin, kidney dialysis, cardiac transplantation, and space in intensive care units have been allocated for specific patients or classes of patients. These decisions are more difficult when an illness is life-threatening and the scarce resource potentially life-saving. The question can become, "Who shall live when not everyone can live?"

Allocation decisions of type 3 and type 4 interact. Type 3 decisions partially determine the necessity and extent of patient selection by determining the availability and supply of a particular resource. Distress in making difficult choices through explicit decisions of type 4 sometimes leads a society to modify its allocation policies at the level of type 3 to increase the supply of a particular resource. For example, when considering difficult allocation decisions about dialysis machines, the U.S. federal government decided to provide funds to ensure near-universal access to kidney dialysis and kidney transplantation without regard for ability to pay.

Setting Priorities

Setting priorities, both in health care and in public health, is one of the most widely discussed and pressing topics about just health policy.[62] Structuring clear priorities in type 3 allocation decisions has been difficult in many countries, and costs continue to rise dramatically as a result of several conditions—in particular, insurance costs, new technology, deteriorating health conditions, and longer life expectancy. These problems of contemporary health policy are extraordinarily complicated. The question in setting priorities is how to determine what ought to be done when resources are inadequate to provide all of the health benefits that it is technically possible to provide. We start with a historical and ongoing example of the problem: the health policy in the state of Oregon.

Lessons from the Oregon plan. Legislators and citizens in the state of Oregon have engaged for years in a closely watched and pioneering effort to set priorities in allocating health care by extending health insurance coverage to uninsured state residents below the poverty line. Oregon's Basic Health Services Act became a focal point for discussion of every major aspect of justice and health policy, including access to care, cost-effectiveness, rationing, and a decent minimum. This Act attempted to put into practice what is often discussed only at the level of theory. Many believed that the Oregon plan would mark the beginning of a new era in coming to grips with problems of rationing in the United States.[63]

The Oregon Health Services Commission (OHSC) was charged with producing a ranked priority list of services that would define a decent minimum of coverage by Medicaid, the state and federal program that provides funds to cover medical needs for financially impoverished citizens. The goal was to expand coverage to those below the poverty level and to fund as many top priority-ranked services as possible. In 1990, the OHSC listed 1,600 ranked medical procedures ranging "from the most important to the least important" services, based in part on data about quality of well-being after treatment and cost-effectiveness analysis. The ranking was widely criticized as unjust and arbitrary. For example, tooth-capping was ranked above appendectomies. Later the list was reduced to 709 ranked services, as it abandoned cost-effectiveness analysis and appealed to citizen values. The goal became to rank items on the prioritized list by *clinical effectiveness* and *social value.* These spare categories need great specificity, although much ingenuity did go into these efforts in Oregon.

Within the state, there was initially a strong endorsement of the list of covered services, because it did succeed in expanding access. However, many procedures (e.g., incapacitating hernias, tonsillectomy, and adenoidectomy) fell below the cut-off line of the priority list.[64] Oregon has had to modify the plan in numerous ways over the years, with the consequence of high rates of coverage loss and disenrollment from the plan, difficulty in meeting the needs of the chronically ill, increased unmet health needs, reduced access to health care services, and financial strain.[65] The history of the plan also demonstrates that Oregon's priority list has trouble managing budget shortfalls, which have repeatedly occurred.

Just strategies for setting priorities.[66] Even before the developments in Oregon, an influential literature on setting priorities had emerged from health economics, as we briefly discussed in Chapter 6. This literature urged use of cost-effectiveness analysis (CEA), the most important version being cost–utility analysis (CUA). In this strategy, health benefits are measured in terms of anticipated health gains, and costs are measured in terms of expenditures of resources. The goal is utilitarian: the greatest health benefits for the money expended. Health benefits are quantified, and an attempt is made to incorporate the outcome directly into public policy by measuring the impact of interventions on both the length and quality of life. QALYs has become a generic name for such measures (see Chapter 6, pp. 230–33).

Libertarians, egalitarians, and communitarians have all raised objections to the QALY strategy for setting limits. Charges of discrimination against infants, the elderly, and the disabled (especially those with permanent incapacitation and the terminally ill), as well as uncertainties about how to judge gains in quality of life, have led many to conclude that appeals to QALYs sometimes allow unjust and impermissible trade-offs in setting priorities. This literature has generated many puzzling cases. For example, will life-saving interventions (e.g., heart transplantation) lose out altogether in the competition for priority if other interventions (e.g., arthritis medication) provide a greater improvement in quality of life?

Many decisions must be made, including whether priority should go to prevention or treatment and whether life-saving procedures take priority over other interventions.[67] Expenditures for treatment, rather than prevention, are far higher in the current health care systems of most industrialized nations, and government officials might justifiably choose, for example, to concentrate on preventing heart disease rather than on providing individuals with heart transplants or artificial hearts. In many cases, preventive care is more effective and more efficient in saving lives, reducing suffering, raising levels of health, and lowering costs. Preventive care typically reduces morbidity and premature mortality for unknown, "statistical lives," whereas critical interventions concentrate on known, "identifiable lives."[68] Many societies have tended to favor identified persons and to allocate resources for critical care, but good evidence exists to show that public health expenditures targeted at poorer communities for preventive measures, such as prenatal care, save many times that amount in future care. Accordingly, our moral intuitions often drive us in conflicting directions: Allocate more to rescue persons in medical need or allocate more to prevent persons from falling into such need.

Although no consensus is found either in health policy or in biomedical ethics, many are now open to the use of utility-driven strategies to generate *data* that the public and policymakers can weigh, together with other considerations. Public preferences, sound arguments for various policy options, and knowledge of the literature of ethics and health policy could help replace or constrain morally objectionable trade-offs suggested by economic analysis.[69] Perhaps the major problem, as we indicated in Chapter 6, is how to establish constraints that are strongly recommended by justice. For example, it seems unfair and unacceptable to allow forms of cost-effective rationing that adversely affect or ignore levels of health among the most disadvantaged populations, in effect worsening the condition of the worse off. This generalization may seem obvious, but it has proved and will continue to prove extremely difficult to implement, especially at the global level.

Procedural strategies for setting priorities. One tempting strategy is to abandon all recourse to theories of justice and instead use the democratic process and democratic legitimacy to reach decisions about priorities. Fair deliberative mechanisms capable of supporting democratic procedures are the anchor of this approach, together with back-up processes of review and appeal.[70]

One option is Erik Nord's proposal that we replace CUA and QALYs with a direct appeal to the public's preferences whenever questions of trade-offs arise. Nord maintains that the answers given by the public are often starkly different from those found in CUAs, because the public weighs factors such as severe incapacity and life-saving technologies more heavily.[71] However, this approach is problematic. It is unclear how to solicit and aggregate preferences—and also unclear why preferences alone should count heavily in the public policy process. There are problems of how to frame a question fairly, so that the question does not itself determine the outcome, and also problems of how to assess the validity of preferences. Any attempt to eliminate unduly biased preferences seems to invoke some appeal to justice beyond the method itself.

Majority preferences, no matter how well informed and fair, will sometimes eventuate in unjust outcomes. A purely procedural solution will return us to the same failures of justice that we have already encountered in health care. The literature remains relatively unclear about how to protect against unfair outcomes, whether citizen deliberators could ever satisfy the demands of true deliberative democracy, and how much real agreement they could reach. The upshot is that at present we lack an acceptable strategy for setting priorities and limits. Although some are ready to forsake traditional theories of justice, these theories likely have staying power. What seems unlikely is that one of these theories will oust the others in the bid to capture fully our sense of justice in the distribution of health care. Moreover, we suggest that several target goals, consistent with justice and national health policies, can be identified. The first objective is unobstructed access to a decent minimum of health care through some form of universal insurance coverage that operationalizes the right to health care. The second objective is to develop acceptable incentives for physicians and consumer-patients. Unless cost consciousness and cost controls are introduced and maintained, expenditures will spiral out of control, and the necessity for rationing at the first tier will threaten the goal of providing a decent minimum. The third objective is to construct a fair system of rationing that does not violate the decent minimum standard. Although rationing is sometimes required at the first tier (e.g., when a new vaccine or drug is in scarce supply or when a public health emergency strikes), frequent rationing at the first tier would sabotage the moral foundations of the enterprise. Finally, the fourth objective is to implement a system that can be put into effect incrementally, without drastic disruption of basic institutions that finance and deliver health care.

Several carefully reasoned proposals attempt, at least partially, to meet these objectives. Despite many differences, these proposals fall into two families: unified systems and pluralist systems. Plans of the first type look primarily to egalitarian justice, with utility a second-level consideration. Plans of the second type look primarily to utility (efficiency and broad coverage), with egalitarian justice a second-level consideration. Typically, pluralist systems incorporate greater freedom of choice for consumers, patients, and providers. Although we cannot consider the details of any one plan or develop an ideal plan, we have argued throughout this chapter in favor of a unitary system at the first tier of health care and a pluralist system at the second tier, thus allowing and indeed strongly endorsing a two-tier system.

Rationing

We have been discussing and now further discuss the types of allocation decision categorized on pp. 267–68 as types 3 and 4. Both are often discussed under the topic of *rationing* and related terms, such as *triage.*[72] The choice of terms is not unimportant, because each term has a different history involving changes in meaning. *Rationing* originally did not suggest harshness or an emergency. It meant a form of allowance, share, or portion, as when food is divided into rations in the military. Only recently has *rationing* been linked to limited resources and the setting of priorities in the health care budget.

Rationing has at least three relevant meanings or types. The first is related to "denial from lack of resources." In a market economy, all types of goods—including health care—are to some extent rationed by ability to pay. A second sense of *rationing* derives not from market limits but from social policy limits: The government determines an allowance or allotment, and individuals are denied access beyond the allotted amount. Rationing gasoline and certain types of food during a war is a well-known example, but national health systems that do not allow purchases of goods or insurance beyond an allotted amount offer an equally good example. Finally, in a third sense of *rationing,* an allowance or allotment is distributed equitably, but those who can afford additional goods are not denied access beyond the allotted amount. In this third form, rationing involves elements of each of the first two forms: Public policy fixes an allowance, and those who cannot afford additional units are thereby effectively denied access beyond the allowance.

We here use "rationing" in each of the three senses, concentrating on the third. Although the term "rationing" often carries a negative connotation, the entire structure of health protection and health care delivery involves some form of rationing. Prioritizing health care resources, as we have seen, is itself an exercise in rationing. We now turn to two case studies in problems of rationing. The first focuses on rationing by age and the second focuses on highly expensive treatments such as heart transplantation.

Rationing by age. Policies sometimes exclude or give a lower priority to persons in a particular age group, but also sometimes provide advantages to the elderly, as in Medicare entitlements in the United States. In the United Kingdom implicit rationing policies have excluded elderly, end-stage kidney patients from kidney dialysis and transplantation because of their age or expected quality of life.[73] In another example, policies for allocating transplantable kidneys in the United States give some priority to very young patients by assigning them additional points in the point system.

Several arguments have been proposed to justify the use of age in allocation policies. Some rest on judgments about the probability of successful treatment (i.e., medical utility). For instance, age may be an indicator of the probability of surviving a major operation. Judgments of the probability of success also can include the length of time that the recipient of an organ is expected to survive, a period that is usually shorter for an older patient than for a younger patient. If anticipated QALYs is a criterion, younger patients will typically do far better than older patients.

Norman Daniels has offered an influential argument for viewing age as different from race and gender for purposes of health care allocation.[74] He appeals to prudential individual decisions about health care from the perspective of an entire lifetime. Each age group represents a stage in a person's life span. The goal is to allocate resources prudently throughout the stages of life within a social system that provides a fair lifetime share of health care for each citizen. As prudent deliberators, he maintains, impartial persons would choose (assuming conditions of scarcity) to distribute health care over a lifetime in a way that improved the chance of attaining at least a normal life span. We would, Daniels argues, reject a pattern that reduced our chances of reaching a normal life span but increased our chances of living beyond a normal life span if we did become elderly. He thinks that an impartial person would choose to shift resources that might otherwise be consumed in prolonging the lives of the elderly to the treatment of younger persons. In this way, we would maximize each person's chances of living at least a normal life span.

Another theory uses a "fair innings" argument. It considers a person's whole lifetime experience and seeks equality. Alan Williams, a proponent, stresses that this conception of intergenerational equity would *require,* not merely *permit,* "greater discrimination against the elderly than would be dictated simply by efficiency objectives."[75]

All calls for age-based rationing face challenges.[76] Such rationing runs the risk of perpetuating injustice by stereotyping the elderly, treating them as scapegoats because of increased health care costs, and creating unnecessary conflicts between generations. Elderly persons in each generation will complain that they did not have access to new technologies that were developed, often using their taxes for funding; and they will claim that it would be unfair to deny them those technologies now. Nonetheless, to protect the health of children and many vulnerable parties, we may find that we have to set a threshold age beyond which funding for various conditions would not be publicly available. This would be a tragic choice, and yet may be an entirely just policy.

Still, we should proceed with caution. Even if age-based allocations of health care do not violate the fair-opportunity rule, they have often been unjust in the way they have been implemented in many countries. These allocations are a prime example of a need for society to take a systematic approach to ensure equitable access to health care.

Rationing heart transplantation. Heart-transplantation controversies began shortly after cardiac transplantation became increasingly effective in the 1980s. The number of heart transplants performed is small, but the cost is large, with first-year cost alone of around $300,000.[77] Changing medical and political circumstances over the years have led to alterations of policy that close one gap in equity only to open other equity issues.

Despite the high cost of coverage for heart transplants, arguments have been offered for publicly funding them. The federal Task Force on Organ Transplantation, appointed by the U.S. Department of Health and Human Services, recommended that "a public program should be set up to cover the costs of people who are medically eligible for organ transplants but who are not covered by private insurance, Medicare, or Medicaid and who are unable to obtain an organ transplant due to the lack of funds."[78] The task force grounded its recommendation on two arguments from justice. The first argument emphasizes the continuity between heart and liver transplants and other forms of medical care (including kidney transplants) that are already accepted as part of the decent minimum of health care that a society as well off as the United States should provide: Heart and liver transplants are comparable to other funded or fundable procedures in terms of their effectiveness in saving lives and enhancing the quality of life. In response to the claim that heart and liver transplants are too expensive, the task force argued that the burden of saving public health funds should be distributed equitably rather than imposed on particular groups of patients, such as those suffering from end-stage heart or liver failure. It would be arbitrary to exclude one life-saving procedure while funding others of comparable life-saving potential and cost.

The task force offered a second argument for equitable access, this time focusing on practices of organ donation and procurement. Various public officials, including the President of the United States, participate in efforts to increase the supply of donated organs by appealing to all citizens to donate organs. It would be unfair and sometimes exploitative to solicit people, rich and poor alike, to donate organs if those organs are then distributed on the basis of ability to pay.[79] Furthermore, it would be morally inconsistent to prohibit the sale of organs, and then to distribute donated organs according to ability to pay. It is morally problematic to distinguish buying an organ for transplantation from buying an organ transplant procedure when a donated organ is the centerpiece of the procedure.

These arguments are attractive appeals to coherence, but they do not establish that justice requires expensive health care irrespective of its cost or that it is arbitrary to use a reasonably structured system of rationing that involves tough choices to set priorities. Once a society has achieved a fair threshold determination of funding at the decent-minimum level, it legitimately may select some procedures while excluding others when they are of equal life-saving potential and of equal cost, as long as it can identify relevant differences through a fair procedure. Substantial public participation along the way would help legitimate these determinations. Just as it would be unfair to solicit people to make gifts of organs and then distribute them on the basis of ability to pay, so it would be unfair to spend in excess of a fairly established level of funding merely because some items are gifts.

In the end, we should situate recommendations about funding heart transplants and all other expensive treatments in the larger context of a just social policy of allocation, which will require that we systematically and fairly set priorities and limits.

Rationing Scarce Treatments to Patients

Health care professionals and policymakers often must decide who will receive an available scarce medical resource that cannot be provided to all needy people. We concentrate here on priority schemes for selecting recipients in urgent circumstances. Two broad approaches vie for primacy: (1) a *utilitarian* strategy that emphasizes maximal benefit to patients and society, and (2) an *egalitarian* strategy that emphasizes the equal worth of persons and fair opportunity. We argue that these approaches can and should be coherently combined.

We defend a system that uses two stages of substantive standards and procedural rules for rationing scarce medical resources: (1) criteria and procedures to determine a qualifying pool of potential recipients, such as patients eligible for heart transplantation; and (2) criteria and procedures for final selection of recipients, such as the patient to receive a particular heart.

The constituency factor. Criteria for screening potential recipients of care fall into three basic categories: constituency, progress of science, and prospect of success.[80] The first criterion uses social rather than medical factors. It is determined by clientele boundaries (e.g., veterans served by medical centers that were constructed for veterans), geographic or jurisdictional boundaries (e.g., citizens of a legal jurisdiction served by a publicly funded hospital), and ability to pay (e.g., the wealthy). These criteria are entirely nonmedical, and they involve moral judgments that often are not impartial (e.g., excluding noncitizens or including only veterans). These clientele boundaries are sometimes acceptable, but often have been dubious. For example, the Task Force on Organ Transplantation in the United States proposed that donated organs be considered national, public resources to be distributed, within limits, according to both the needs of patients and the probability of successful transplantation.[81] The task force judged that foreign nationals do not have the same moral claim on organs donated in the United States as its own citizens and residents do. The judgment apparently is that citizenship and residency are *morally relevant* properties for distribution, but the task force also determined that compassion should lead to the admission of some nonresident aliens. In a split vote, it recommended that nonresident aliens comprise no more than 10% of the waiting list for cadaver kidneys donated for transplantation and that all patients on the waiting list, including nonresident aliens, have access to organs according to the same criteria of need, probability of success, and time on the waiting list.[82]

Progress of science. The second criterion is relevant during an experimental phase in the development of a treatment. For example, physician-investigators may justifiably exclude patients who suffer from other diseases that might obscure the research result. The whole point is to determine whether an experimental treatment is effective and how it can be improved. This criterion of scientific progress is research-oriented, and its use rests on moral and prudential judgments about the efficient use of resources. The factors used to include or to exclude patients for participation in such research can be controversial, especially if persons who potentially could benefit are excluded for reasons of scientific efficiency or persons who are very unlikely to benefit are continued in a clinical trial to make trial results acceptable to the scientific community. Clearly, the factors used to select patients for participation in such research will require reassessment when a treatment developed through the research becomes accepted.

Prospect of success. Whether a treatment is experimental or routine, the likelihood of success in treating the patient is a relevant criterion because scarce medical resources should be distributed only to patients who have a reasonable chance of benefit. Ignoring this factor is unjust, because it wastes resources, as in the case of organs that can be transplanted only once. Heart-transplant surgeons sometimes list their patients as urgent priority candidates for an available heart because the patients will soon die if they do not receive a transplant, but some of these patients are virtually certain to die even if they do receive the heart. Good candidates are passed over in the process. A classification and queuing system that permits the urgency of a situation alone to determine priority is as unjust as it is inefficient.

Medical utility. We turn now to standards proposed for *final selection* of patients. Controversy about these standards centered on standards of medical utility and social utility, and on impersonal mechanisms such as lotteries and queuing.

We assume the generally accepted rule that judgments about medical utility should figure into decisions to ration scarce medical resources. Differences in patients' prospects for successful treatment are relevant considerations, as is maximizing the number of lives saved.

However, both need and prospect of success are value-laden concepts, and uncertainty often exists about likely outcomes and about the factors that contribute to success. For example, kidney transplant surgeons dispute the importance of having a good tissue match, because minor tissue mismatches can be managed by immunosuppressant medications that reduce the body's tendency to reject transplanted organs. Insisting on the seemingly objective criterion of tissue type in distributing organs also can disadvantage persons with a rare tissue type and racial minorities, as we saw earlier in this chapter.

The criteria of medical need and prospect of success sometimes come into conflict. In intensive care units, trying to save a patient whose need is medically urgent sometimes inappropriately consumes resources that could be used to save more people.[83] A rule of giving priority to the sickest patients or those with the most urgent medical needs will produce unfairness, because it will lead in some cases to inefficient uses of resources. Rationing schemes that altogether exclude considerations of medical utility are indefensible, but judgments of medical utility are not sufficient by themselves. This problem takes us to the subject of chance and queuing.

Impersonal mechanisms of chance and queuing. We began this chapter by noting the oddity and unacceptability of using a lottery to distribute all social positions. However, a lottery or another system of chance is not always odd and unacceptable.[84] If medical resources are scarce and not divisible into portions, and if no major disparities exist in medical utility for patients (particularly when selection determines life or death), then considerations of fair opportunity and equal respect may justify queuing, a lottery, or randomization—depending on which procedure is the most appropriate and feasible in the circumstances.

Similar judgments have supported the use of lotteries to determine who would gain access to new drugs available only in limited supply, either because they had only recently been approved or because they remained experimental. For instance, Berlex Laboratories held a lottery to distribute Betaseron, a new genetically engineered drug that appeared to slow the deterioration caused by multiple sclerosis, and several drug companies held lotteries to distribute a new class of compounds to patients with AIDS. The symbolic value of the lotteries also can be morally significant. "Lotteries say that after you meet medical criteria, all persons should have an equal shot at the good of society. Lotteries celebrate an understanding that all humans are endowed with equal dignity."[85] These methods also make the selection with little investment of time and financial resources and can create less stress for all involved, including patients.[86]

Even by-passed candidates may feel less distress at being rejected by chance than by judgments of comparative merit.

However, there are both theoretical and practical problems with some impersonal selection procedures. For example, the rule "first come, first served" carries the potential for injustice. Under some conditions a patient already receiving a particular treatment has a severely limited chance of survival (virtually to the point of futility), whereas other patients who need the treatment have a far better chance of survival. Does "first come, first served" imply that those already receiving treatment have absolute priority over those who arrive later but have either more urgent needs or better prospects of success? Intensive care units again provide a good example. Although admission to the ICU establishes a presumption in favor of continued treatment, it does not give a person an absolute claim. In decisions in neonatal intensive care about the use of extracorporeal membrane oxygenation (ECMO), a form of cardiopulmonary bypass used to support newborns with life-threatening respiratory failure, a truly scarce resource is being provided, because it is not widely available and requires the full-time presence of well-trained personnel. Robert Truog argues, rightly in our judgment, that ECMO should be withdrawn from a newborn with a poor prognosis in favor of another with a good prognosis if the latter is far more likely to survive, requires the therapy, and cannot be safely transferred to another facility.[87] Such displacement of a child from the ICU requires justification, but it need not constitute abandonment or injustice if other forms of care are provided.

Which mechanism, queuing or chance, is preferable will depend largely on practical considerations, but queuing appears to be feasible and acceptable in many health care settings, including emergency medicine, ICUs, and organ transplant lists. A complicating factor is that some people do not enter the queue (or the lottery) in time because of factors such as slowness in seeking help, inadequate or incompetent medical attention, delay in referral, or overt discrimination. A system is unfair if some people gain an advantage in access over others because they are better educated, better connected, or have more money for frequent visits to physicians.

Social utility. Although criteria of social utility are controversial, the comparative social value of potential recipients is, under some conditions, a relevant and even decisive consideration. An often-used analogy comes from World War II, when, according to some reports, the scarce resource of penicillin was distributed to U.S. soldiers suffering from venereal disease rather than to those suffering from battle wounds. The rationale was military need: The soldiers suffering from venereal disease could be restored to battle more quickly.[88]

An argument in favor of social-utilitarian selection is that medical institutions and personnel are trustees of society and must consider the probable future contributions of patients. We argue later that, in certain rare and exceptional cases involving persons of critical social importance, criteria of social value—narrow and specific as opposed to broad and general social utility—are appropriately overriding. However, in general we need to protect the relationship of personal care and trust between patients and physicians, and it would be threatened if physicians were trained to look beyond their patients' needs to society's needs.

Triage: Medical utility and narrow social utility. Some have invoked the model of *triage,* a French term meaning "sorting," "picking," or "choosing." It has been applied to sorting items such as wool and coffee beans according to their quality. In the delivery of health care, triage is a process of developing and using criteria for prioritization. It has been used in war, in community disasters, and in emergency rooms where injured persons have been sorted for medical attention according to their needs and prospects. Decisions to admit and to discharge patients from ICUs often involve triage. The objective is to use available medical resources as effectively and as efficiently as possible, a utilitarian rationale.[89]

Triage decisions usually appeal to medical utility rather than social utility. For example, disaster victims are generally sorted according to medical need. Those who have major injuries and will die without immediate help, but who can be salvaged, are ranked first; those whose treatment can be delayed without immediate danger are ranked second; those with minor injuries are ranked third; and those for whom no treatment will be efficacious are ranked fourth. This priority scheme is fair and does not involve judgments about individuals' comparative social worth.

However, narrow or specific judgments of comparative social worth are inescapable and acceptable in some situations.[90] For example, in an earthquake disaster in which some injured survivors are medical personnel who suffer only minor injuries, they justifiably receive priority of treatment if they are needed to help others. Similarly, in an outbreak of infectious disease, it is justifiable to inoculate physicians and nurses first to enable them to care for others. Under such conditions, a person may receive priority for treatment on grounds of social utility if and only if his or her contribution is indispensable to attaining a major social goal. As in analogous lifeboat cases, we should limit judgments of comparative social value to the *specific* qualities and skills that are essential to the community's immediate protection, without assessing the *general* social worth of persons.

It is legitimate to invoke medical utility followed by the use of chance or queuing for scarce resources when medical utility is roughly equal for eligible patients. It is also legitimate to invoke narrow considerations of social utility to give priority to individuals who fill social roles that are essential in achieving a better overall outcome. This nexus of standards should prove to be both coherent and stable, despite our mixed appeals to egalitarian justice and utility.

CONCLUSION

In this chapter we have examined several approaches to justice, including egalitarian, communitarian, libertarian, and utilitarian theories. Although we have primarily sided with egalitarian and utilitarian theories, we have maintained that no single theory of justice or system of distributing health care is necessary, or sufficient, for constructive reflection on health policy. Our discussions in Chapter 1 (and in Chapters 9 and 10 as well) expose several limitations in the use of general ethical theories, and those limitations are prominent in debates about allocation decisions. Each general theory of justice provides a valuable perspective on the moral life, but only partially captures the rich diversity of that life.

The richness of our traditional moral practices and theories helps explain why diverse theories of justice have all received skillful defenses. Absent a social consensus about these competing theories of justice, we can expect that public policies will sometimes emphasize elements of one theory and at other times elements of another theory. We have done so ourselves in this chapter. However, the existence of several theories does not justify the piecemeal approach that many countries, including the United States, have taken to their health care systems. A piecemeal approach may only be a way of avoiding larger questions of justice about what the people of a nation and the global community should expect from their health care system and how nations can address needs for increased resources and the like.

Countries lacking a comprehensive and coherent system of health care financing and delivery—the United States being a prime example—are destined to continue on the trail of higher costs and larger numbers of unprotected citizens unless they make significant changes. They must improve both utility (efficiency) and justice (fairness and equality). Although justice and utility may appear to be opposing values, and have often been presented as such, both are indispensable in shaping a health care system. Creating a more efficient system by cutting costs and providing appropriate incentives can conflict with the goal of universal access to health care, and justice-based goals of universal coverage also may make the system inefficient. Clearly there must be trade-offs between equality and efficiency.

Policies of just access to health care, strategies of efficiency in health care institutions, and global needs for the reduction of health-impairing conditions dwarf in social importance every other issue considered in this book. Many barriers exist to achieving these goals. For millions who encounter these barriers, global justice and a just health care system are distant goals. Although every society must ration its resources, many societies can close gaps in fair rationing more conscientiously than they have to date. We have suggested a general perspective from which to approach these problems. In particular we have proposed that society recognize global rights to health and enforceable rights to a decent minimum of health care within a framework for allocation that incorporates both utilitarian and egalitarian standards. This perspective recognizes the legitimacy of trade-offs between efficiency and justice, a position that mirrors our insistence throughout this book on the possibility of contingent conflicts between beneficence and justice.

NOTES

1. Jorge Luis Borges, *Labyrinths* (New York: New Directions, 1962), pp. 30–35.

2. For example, see the subtle connections between justice, nonmaleficence, and beneficence in Onora O'Neill, *Towards Justice and Virtue: A Constructive Account of Practical Reasoning* (Cambridge: Cambridge University Press, 1996); Martha C. Nussbaum, *Frontiers of Justice: Disability, Nationality, Species Membership* (Cambridge, MA: Harvard University Press, 2006); Thomas Pogge, *World Poverty and Human Rights* (Malden, MA: Polity Press, 2002); and Madison Powers and Ruth Faden, *Social Justice: The Moral Foundations of Public Health and Health Policy* (New York: Oxford University Press, 2006).

3. See Samuel Fleishacker, *A Short History of Distributive Justice* (Cambridge, MA: Harvard University Press, 2005).

4. See Carol Levine, "Changing Views of Justice after Belmont: AIDS and the Inclusion of 'Vulnerable' Subjects," in *The Ethics of Research Involving Human Subjects: Facing the 21st Century,* ed. Harold Y. Vanderpool (Frederick, MD: University Publishing Group, 1996); Jeffrey P. Kahn, Anna C. Mastroianni, and Jeremy Sugarman, eds., *Beyond Consent: Seeking Justice in Research* (New York: Oxford University Press, 1998); and Leslie Meltzer and James F. Childress, "What Is Fair Subject Selection?" in *Oxford Textbook for Clinical Trials,* ed. Ezekiel Emanuel et al. (New York: Oxford University Press, forthcoming).

5. See, for example, Guido Calabresi and Philip Bobbitt, *Tragic Choices* (New York: Norton, 1978).

6. See, e.g., Nicholas Rescher, *Distributive Justice* (Indianapolis, IN: Bobbs-Merrill, 1966), chap. 4. Rescher's list is indebted to John A. Ryan, *Distributive Justice: The Right and Wrong of Our Present Distribution of Wealth* (New York: Macmillan, 1922).

7. *International Union, UAW v. Johnson Controls,* 111 S.Ct. 1196 (1991).

8. Robert Nozick, *Anarchy, State, and Utopia* (New York: Basic Books, 1974), esp. pp. 149–82.

9. Two instructive theories are Alasdair MacIntyre, *Whose Justice? Which Rationality?* (Notre Dame, IN: University of Notre Dame Press, 1988), esp. pp. 1, 390–403; and Michael Walzer, *Spheres of Justice: A Defense of Pluralism and Equality* (New York: Basic Books, 1983), esp. pp. 86–94.

10. See Henk ten Have and Helen Keasberry, "Equity and Solidarity: The Context of Health Care in the Netherlands," *Journal of Medicine and Philosophy* 17 (August 1992): 463–77, esp. 474–76.

11. Ezekiel J. Emanuel, *The Ends of Human Life: Medical Ethics in a Liberal Polity* (Cambridge, MA: Harvard University Press, 1991).

12. Rawls, "Kantian Constructivism in Moral Theory" (The Dewey Lectures), *Journal of Philosophy* 77 (1980): 519. Rawls progressively deemphasized Kantian conceptions of rationality and emphasized political conceptions in modern constitutional democracies. See his *Political Liberalism* (New York: Columbia University Press, 1996).

13. Daniels, *Just Health Care* (New York: Cambridge University Press, 1985), pp. 34–58; and *Just Health: Meeting Health Needs Fairly* (New York: Cambridge University Press, 2007).

14. Rawls, *A Theory of Justice* (Cambridge, MA: Harvard University Press, 1971; rev. ed., 1999), pp. 73ff (1999: pp. 63–65).

15. See Bernard Williams, "The Idea of Equality," in *Justice and Equality*, ed. Hugo Bedau (Englewood Cliffs, NJ: Prentice Hall, 1971), p. 135; Jeff McMahan, "Cognitive Disability, Misfortune, and Justice," *Philosophy and Public Affairs* 25 (1996): 3–35; and Janet Radcliffe Richards, "Equality of Opportunity," *Ratio* 10 (1997): 253–79.

16. H. Tristram Engelhardt, Jr., *The Foundations of Bioethics*, 2nd ed. (New York: Oxford University Press, 1996), chap. 8; and Gert Jan van der Wilt, "Health Care and the Principle of Fair Equality of Opportunity," *Bioethics* 8 (1994): 329–49.

17. See Brian D. Smedley, Adrienne Y. Stith, and Alan R. Nelson, eds., for the Committee on Understanding and Eliminating Racial and Ethnic Disparities in Health Care, Institute of Medicine, *Unequal Treatment: Confronting Racial and Ethnic Disparities in Health Care* (Washington, D.C.: National Academies Press, 2003).

18. Nancy S. Jecker, "Can an Employer-Based Health Insurance System Be Just?" *Journal of Health Politics, Policy and Law* 18 (1993): 657–73; Lisa Cooper-Patrick et al., "Race, Gender, and Partnership in the Patient–Physician Relationship," *Journal of the American Medical Association* 282 (August 11, 1999): 583–89.

19. Ivor L. Livingston, ed., *Praeger Handbook of Black American Health: Policies and Issues behind Disparities in Health* (Westport, CT: Praeger, 2004), 2 vols.; Kathryn S. Ratcliff, *Women and Health: Power, Technology, Inequality, and Conflict in a Gendered World* (Boston: Allyn & Bacon, 2002); and Nicole Lurie, "Health Disparities—Less Talk, More Action," *New England Journal of Medicine* 353 (August 18, 2005): 727–28.

20. Kenneth C. Goldberg, Arthur J. Hartz, Steven J. Jacobsen, et al., "Racial and Community Factors Influencing Coronary Artery Bypass Graft Surgery Rates for All 1986 Medicare Patients," *Journal of the American Medical Association* 267 (March 18, 1992): 1473–77; and Lucian L. Leape et al., "Underuse of Cardiac Procedures: Do Women, Ethnic Minorities, and the Uninsured Fail to Receive Needed Revascularization?" *Annals of Internal Medicine* 130 (February 2, 1999): 183–92.

21. See Edward L. Hannan et al., "Access to Coronary Artery Bypass Surgery by Race/Ethnicity and Gender Among Patients who are Appropriate for Surgery," *Medical Care* 37 (1999): 68–77; and Ashish K. Jha et al., "Racial Trends in the Use of Major Procedures among the Elderly," *New England Journal of Medicine* 353 (August 18, 2005): 683–91.

22. Viola Vaccarino et al., "Sex and Racial Differences in the Management of Acute Myocardial Infarction, 1994 through 2002," *New England Journal of Medicine* 353 (August 18, 2005): 671–82.

23. Amal N. Trivedi et al., "Trends in the Quality of Care and Racial Disparities in Medicare Managed Care," *New England Journal of Medicine* 353 (August 18, 2005): 692–700.

24. Smedley, Stith, and Nelson, eds., *Unequal Treatment*.

25. Smedley, Stith, and Nelson, eds., *Unequal Treatment*. For critical analyses of this report, see the special issue of *Perspectives in Biology and Medicine* 48, no. 1 suppl. (Winter 2005).

26. Katrina Armstrong, Chanita Hughes-Halbert, and David A. Asch, "Patient Preferences Can be Misleading as Explanations for Racial Disparities in Health Care," *Archives of Internal Medicine* 166 (May 8, 2006): 950–54; and Norman G. Levinsky, "Quality and Equity in Dialysis and Renal Transplantation," *New England Journal of Medicine* 341 (November 25, 1999): 1691–93. See also

Office of Inspector General, *Racial and Geographic Disparity in the Distribution of Organs for Transplantation,* OEI-01–98–00360 (Washington, D.C.: U.S. Department of Health and Human Services, June 1998).

27. John P. Roberts et al., "Effect of Changing the Priority for HLA Matching on the Rates and Outcomes of Kidney Transplantation in Minority Groups," *New England Journal of Medicine* 350 (February 5, 2004): 545–51, at 551. See also Jon J. van Rood, "Weighing Optima Graft Survival through HLA Matching against the Equitable Distribution of Kidney Allografts," *New England Journal of Medicine* 350 (February 5, 2004): 535–36. Other analysts argue that "[p]olicies to increase minority transplants by increasing donation rates [among Caucasians or African-Americans] may prove more cost effective than the elimination of HLA-B matching from deceased donor kidney allocation." *American Journal of Transplantation* 5 (2006): 1090–98, at 1090.

28. See Robert Bornholz and James J. Heckman, "Measuring Disparate Impacts and Extending Disparate Impact Doctrine to Organ Transplantation," *Perspectives in Biology and Medicine* 48, no. 1 suppl (Winter 2005): S95–S122.

29. Council on Ethical and Judicial Affairs, American Medical Association, "Gender Disparities in Clinical Decision Making," *Journal of the American Medical Association* 266 (July 24, 1991): 559–662.

30. Catherine Kim et al., "Review of Evidence and Explanations for Suboptimal Screening and Treatment of Dyslipidemia in Women," *Journal of General Internal Medicine* 18 (October 2003): 854–63.

31. "Progress in Eliminating Gender Disparities in Health Care Quality Is Mixed," *AHRQ News and Numbers,* May 9, 2007, http://www.ahrq.gov/news/nn/nn050907.htm. Contrast Vaccarino et al., "Sex and Racial Differences in the Management of Acute Myocardial Infarction, 1994 through 2002."

32. Lisa R. Hirschhorn et al., "Gender Differences in Quality of HIV Care in Ryan White CARE Act-Funded Clinics," *Women's Health Issues* 16 (May–June 2006): 104–12.

33. Carl Tishler and Suzanne Bartholomae, "The Recruitment of Normal Healthy Volunteers," *Journal of Clinical Pharmacology* 42 (2002): 365–75.

34. Tom L. Beauchamp, Bruce Jennings, Eleanor Kinney, and Robert Levine, "Pharmaceutical Research Involving the Homeless," *Journal of Medicine and Philosophy* (2002), 547–64; M. H. Kottow, "The Vulnerable and the Susceptible," *Bioethics* 17 (2003): 460–71; Toby L. Schonfeld, Joseph S. Brown, Meaghann Weniger, and Bruce Gordon, "Research Involving the Homeless," *IRB* 25 (September–October 2003): 17–20.

35. For analysis of the concept of exploitation, see Alan Wertheimer, *Exploitation* (Princeton, NJ: Princeton University Press, 1996), which focuses on "mutually advantageous and consensual exploitation," in which one party takes advantage of the other.

36. See Carol Levine, Ruth Faden, Christine Grady, et al. (for the Consortium to Examine Clinical Research Ethics), "The Limitations of 'Vulnerabililty' as a Protection for Human Research Participants," *American Journal of Bioethics* 4 (2004): 44–49; Debra A. DeBruin, "Reflections on Vulnerability," *Bioethics Examiner* 5 (2001): 1, 4, 7; Ruth Macklin, "Bioethics, Vulnerability, and Protection," *Bioethics* 17 (2003): 472–86.

37. See Debra A. DeBruin, "Looking Beyond the Limitations of 'Vulnerability': Reforming Safeguards in Research," *The American Journal of Bioethics* 4 (2004): 76–78; National Bioethics Advisory Commission, *Ethical and Policy Issues in Research Involving Human Participants,* vol. 1 (Bethesda, MD: Government Printing Office, 2001); Kenneth Kipnis, "Vulnerability in Research Subjects: A Bioethical Taxonomy," in National Bioethics Advisory Commission, *Ethical and Policy Issues in Research Involving Human Participants,* vol. 2 (Bethesda, MD: Government Printing Office, 2002), G1–13.

38. Gail E. Henderson, Arlene M. Davis, and Nancy M. P. King, "Vulnerability to Influence: A Two-Way Street," *American Journal of Bioethics* 4 (2004): 50–53.

39. Cf. Anita Silvers, "Historical Vulnerability and Special Scrutiny: Precautions against Discrimination in Medical Research," *American Journal of Bioethics* 4 (2004): 56–57.

40. A report from a National Academy of Sciences committee argues for loosening some of the restrictions on the use of prisoners in research. See Lawrence O. Gostin, Cori Vanchieri, and Andrew Pope, eds., *Ethical Considerations for Research Involving Prisoners* (Washington, D.C.: The National Academies Press, 2007).

41. See Sarah E. Hewlett, "Is Consent to Participate in Research Voluntary?" *Arthritis Care and Research* 9 (1996): 400–04; Hewlett, "Consent to Clinical Research—Adequately Voluntary or Substantially Influenced?" *Journal of Medical Ethics* 22 (1996): 232–36; Robert M. Nelson and Jon F. Merz, "Voluntariness of Consent for Research: An Empirical and Conceptual Review," *Medical Care* 40 (2002), Suppl., V69–80.

42. Common Rule for the Protection of Human Subjects, U.S. Code of Federal Regulations, 45 CFR 46.116 (as revised October 1, 2003); and see Ezekiel Emanuel, "Ending Concerns about Undue Inducement," *Journal of Law, Medicine, & Ethics* 32 (2004): 100–05, esp. p. 101.

43. The justification of monetary inducement in terms of mutual benefit is defended by Martin Wilkinson and Andrew Moore, "Inducement in Research," *Bioethics* 11 (1997), 373–89; and Wilkinson and Moore, "Inducements Revisited," *Bioethics* 13 (1999): 114–30. See also Christine Grady, "Money for Research Participation: Does It Jeopardize Informed Consent?" *American Journal of Bioethics* 1 (2001): 40–44.

44. See Neal Dickert and Christine Grady, "What's the Price of a Research Subject?: Approaches to Payment for Research Participation," *New England Journal of Medicine* 341 (1999): 198–203; David Resnick, "Research Participation and Financial Inducements," *American Journal of Bioethics* 1 (2001): 54–56.

45. See Beauchamp, Jennings, Kinney, and Levine, "Pharmaceutical Research Involving the Homeless."

46. See Nik Theodore, Edwin Melendez, and Ana Luz Gonzalez, "On the Corner: Day Labor in the United States," http://www.sscnet.ucla.edu/issr/csup/uploaded_files/Natl_DayLabor-On_the_Corner1.pdf.

47. For figures, see U.S. Census information on health insurance: http://www.census.gov/hhes/www/hlthins/hlthin05/hlth05asc.html.

48. See Daniels, *Just Health Care,* chaps. 3 and 4.

49. Cf. Allen Buchanan, "The Right to a Decent Minimum of Health Care," *Philosophy and Public Affairs* 13 (Winter 1984): 55–78; and Buchanan, "Health-Care Delivery and Resource Allocation," in *Medical Ethics,* 2nd ed., ed. Robert M. Veatch (Boston: Jones & Bartlett, 1997), esp. pp. 337–59.

50. Compare Peter A. Ubel et al., "Cost-Effectiveness Analysis in a Setting of Budget Constraints—Is It Equitable?" *New England Journal of Medicine* 334 (May 2, 1996): 1174–77; and Paul T. Menzel, "Justice and the Basic Structure of Health-Care Systems," in *Medicine and Social Justice,* ed. R. Rhodes, M. P. Battin, and A. Silvers (New York: Oxford University Press, 2002), pp. 24–37.

51. This discussion of Dworkin's position draws from his *Sovereign Virtue: The Theory and Practice of Equality* (Cambridge, MA: Harvard University Press, 2000), chap. 8; and "Justice in the Distribution of Health Care," *McGill Law Journal* 38 (1993): 883–98.

52. Robert M. Veatch, "Voluntary Risks to Health: The Ethical Issues," *Journal of the American Medical Association* 243 (January 4, 1980): 50–55.

53. Abdou S. Gueye et al., "The Association between Recipient Alcohol Dependency and Long-Term Graft and Recipient Survival," *Nephrology Dialysis Transplantation* 22 (2007): 891–98; J. Dumortier et al., "Negative Impact of De Novo Malignancies Rather than Alcohol Relapse on Survival after Liver Transplantation for Alcoholic Cirrhosis," *American Journal of Gastroenterology* 102 (2007): 1032–41; and Robert Pfitzmann et al., "Long-Term Survival and Predictors of Relapse after Orthotopic Liver Transplantation for Alcoholic Liver Disease," *Liver Transplantation* 13 (2007): 197–205.

54. Alvin H. Moss and Mark Siegler, "Should Alcoholics Compete Equally for Liver Transplantation?" *Journal of the American Medical Association* 265 (March 13, 1991): 1295–98. See also Robert M. Veatch, *Transplantation Ethics* (Washington, D.C.: Georgetown University Press, 2000); and Walter Glannon, "Responsibility, Alcoholism, and Liver Transplantation," *Journal of Medicine and Philosophy* 23 (1998): 31–49.

55. On this distinction and egalitarian justice, see John E. Roemer, *Equality of Opportunity* (Cambridge, MA: Harvard University Press, 1998).

56. An argument based on justice against the total exclusion of alcoholics from liver transplantation appears in Carl Cohen, Martin Benjamin, and the Ethics and Social Impact Committee of the [Michigan] Transplant and Health Policy Center, "Alcoholics and Liver Transplantation," *Journal of the American Medical Association* 265 (March 13, 1991): 1299–1301.

57. United Nations Office of the High Commissioner for Human Rights, "The Right of Everyone to the Enjoyment of the Highest Attainable Standard of Physical and Mental Health," United Nations Commission on Human Rights Resolution 2004/27 (New York: United Nations, 2004).

58. Thomas Pogge, ed., *Freedom from Poverty as a Human Right: Who Owes What to the Very Poor?* (Oxford: Oxford University Press, 2007); Pogge, "Human Rights and Global Health: A Research Program," *Metaphilosophy* 36 (2005): 182–209.

59. For an expansive list focused on capabilities, see Martha Nussbaum's writings, including *Frontiers of Justice: Disability, Nationality, Species Membership*; *Sex and Social Justice* (New York: Oxford University Press, 1999); and *Women and Human Development* (Cambridge: Cambridge University Press, 2000). In part, she is extending Amartya Sen's work—see, for example, his *Development as Freedom* (New York: Random House, 1999).

60. Powers and Faden, *Social Justice: The Moral Foundations of Public Health and Health Policy*, esp. pp. 64–79.

61. In contrast to some societies, the United States does not have a closed system, but a pluralistic system, only some portions of which are closed so that trade-offs can be clearly made.

62. See Norman Daniels and James Sabin, *Setting Limits Fairly: Can We Learn to Share Medical Resources?* (New York: Oxford University Press, 2002); Powers and Faden, *Social Justice*, chap. 6, "Setting Limits."

63. Oregon Senate Bill 27 (March 31, 1989). See also Lawrence Jacobs, Theodore Marmor, and Jonathan Oberlander, "The Oregon Health Plan and the Political Paradox of Rationing: What Advocates and Critics Have Claimed and What Oregon Did," *Journal of Health Politics, Policy and Law* 24 (1999): 161–80.

64. Health Economics Research, Inc., for the Health Care Financing Administration, *Evolution of the Oregon Plan* (Washington, D.C.: NTIS No. PB98–135916 INZ, Dec. 12, 1997, as updated Jan. 19, 1999). Oregon Department of Administrative Services, *Assessment of the Oregon Health Plan Medicaid Demonstration* (Salem, OR: Office for Oregon Health Plan Policy and Research, 1999).

65. Jonathan Oberlander, "Health Reform Interrupted: The Unraveling of the Oregon Health Plan," *Health Affairs* 26 (January–February 2007): w96–w105; Rachel Solotaroff et al., "Medicaid Programme Changes and the Chronically Ill: Early Results from a Prospective Cohort Study of the Oregon Health

Plan," *Chronic Illness* 1 (2005): 191–205; Matthew J. Carlson, Jennifer DeVoe, and Bill J. Wright, "Short-Term Impacts of Coverage Loss in a Medicaid Population: Early Results from a Prospective Cohort Study of the Oregon Health Plan," *Annals of Family Medicine* 4 (2006): 391–98.

66. This section is indebted to Powers and Faden, *Social Justice,* chap. 6.

67. See Paul T. Menzel, *Medical Costs, Moral Choices* (New Haven, CT: Yale University Press, 1983), chap. 7.

68. A classic article on this now commonplace distinction is Thomas C. Schelling, "The Life You Save May Be Your Own," in *Problems in Public Expenditure Analysis,* ed. Samuel B. Chase, Jr. (Washington, D.C.: Brookings Institution, 1966), pp. 127–76.

69. L. B. Russell et al., "The Role of Cost-Effectiveness Analysis in Health and Medicine," *Journal of the American Medical Association* 276 (1996): 1172–77; Dan Brock, "Ethical Issues in the Use of Cost-Effectiveness Analysis," in *Public Health, Ethics, and Equity,* ed. Sudhir Anand, Fabienne Peter, and Amartya Sen (Oxford: Oxford University Press, 2004), pp. 201–23.

70. See Norman Daniels and James E. Sabin, "Last Chance Therapies and Managed Care: Pluralism, Fair Procedures, and Legitimacy," *Hastings Center Report* 28 (1998): 27–41; Dennis Thompson and Amy Gutmann, *Democracy and Disagreement* (Cambridge, MA: The Belknap Press of Harvard University Press, 1996).

71. Erik Nord, *Cost-Value Analysis in Health Care: Making Sense out of QALY's* (Cambridge: Cambridge University Press, 1999); Paul Menzel, "How Should What Economists Call 'Social Values' Be Measured?" *Journal of Ethics* 3 (1999): 249–73; and Christopher Murray and Arnab Acharya, "Understanding DALYs," *Journal of Health Economics* 16 (1997): 703–30.

72. For a discussion of "rationing" and a defense of its broad use, see Peter A. Ubel, *Pricing Life: Why It's Time for Health Care Rationing* (Cambridge, MA: The MIT Press, 2000).

73. John McKenzie et al., "Dialysis Decision Making in Canada, the United Kingdom, and the United States," *American Journal of Kidney Diseases* 31 (1998): 12–18; Adrian Furnham and Abigail Ofstein, "Ethical Ideology and the Allocation of Scarce Medical Resources," *British Journal of Medical Psychology* 70 (1997): 51–63.

74. Daniels, *Just Health* and *Am I My Parents' Keeper?* (New York: Oxford University Press, 1988).

75. Alan Williams, "Intergenerational Equity: An Exploration of the 'Fair Innings' Argument," *Health Economics* 6 (1997): 117–32.

76. For criticism, see Dan W. Brock, "Justice, Health Care, and the Elderly," *Philosophy and Public Affairs* 18 (1989): 297–312.

77. Nicholas G. Smedira, "Allocating Hearts," *Journal of Thoracic and Cardiovascular Surgery* 131 (2006): 775–76; National Kidney Foundation, "Getting a Heart Transplant," http://www.kidney.org/atoz/atozItem.cfm?id=158 (accessed July 9, 2007).

78. U.S. Department of Health and Human Services, *Report of Task Force on Organ Transplantation, Organ Transplantation: Issues and Recommendations* (Washington, D.C.: DHHS, 1986), pp. 105, 111. See also Institute of Medicine, "Improving the Nation's Organ Transplantation System," http://www.iom.edu/iom/iomhome.nsf/pages/1999+reports.

79. Contrast Norman Daniels, "Comment: Ability to Pay and Access to Transplantation," *Transplantation Proceedings* 21 (June 1989): 3434; and F. M. Kamm, "The Report of the U.S. Task Force on Organ Transplantation: Criticisms and Alternatives," *Mount Sinai Journal of Medicine* 56 (May 1989): 207–20.

80. Originally proposed by Nicholas Rescher, "The Allocation of Exotic Medical Lifesaving Therapy," *Ethics* 79 (1969): 173–86.

81. Task Force, *Organ Transplantation*. On the evolution of U.S. organ transplant policies, see Jeffrey Prottas, *The Most Useful Gift: Altruism and the Public Policy of Organ Transplants* (San Francisco: Jossey-Boss, 1994).

82. Task Force, *Organ Transplantation*, p. 95.

83. Compare and contrast Robert M. Veatch, "The Ethics of Resource Allocation in Critical Care," *Critical Care Clinics* 2 (January 1986): 73–89; Richard Wenstone, "Resource Allocation in Critical Care," in *Ethics in Anaesthesia and Intensive Care,* ed. Heather Draper and Wendy E. Scott (New York: Butterworth-Heinemann, 2003): 145–62; Gerald Winslow, *Triage and Justice: The Ethics of Rationing Life-Saving Medical Resources* (Berkeley, CA: University of California Press, 1982); and John Kilner, *Who Lives? Who Dies? Ethical Criteria in Patient Selection* (New Haven, CT: Yale University Press, 1990).

84. See Duff R. Waring, *Medical Benefit and the Human Lottery* (Dordrecht, Netherlands: Springer, 2004) and, more broadly, Barbara Goodwin, *Justice by Lottery* (Chicago: The University of Chicago Press, 1992).

85. The statement derives from Evan DeRenzo. It appeared in Diane Naughton, "Drug Lotteries Raise Questions: Some Experts Say System of Distribution May Be Unfair," *Washington Post,* Health Section, September 26, 1995, pp. 14–15.

86. In Seattle, members of a closely watched committee that selected patients for dialysis felt intense pressure and stress, often accompanied by guilt. See John Broome, "Selecting People Randomly," *Ethics* 95 (1984): 41.

87. Robert D. Truog, "Triage in the ICU," *Hastings Center Report* 22 (May–June 1992): 13–17.

88. See Ramsey, *The Patient as Person* (New Haven, CT: Yale University Press, 1970), pp. 257–58. For the controversy about this example, see Robert Baker and Martin Strosberg, "Triage and Equality: An Historical Reassessment of Utilitarian Analyses of Triage," *Kennedy Institute of Ethics Journal* 2 (1992): 101–23.

89. Winslow, *Triage and Justice*; but contrast Baker and Strosberg, "Triage and Equality: An Historical Reassessment." See also Robert A. Gatter and John C. Moskop, "From Futility to Triage," *Journal of Medicine and Philosophy* 20 (1995): 191–205; Society of Critical Care Medicine—Ethics Committee, "Consensus Statement on the Triage of Critically Ill Patients," *Journal of the American Medical Association* 271 (April 20, 1994): 1200–03. See also the utilitarian rationale in U.S. penicillin rationing examined in David P. Adams, *"The Greatest Good to the Greatest Number": Penicillin Rationing on the American Home Front, 1940–1945* (New York: Peter Lang, 1991).

90. See James F. Childress, "Triage in Response to a Bioterrorist Attack," in *In the Wake of Terror: Medicine and Morality in a Time of Crisis,* ed. Jonathan D. Moreno (Cambridge, MA: The MIT Press, 2003), pp. 77–93.

8
Professional–Patient Relationships

The previous four chapters presented moral principles relevant to medicine, health care, and research with human subjects. In this chapter we specify these principles in the form of rules of veracity, privacy, confidentiality, and fidelity. Some rules specify a single principle, and others specify more than one principle.

VERACITY

Codes of medical ethics have traditionally ignored obligations and virtues of veracity. The Hippocratic Oath does not recommend veracity, nor does the Declaration of Geneva of the World Medical Association. The Principles of Medical Ethics of the American Medical Association (AMA) from its origins until 1980 made no mention of an obligation or virtue of veracity, giving physicians unrestricted discretion about what to divulge to patients. The 1980 revision recommended, without elaboration, that physicians "deal honestly with patients and colleagues," and the 2001 revision indicates that physicians shall "be honest in all professional interactions."[1]

Despite this traditional neglect of veracity, the virtues of candor, honesty, and truthfulness are among widely and deservedly praised character traits of health professionals and researchers. However, the nature and status of norms and virtues of veracity are unclear. Henry Sidgwick's nineteenth-century observation still holds: "It does not seem clearly agreed whether Veracity is an absolute and independent obligation, or a special application of some higher principle."[2] G. J. Warnock's later assessment was that veracity is an independent principle and virtue that ranks in importance with beneficence, nonmaleficence, and justice.[3] We view obligations of veracity as specifications of more than one principle.

Obligations of Veracity

Veracity in the health care setting refers to comprehensive, accurate, and objective transmission of information, as well as to the way the professional fosters the patient's or subject's understanding. In this regard, veracity is closely connected to respect for autonomy. However, three arguments support obligations of veracity, and they are not entirely derivable from respect for autonomy.

First, obligations of veracity are based on respect owed to others. Even if consent is not at issue, the obligation to respect others' autonomy supports obligations of veracity in many contexts. Second, obligations of veracity are connected to obligations of fidelity, promise-keeping, and contract.[4] When we communicate with others, we implicitly promise that we will speak truthfully and that we will not deceive listeners. By entering into a relationship in health care or research, the patient or subject enters into a contract that includes a right to truthful information regarding diagnosis, prognosis, procedures, and the like, just as the professional gains a right to truthful disclosures from patients and subjects. Third, relationships between health professionals and patients and subjects depend on trust, and adherence to rules of veracity is essential to foster trust.

Like other obligations discussed in this volume, veracity is prima facie binding, not absolute. Careful management of medical information—including limited disclosure, nondisclosure, deception, and even lying—is occasionally justified when veracity conflicts with other obligations. Although the weight of various obligations of veracity is difficult to determine outside of specific contexts, some generalizations may be tendered: Deception that does not involve lying is usually less difficult to justify than lying, in part because in many contexts in health care it does not threaten as deeply the relationship of trust. Deception involves intentionally leading, or attempting to lead, someone to believe what is false, while lying seeks the same aim through statements.[5] Underdisclosure and nondisclosure of information are usually still less difficult to justify.[6]

The Disclosure of Bad News to Patients

An example of these problems is intentional nondisclosure to patients of a diagnosis of cancer or a prognosis of imminent death. Various views exist, often rooted in different cultural traditions, about when nondisclosure can be justified.[7] In a striking case, Mr. X, a fifty-four-year-old male patient, consented to surgery for probable malignancy in his thyroid gland. After the surgery, the physician told him that the diagnosis had been confirmed and that the tumor had been successfully removed, but did not inform him of the likelihood of lung metastases and death within a few months. The physician did, however, inform Mr. X's wife, son, and daughter-in-law about the fuller diagnosis and about the prognosis for Mr. X, but all parties agreed to conceal the diagnosis and prognosis from Mr. X. The physician told Mr. X only that he needed "preventive" treatment, and Mr. X consented to irradiation and chemotherapy. The physician did not inform Mr. X of the probable causes of his subsequent shortness of breath and back pain. Unaware of his impending death, Mr. X died three months later.[8]

Shifts in policies of disclosure. Over a couple of decades, a dramatic shift occurred in U.S. physicians' stated policies of disclosure of the diagnosis of cancer to patients. In 1961, 88% of physicians surveyed indicated that they sought to avoid disclosing a diagnosis of cancer to patients, but by 1979, 98% of those surveyed reported a policy of disclosure to cancer patients.[9] In the 1979 survey physicians identified the four factors they most frequently considered in deciding whether to tell the patient: age (56% of respondents), a relative's wishes regarding disclosure to the patient (51%), emotional stability (47%), and intelligence (44%).

Although veracity in the disclosure of bad news has increased still further since 1979, some oncology communities remain reluctant to disclose bad news and choose to withhold certain types of information.[10] It is unfortunate that, as in the case of Mr. X, familial preferences often unjustifiably influence clinicians' decisions about disclosure of diagnosis and prognosis to patients. Some physicians might counter that the family can help the physician determine whether the patient is autonomous and capable of receiving information about serious risk. Although true, this point begs the most important question: By what right does a physician initially disclose information to a family without the patient's consent? Families provide important care and support for many patients, but an autonomous patient has the right to veto familial involvement altogether. It is unethical for the physician to first disclose information to a patient's family without the patient's authorization. The best policy is to ask the patient both at the outset and as the illness progresses about the extent to which he or she wants to involve others. This generalization holds irrespective of the patient's cultural background, which often serves as an inappropriate excuse for going around the patient to another party.

Arguments for noncommunication or limited communication of bad news. Four arguments support some measure of noncommunication, limited disclosure, or deception in health care, particularly when there is "bad news."

The first argument rests on what Henry Sidgwick and others have called "benevolent deception." Such deception has long been a part of medical tradition and practice. Its defenders hold that disclosure, particularly of a prognosis of death, sometimes violates obligations of beneficence and nonmaleficence by causing the patient anxiety, by destroying the patient's hope, by retarding or erasing a therapeutic outcome, by leading the patient to commit suicide, and the like.

This first line of argument—"What you don't know can't hurt and may help you"—is consequentialist. One objection to this argument rests on the uncertainty of predicting consequences. Samuel Johnson said, "I deny the lawfulness of telling a lie to a sick man for fear of alarming him. You have no business with consequences; you are to tell the truth. Besides, you are not sure what effects your telling him that he is in danger may have."[11] Lies may increase rather than relieve suffering.[12]

Staged disclosure and cautious language about prognosis, with the aspiration of maintaining a patient's hope, can be justified in some cases, despite their threat to trust between clinicians and patients. Professional norms generally support the frank and direct sharing of information about diagnosis and about therapeutic options, but they often tend to discourage these same qualities in sharing prognostic information.[13] For prognosis, professional norms incorporate the therapeutic value of hope for patients, and virtues of compassion, gentleness, and sensitivity often displace veracity. These norms encourage disclosure of "bad news" over time rather than all at once. Staged disclosure and cautious language are illustrated in the following case from rehabilitation medicine.[14] For close to a month, a physician in a stroke rehabilitation unit carefully managed information in his interactions with a patient who had suffered a stroke and who asked during a first session how long it would take for his arm to improve. From the beginning the doctor knew that the patient was unlikely to recover significant use of his arm, and he offered caveats and uncertainty that did not fully match what he believed or felt. He stressed the limitations of prognostication, the unpredictability of recovery, and the need to give the brain a chance to heal. The patient received these answers well at the time, apparently preferring the physician's "ambiguous statements about the future to the alternative judgment of the permanent paralysis he fears." This indefinite, but caring and supportive, exchange continued, with the physician praising the patient's progress in walking and performing daily activities, despite residual weakness. After two weeks, the patient was enthusiastic about his progress and asked, "How about my arm?" The physician responded, "The arm may not recover as much as the leg." Although this statement confirmed his fears, the patient focused on his overall progress. He had a strong hope that the physician might be mistaken, since he had repeatedly stressed his inability to prognosticate accurately.

Commenting on this case later, the physician noted that, having been trained in the era of "patient autonomy," he once felt that he "should share all available information [he] could provide about prognosis as early as possible," trying to temper unfavorable news, for instance, about arm recovery, with positive predictions of restored walking and independent living. However, because his patients hoped for a return to their earlier lives, the bad news at any early stage tended to overwhelm the good news. Thus, he became convinced that most of his "patients were not ready for the cold hard facts the minute they arrived at the rehabilitation hospital. They needed time to come to terms with the reality of their disabilities, while simultaneously regaining lost function." Staged disclosures clearly help to sustain patients' hopes.

The second argument for limited disclosure, nondisclosure, and deception is that health care professionals cannot know the "whole truth": "you can never tell what will happen," "each patient is unique," and so on. Disclosure of the whole truth about a complex situation is an ideal against which health care professionals can measure their performance, but it can only be approximated. We can best use this ideal to help formulate a standard of *substantial* completeness that is realistic and appropriate for health care professionals (as we discussed thoroughly in Chapter 4).

The third argument is that, even if professionals could know the whole truth, patients—or at least many patients—would not be able to understand and appreciate the scope and implications of the information provided. Communication can be complex, especially if the patient has limited capacity to understand, and sometimes, as in the following case, intentional verbal inaccuracy can be justified: Over the years, a ninety-year-old patient, who as a young man had been decorated for courageous actions in battle, had become fearful that he would develop cancer, which, for him, meant a shameful, painful, and fatal disease that would spread inexorably. He was referred for an ulcer on his lip; a biopsy established the diagnosis of squamous cell carcinoma, which would require only a short course of radiotherapy to cure, without any need for surgery or even admission to the hospital. The elderly patient, tears in his eyes, asked, "It's not cancer, is it?" The physician emphatically denied that it was cancer.[15]

The physician justified his action on several grounds. First, he pointed to the patient's deep need for "effective reassurance." Second, he argued that it was "more truthful" to tell this patient that he did not have cancer than to tell him that he did, because it would have been impossible to inform him that he had a curable cancer "without leaving him with a false and untrue impression" because of his enduring and unchangeable beliefs. Third, addressing this patient and his concerns in his own language expressed respect rather than paternalistic arrogance. Implicit in these justifications is the conviction that, because of his apparently unalterable false beliefs, this patient lacked the capacity to understand the diagnosis of cancer, which, *for him,* entailed the prognosis of death. In our judgment the physician's decision was warranted. (See our discussion of false belief in Chapter 4 and of weak paternalism in Chapter 6.)

A fourth argument is that some patients, particularly the very sick and the dying, do not want to know the truth about their condition. Despite surveys that almost universally indicate that the majority of patients in the United States want to know, physicians and others maintain that some patients indicate by signals, if not actual words, that they do not, in fact, want the truth. However, claims about what patients genuinely want are inherently dubious when they contradict the patients' own reports, and this fourth argument sets dangerous precedents for patently paternalistic actions, masquerading as respect for autonomy.

Relying heavily on the family's judgment that the patient would not want to receive "bad news" also sets dangerous precedents. An Italian oncologist reports that she tries to tell her patients "the complete truth," but sometimes the patient's family asks her not to use the word "cancer."[16] She then relies, in a manner traditionally honored as Italian medical beneficence, on *nonverbal communication* to establish truthful therapeutic relationships with patients, listening to them and respecting their need for information. Although this is a dangerous position, we should not conclude that such traditional social practices necessarily fail to respect individual autonomy. The ways in which patients exercise their autonomy will reflect their self-understandings, including sociocultural expectations and religious or other beliefs. A choice not to know can be as autonomous and as worthy of respect as a choice to know. Accordingly, a physician needs care and sensitivity to understand a particular patient's preferences and to respect that patient by managing the information according to those preferences.

Nevertheless, attending to a particular patient's desire for information about prognosis is often complicated, and it may be unclear at the time, or even at the end, whether a moral mistake was made. In one case, a twenty-six-year-old woman, the mother of two young children, had an aggressive adenocarcinoma. Following radiation therapy and two different chemotherapeutic combinations, she was fragile, but stable.[17] She was on oxygen continuously and took long-acting morphine (60 mg) three times a day. Yet, she was energetic and life-affirming. She told the new hematology/oncology fellow that she had "a feeling" (based on her increased hip pain and enlarged nodules) that "things aren't going as well as people tell me they are" and hoped he had some new "tricks" up his sleeve. She promptly consented to a new drug after he explained its administration, its potential adverse effects, and the ways they would try to prevent those effects, as well as his "hope that we would begin to see the long-sought-for response that might begin to heal her."

However, on the way to the chemotherapy unit, she said that she had heard about a woman dying of leukemia who had written several stories for her children to remember her by. She continued, "My girlfriend said I should do the same thing for my kids, but I don't think I'm *that* far gone, am I, Doctor Dan?" Her physician reports his "stunned silence." Unprepared for such a question, he was unsure how to respond in the hall of a busy clinic, hardly the ideal setting in which to break bad news. Faced with her radiant smile, he replied: "No, Lisa, I don't think you're at that point. I'm hopeful that this new treatment will work and that you will be able to spend a lot more time with your kids." "That's what I thought, Doctor Dan," she responded. "Thanks. Now on to round three." Fourteen days later, she died, without having written her stories for her children. Years later, the physician continued to hear the echo of his last words to her, wondering whether conveying a different message, with its bad news, would have allowed her to pen a few words or poems or to record thoughts or messages that would provide her children a living memory of their dynamic, carefree mother.

Disclosure of medical errors. "Preventable adverse events are a leading cause of death" in U.S. hospitals, according to a report from the Institute of Medicine, which claims that "at least 44,000, and perhaps as many as 98,000, Americans die in hospitals each year as a result of medical errors."[18] There are disputes about the classification of preventable adverse events, their numbers, their causes, and potential solutions.[19] For instance, not all preventable adverse events—whether lethal or nonlethal, in the hospital or in other settings—are the result of medical errors or mistakes. One primary moral responsibility is to develop systems, including training programs, to reduce medical errors and other causes of preventable adverse events. A related moral responsibility is to disclose specific medical errors to patients and their families. Adequate disclosure often does not occur and is rarely documented.[20] Evasive formulations, including the use of the passive voice, ambiguous language, and euphemisms, frequently mark disclosures that do occur.[21]

According to recent codes and guidelines—and according to our arguments about respect for autonomy in Chapter 4—individual clinicians and institutions have an ethical responsibility to disclose unanticipated negative outcomes.[22] Respect for personal autonomy entails disclosure of what occurred—even if no further medical decisions are involved—and of options to take nonmedical actions, including legal actions, if appropriate.

The disclosure of medical error is a subset of the provision of bad news, but it is more difficult to undertake, because clinicians or institutions caused or exacerbated the harms. Fears of malpractice suits regularly deter disclosure of medical errors. Although these fears are understandable, nondisclosure is morally wrong. Moreover, available evidence indicates that these fears are often overblown, and some evidence shows that disclosure is the best policy for reducing the likelihood of malpractice suits.[23] Other reasons for nondisclosure or limited disclosure of medical errors include concerns about harming patients and damaging patient and public trust, as well as facing staff opposition. None of these reasons justifies secrecy regarding medical errors.

The wall of almost collusive silence that often surrounds medical mistakes is a troublesome feature of medical cultures. In one case, a young boy's parents took him to a medical center for treatment of a respiratory problem. After being placed in the adult intensive care unit, he received ten times the normal dosage of muscle relaxant, and the respirator tube slipped and pumped oxygen into his stomach for several minutes. He suffered cardiac arrest and permanent brain damage. His parents accidentally overheard a conversation that mentioned the overdose. The physician involved had decided not to inform the parents of the mistake because they "had enough on [their] minds already," but the parents felt that their tragedy was compounded by the duplicity of the physician, whom they had, until this point, trusted.

Deception of Third-Party Payers

Vigorous efforts to contain the costs of health care in the United States, particularly through managed care organizations, have led some physicians to use and to justify deception to secure third-party coverage. A physician in obstetrics and gynecology presented the following example: A forty-year-old woman underwent a diagnostic laparoscopy for primary infertility. Because the woman's private insurance policy did not cover this procedure for this indication, the attending surgeon instructed the resident not to write anything about infertility in the operative notes, but rather to stress the two or three fine adhesions found in the pelvic area; if these pelvic adhesions were the indication for the procedure, the patient's insurance would then cover it. When the resident refused, the attending prepared the operative note.[24]

Several studies have attempted to determine the extent to which physicians use, or would be willing to use, deception on behalf of their patients. According to one study, close to 50% of the physicians surveyed admitted that they had exaggerated the severity of their patients' medical condition so that those patients would be covered for the medical care the physicians believed they needed.[25] In another survey, 39% of physicians indicated that they had exaggerated the severity of patients' conditions, altered patients' diagnoses, or reported signs or symptoms that patients did not have, with the intent to help patients obtain coverage for needed care.[26] Other studies have used vignettes to determine the extent to which physicians are willing to deceive or allow deception of a third-party payer to secure approval for procedures for patients. In one study, over half of the internists surveyed sanctioned the use of deception for clinically severe vignettes in which the patients were at immediate risk and needed coronary bypass surgery or arterial revascularization.[27] A survey of physicians and the general public found that "the public was more than twice as likely as physicians to sanction deception (26% versus 11%) and half as likely to believe that physicians have adequate time to appeal coverage decisions (22% versus 59%)."[28]

Physicians confront a tension between their traditional roles as patient advocates and their roles within institutional structures that control financial resources. We do not maintain that deception can never be justified, but physicians should seek alternative, nondeceptive courses of action, such as formal appeals, and should work to alter unduly restrictive systems. The understandable temptations of deception in these systems pose a threat to physician integrity as well as to fairness in the distribution of benefits in these systems.

Privacy

Concerns about privacy and confidentiality pervade much of medicine, health care, and research. Privacy became a major concern more recently than confidentiality, which has a long history in medical ethics.

Privacy in Law and Legal Theory

In the 1920s the U.S. Supreme Court employed an expansive "liberty" interest to protect family decision making about child rearing, education, and the like. It later adopted the term *privacy* and expanded the individual's and the family's interests in family life, child rearing, and other areas of personal choice. The Court's famous family-planning decisions articulate this privacy right. *Griswold v. Connecticut* (1965), a contraception case, was the first to construe the right to privacy not only as shielding information from others, but as protecting an area of individual and familial freedom from governmental interference. The Court's decision overturned state legislation that prohibited the use or dissemination of contraceptives. It indicated that the right to privacy protects liberty by exempting a zone of private life from public regulation.[29]

It may seem inappropriate to make a right that protects individual or familial interests one of privacy rather than liberty or autonomy. However that difficult issue is decided, the right to privacy in American law encompasses rights of limited physical and informational access, as well as rights of decisional freedom. Reducing this right to a right to be free to do something or a right to act autonomously creates confusion for reasons we now explore.

The Concept of Privacy

Some definitions of "privacy" focus on an agent's *control* over access to himself or herself, but these definitions confuse privacy, which is a state or condition of limited access, with an agent's control over privacy or a right to privacy, which involves the agent's right to control access. These definitions focus on powers or rights rather than privacy itself. A person can have privacy without having any *control* over access by others. Privacy exists, for example, in some long-term care facilities that render patients inaccessible.

Anita Allen has identified four forms of privacy that involve limited access to the person: *informational privacy,* which biomedical ethics often emphasizes; *physical privacy,* which focuses on persons and their personal spaces; *decisional privacy,* which concerns personal choices; and *proprietary privacy,* which highlights property interests in the human person.[30] We propose a fifth form of privacy—*relational* or *associational privacy.* It includes the family and similarly intimate relations, within which individuals make decisions in conjunction with others. This form of privacy recognizes that often individuals make private decisions within intimate relationships.

As these different forms of privacy suggest, definitions of privacy are too narrow if presented solely in terms of limited access to *information* about a person. A loss of privacy occurs if others use any of several forms of access, including intervening in zones of secrecy, anonymity, seclusion, or solitude.[31] Privacy, as limited access, extends to bodily products and objects intimately associated with the person, as well as to the person's intimate relationships with friends, lovers, spouses, physicians, and others.

In some contexts it is desirable to provide a tighter definition of "privacy," especially when developing policies about which forms of access to which aspects of persons will constitute losses and violations of privacy. We are, however, reluctant to tinker with the concept to make it more serviceable for certain types of policy. Instead, we recommend that policymakers who construct privacy policies carefully specify the conditions of access that will and will not count as a loss of privacy or a violation of the right to privacy. The policy should define the zones that are considered private and not to be invaded and should also identify interests that legitimately may be balanced against privacy interests. Often the focus will be informational privacy, but the strategy we recommend applies to the range of privacy interests.

Finally, the value we place on a condition of limited access or nonaccess explains how it comes to be categorized as private. Concerns about a loss of privacy may depend not only on the kind and extent of access, but also on who has access, through what means, to which aspect of the person. As Charles Fried notes, "We may not mind that a person knows a general fact about us, and yet feel our privacy invaded if he knows the details. For instance, a casual acquaintance may comfortably know that I am sick, but it would violate my privacy if he knew the nature of the illness."[32]

Justifications of the Right to Privacy

In their celebrated 1890 article "The Right to Privacy," Samuel Warren and Louis Brandeis argued that a legal right to privacy flows from fundamental rights to life, liberty, and property.[33] They derived it largely from "the right to enjoy life—the right to be let alone." But this near-vacuous right needs more content. In recent discussions, several alternative justifications of the right to privacy have been proposed, three of which deserve attention here.

One approach reduces the right to privacy to a cluster of other rights from which this right derives. Judith Thomson argues that this cluster of personal and property rights includes rights not to be looked at, not to be listened to, not to be caused distress (e.g., by the publication of certain information), not to be harmed, hurt, or tortured (in an effort to obtain certain information, say), and so on. Her argument relies on several allegedly foundational rights that have an uncertain status, such as the right not to be looked at. We are not convinced that each of these alleged rights is a right, and some of these rights may have the right to privacy as their basis, rather than the converse.[34] One might plausibly argue that each violation of these "basic" rights is wrong because it wrongfully gains access to a person, thereby violating a right to privacy.

A second approach emphasizes the instrumental value of privacy and the right to privacy by identifying various ends that rules of privacy promote. Consequentialist theories justify rules of privacy according to their instrumental value for such ends as personal development, creating and maintaining intimate social relations, and expressing personal freedom.[35] Fried, for example, argues that privacy is a necessary condition for creating and maintaining intimate relationships of respect, love, friendship, and trust.[36]

Clearly, we build and maintain various relationships by granting some and denying others certain kinds of access to ourselves. However, we question whether the instrumental value of privacy is the primary justification of rights to privacy. Instead, the primary justification seems closer to respect for autonomy, the third justification commonly offered. We owe respect in the sense of deference to persons' autonomous wishes not to be observed, touched, intruded on, and the like. The right to authorize or decline access is basic. In this respect, the justification of the right to privacy parallels the justification of the right to give an informed consent that we developed in Chapter 4.

Joel Feinberg has observed that, historically, the language of autonomy has functioned as a political metaphor for a domain or territory in which a state is sovereign. Personal autonomy carries over the idea of a region of sovereignty for the self and a right to protect it by restricting access, an idea closely linked to the concepts of privacy and the right to privacy.[37] Other metaphors expressing privacy in the personal domain include zones and spheres of privacy that protect autonomy.

Specifying and Balancing Rules of Privacy for Public Policy

Three examples will indicate how to specify rules and rights of privacy, while allowing for justified intrusions on privacy that balance privacy interests against other interests. These examples concern privacy in (1) screening and testing for HIV infection, (2) ensuring effective treatment for patients with active tuberculosis, and (3) applied human genetics. The first two are issues in public health ethics.[38]

Compulsory and voluntary screening for HIV. The HIV/AIDS epidemic has caused many millions of deaths and vast suffering around the world. Many people do not know that they are infected. At first glance, testing and screening appear to be a good public health strategy to reduce the spread of HIV infection.[39] However, as HIV testing and screening expand, it becomes urgent to ask what social institutions and health care professionals plan to do with information about a person who tests positive for HIV infection. Screening that identifies the individual screened involves some loss of privacy, because others gain access to private information. If testing is anonymous, no loss of privacy occurs. The following chart depicts possible policies toward screening with identifiers for HIV infection:

		Form of Authorization	
		Voluntary	*Compulsory*
	Universal	1	2
Scope of Screening			
	Selective	3	4

Voluntary-universal screening (1), in contrast to compulsory-universal screening (2), rests on encouragement and choice, rather than coercion, and consequently does not in itself violate any moral rights of privacy or autonomy. However, neither voluntary- nor compulsory-universal screening is justified by current evidence. Universal screening is not necessary to protect the public health. HIV infection is not widespread outside groups engaging in high-risk activities. Screening in groups or areas with low prevalence of HIV infection produces false positives, especially without confirmatory testing. Universal screening would be very costly and cost-ineffective, and it would have to be repeated often.

In the fifth edition of this book, we indicated that our rejection of (1) and (2) is subject to reversal if various conditions change. Several circumstances have recently changed, particularly the development and use of increasingly effective antiretroviral drugs that, combined with other medical developments, have made HIV/AIDS more of a chronic condition. Nevertheless, it is still difficult to justify voluntary-universal screening in terms of cost-effectiveness and cost-benefit assessments, and it is impossible, in our judgment, to justify mandatory universal HIV screening.

However, voluntary-selective screening (3) can be justified, especially for people who engage in unsafe sexual practices, for people who share needles in intravenous drug use, and for pregnant women and newborns. But many unresolved questions remain, including who should be encouraged to be tested, who should bear the costs, which sorts of pre- and posttest counseling should be provided, and which conditions make the decision to undergo the test reasonable for individuals. Because of the current medical and public health consensus that the benefits of HIV testing outweigh the risks for individuals, there has been a move toward routine testing in health-care settings, with notification and the option to refuse testing (see the discussion in Chapter 4, pp. 108–9).

If we assume the accuracy of the test results, the possible benefits of testing to those who test negative include reassurance, the opportunity to make future plans, and the motivation to make behavioral changes to prevent infection. Possible benefits to those who test positive include closer medical follow-up, earlier use of antiretroviral agents, prophylaxis or other treatment of associated diseases, a clearer sense of future options, and protection of loved ones. No significant risks of HIV testing exist for individuals with negative tests, but there are psychological and social risks to individuals with positive tests. The psychological risks include anxiety and depression. The social risks include stigmatization, discrimination, and breaches of confidentiality. Society can further reduce these risks by establishing or enforcing firm rules to protect individuals against breaches of confidentiality and against discrimination in housing, employment, and insurance.

Finally, several policies of compulsory-selective screening (4) are justifiable. For example, conditionally mandatory screening is justifiable whenever persons engage in actions or are involved in procedures that impose risks on others who cannot avoid those risks. Examples include blood donation, sperm donation, and organ donation. But ethical difficulties arise in certain institutional settings. For example, mandatory screening in the workplace is inappropriate, except where exposure to bodily fluids could transmit the virus. Mandatory HIV screening in prisons, where there is a high rate of HIV infection, could be more justifiable, but a better policy may be to protect prisoners from sexual assaults and the like.

The use of antiretroviral treatments by HIV-infected pregnant women has greatly reduced the transmission of HIV infection to their offspring. Efforts to mandate HIV testing for all pregnant women or a targeted subset of pregnant women would probably be ineffective and even counterproductive. Under mandatory HIV testing, some pregnant women, including those most at risk, would probably not seek prenatal care. A policy of voluntary screening most respects pregnant women's autonomy and privacy, and probably would be the most effective in producing the desired public health results.

Mandatory treatment and detention of patients with tuberculosis. By contrast to HIV infection, tuberculosis (TB) is spread by airborne transmission. Obligations to respect privacy and autonomy dictate a priority for policies of voluntary compliance to control the TB epidemic, as in the AIDS epidemic. However, TB's different mode of transmission makes it easier to justify infringements of both privacy and autonomy. Mandatory TB screening is readily justifiable if substantial risk of transmission exists (e.g., in crowded workplaces and prisons) and coercive police powers are justified to protect the public from persons shown to have active TB. Quarantine, isolation, and mandatory, directly observed treatment (DOT, which entails directly observing patients take their medication) are all justified in some circumstances.

A continuing moral problem concerns how to handle noncompliant patients who lack either the capacity or the will to complete the recommended treatments. Although treatment regimens for TB vary, the initial phase often requires daily medications for one to two months, followed by twice-weekly medications for a total of six to nine months. The incidence of multidrug-resistant TB is much higher among previous recipients of anti-TB therapy, mainly because of their failure to continue the prescribed treatment until cured. Their noncompliance or partial compliance with prescribed treatment regimens is the major cause of multidrug-resistant TB.

According to some studies, about one-third of patients with TB fail to adhere to treatment. Their noncompliance stems from the conditions that foster TB, as well as from other social and psychological factors. Health care professionals lack clear and reliable ways to identify noncompliant patients in advance. Critics of mandatory DOT contend that, because the majority of TB patients comply, it would be "wasteful, inefficient, and gratuitously annoying" to mandate DOT for all patients with TB. Moreover, to opt for DOT would be to fail to select the least restrictive and intrusive intervention for particular patients. However, the risks of not implementing DOT include the further spread of TB, particularly its multidrug-resistant forms, and the escalation of treatment costs.[40]

An effective public health strategy in response to the TB epidemic should pay careful attention to the conditions that cause TB and noncompliance with therapy, and it should give priority to effective policies that adequately protect privacy and freedom of choice. How a society ensures compliance often reflects its attitudes toward its vulnerable members, and calls for coercive measures need to be tempered by a coordinated approach that supports individuals with TB.[41] Nevertheless, coercive measures, including mandated DOT that intrudes on privacy, are justified when necessary to protect the public health, as long as priority is assigned to the least restrictive and least intrusive measures.

Genetic privacy. In addition to long-standing concerns about the privacy (and confidentiality) of medical records, concerns have increased about the protection of genetic information. Genetic privacy involves informational privacy, on which we here concentrate, but it also encompasses decisional, physical, and proprietary privacy.[42]

Arguments for the importance of genetic informational privacy often claim that genetic information is uniquely personal and powerful. These features have been expressed in the problematic metaphor of a "future diary." Even when the future diary is viewed as probabilistic, it still tends to underwrite both genetic determinism—"We are our genes"—and genetic exceptionalism—"Genetic information is unique and merits special protection."[43] However, the differences between genetic information and other medical and health information are matters of degree, not of kind. Much health and medical information is "inferentially fertile"[44] and provides information similar to what would be gained by genetic tests. In addition, other medical and health information is often sensitive and may be stigmatizing.

In view of these considerations, public policies should address the privacy of medical and health information in general, and then add protections for genetic information only if needed.[45] In particular circumstances, both ethical and practical reasons may support separate, special legal and other protections of individuals' genetic information, as long as these protections meet certain stringent conditions. Specifically, they must effectively address a demonstrated need, avoid undue interference with medical research, and not delay better and broader legislation.[46]

Public policies should address both *access* to and *uses* of a person's genetic information. On the one hand, there are widespread concerns about uses of a person's genetic information by employers, insurance companies, and others for discriminatory purposes. For example, women with a family history of breast cancer reportedly sometimes refrain from undergoing potentially valuable genetic testing from fear that the information will be used to discriminate against them in employment or health insurance. Public policies that prohibit genetic discrimination can partially address such concerns. On the other hand, even if certain uses of genetic information are prohibited, or at least regulated, concerns will still remain about third-party access to a person's genetic information. While adequate protections for "genetic secrets" are vital, those protections should not have unlimited scope or rigidity. Finding the right balance in public policy is difficult.[47]

CONFIDENTIALITY

We surrender some of our privacy when we grant others access to our personal information or our bodies, but we usually retain some control over information generated about us in diagnostic and therapeutic contexts and in research. For example, physicians are obligated not to grant an insurance company or a prospective employer access to information about patients, unless the patients authorize its release. When others gain access to protected information without authorization, they infringe our right to confidentiality, our right to privacy, or both.

From one standpoint, confidentiality is a branch or subset of informational privacy. It prevents *redisclosure* of information originally disclosed within a confidential relationship; that is, a relationship in which the confider has a reasonable and legitimate expectation that the confidant will not further disclose the information without the confider's authorization.[48] The basic difference between privacy and confidentiality is this: An infringement of a person's right to confidentiality occurs only if the person (or institution) to whom the information was disclosed in confidence fails to protect the information or deliberately discloses it to someone without first-party consent. By contrast, a person who, without authorization, enters a hospital record room or computer database violates rights of privacy, although he or she may also obtain confidential information. Only the person or institution who obtains information in a confidential relationship can be charged with violating rights of confidentiality.

Traditional Rules and Contemporary Practices

Rules of confidentiality appear as early as the Hippocratic Oath and continue today in national and international codes. However, some commentators ridicule these confidentiality rules as little more than a convenient fiction, publicly acknowledged by health care professionals and their professional organizations, but widely ignored and violated in practice. We agree that, unless there is a medical culture that values the protection of health information, the rules are merely ceremonial.

Mark Siegler has argued that "confidentiality in medicine" is a "decrepit concept," because what both physicians and patients have traditionally understood as medical confidentiality no longer exists. Rather, it is "compromised systematically in the course of routine medical care." To make his point graphic, Siegler presents the case of a patient who became concerned about the number of people in the hospital with apparent access to his record and threatened to leave prematurely unless the hospital would guarantee confidentiality. Upon inquiry, Siegler discovered that many more people than he suspected had responsibilities to examine the patient's chart. When he informed the patient of the number—approximately seventy-five—he assured the patient that "these people were all involved in providing or supporting his health care services." The patient retorted, "I always believed that medical confidentiality was part of doctors' code of ethics. Perhaps you should tell me just what you people mean by 'confidentiality.'"[49]

This reaction is reasonable, and it raises important questions about the seriousness of many putative institutional protections. When William Behringer tested positive for HIV at the medical center in New Jersey where he worked as an otolaryngologist and plastic surgeon, he received numerous phone calls of sympathy within just a few hours from members of the medical staff. Within a few days, he received similar calls from his patients, and, shortly thereafter, his surgical privileges at the medical center were suspended and his practice ruined. Despite his expectation of and request for confidentiality, the medical center took no serious precautions to protect his medical records.[50]

According to one survey of patients, medical students, and house staff about expectations and practices of confidentiality, "patients expect a more rigorous

standard of confidentiality than actually exists." Virtually all patients (96%) recognized the common practice of informally discussing patients' cases for second
opinions. Most (69%) expected cases to be discussed openly in professional settings to receive other opinions. A majority (51%) expected cases to be discussed
in professional settings simply because they were medically interesting, and half
of the patients expected cases to be discussed with office nursing staff. However,
they did not expect cases to be discussed in other contexts, such as in medical
journals, at parties, or with spouses or friends. To take two examples, house staff
and medical students reported that cases were frequently discussed with physicians' spouses (57%) and at parties (70%).[51]

Threats to confidentiality emerge in many institutions with a capacity
to store and disseminate confidential medical information, such as medical
records on file, drugs prescribed, medical tests administered, and reimbursement
records. In occupational medicine, computer records in corporations are growing rapidly, and data in these records can be searched quickly and thoroughly.
If the company routinely offers medical examinations by a corporate physician,
records can be computerized and merged with all claims filed by an employee's
private physician for reimbursement under corporate insurance policies. Many
employees (especially in industries with hazardous work environments) are concerned that this extensive, two-track medical history will be used against them if
a question of continued employment arises.

It may be possible to alter current health care practices to approximate
more closely the traditional ideal of confidentiality, but a gap will almost certainly remain because of the need for quick and efficient access to information
in medicine. Improved security of information through technological measures
will likely address only a few of the interests traditionally protected by rules of
confidentiality.

The Nature of Medical Confidentiality

Confidentiality is present when one person discloses information to another,
whether through words or other means, and the person to whom the information
is disclosed pledges (implicitly or explicitly) not to divulge that information to a
third party without the confider's permission. Confidential information is private
and is voluntarily imparted in confidence and trust. If a patient or research subject authorizes release of the information to others, then *no violation* of rights of
confidentiality occurs, although a *loss* of both confidentiality and privacy may
occur.

There exist acknowledged and justifiable exceptions to the kind of information that can be considered confidential in policy and practice. For example, legal
rules may set external limits to confidentiality, as when they require practitioners
to report gunshot wounds and venereal diseases. Some unwanted disclosures

of information to third parties may not breach confidentiality because of the arrangement in which the information was originally gathered. For example, IBM physician Martha Nugent informed her employer of her belief that an employee, Robert Bratt, had a problem of paranoia that affected his behavior on the job.[52] Bratt knew that Nugent had been retained by IBM to examine him, but expected conventional medical confidentiality. The company held that the facts disclosed by Nugent were necessary for evaluating Bratt's request for a job transfer and, under law, were a legitimate business communication. In our view, it is a reasonable conclusion that such information is not confidential by the standards of medical confidentiality and that Nugent was not bound by obligations of confidentiality in the same way a private physician would be.

Contracts for at least limited disclosures are not illegitimate as long as employees are aware of provisions in the contract. A similar point applies to military physicians who have a dual responsibility—to the soldier as patient and to the military. Nevertheless, the company and the military, along with the physicians in each context, have a moral responsibility to ensure that employees and soldiers understand, at the outset, the conditions under which rules of confidentiality apply.

The Justification of Obligations of Confidentiality

It is easy to imagine a society that recognizes no obligations of confidentiality. Many of the goods of medicine and research could be realized without rules of confidentiality. On what basis, then, can we justify a system of extensive, often expensive, protections of confidentiality? We believe that two types of argument justify (prima facie) rules to protect confidentiality: (1) consequence-based arguments and (2) rights-based autonomy and privacy arguments. These arguments will also help us address the topic of legitimate exceptions to rules of confidentiality.

Consequentialist arguments. If they could not trust physicians to conceal some information from third parties, patients would be reluctant to disclose full and forthright information or authorize a complete examination and a full battery of tests. Without such information, physicians would not be able to make accurate diagnoses and prognoses or recommend the best course of treatment. Although such consequence-based reasons establish a need for some rule of confidentiality, consequentialists disagree among themselves about which rule should be adopted, and about the rule's scope and weight.

In the famous *Tarasoff* case, a patient told his therapist about his desire to kill a young woman who had spurned his attention. The therapist alerted the university police but did not warn the intended victim. After the patient killed the young woman, the family brought a suit alleging that the therapist should have warned the intended victim. In this case, the California Supreme Court examined the basis and limits of confidentiality.[53] Both the majority opinion, which affirmed that therapists have an obligation to warn third parties of their patients' threatened violence, and the dissenting opinion, which denied such an obligation, used consequentialist arguments. Their debate hinged on different predictions and assessments of the consequences of a rule that *requires* therapists to breach confidentiality by warning intended victims of a client's threatened violence and a rule that *allows* therapists to breach confidentiality when a member of the public is endangered. The majority opinion pointed to the victims who would be saved, such as the young woman who had been killed in this case, and contended that a professional's obligation to disclose information to third parties could be justified by the need to protect such potential victims. By contrast, the minority opinion contended that if it were common practice to override obligations of confidentiality, the fiduciary relation between the patient and the doctor would soon erode and collapse. Patients would lose confidence in psychotherapists and would refrain from disclosing information crucial to effective therapy. As a result, violent assaults would increase because dangerous persons would refuse to seek psychiatric aid or to disclose relevant information, such as their violent fantasies. Hence, the debate about different rules of confidentiality hinges, in part, on empirical claims about which rule more effectively protects the interests of other persons.

In cases of other legally accepted and mandated exceptions to confidentiality—such as requirements to report contagious diseases, child abuse, and gunshot wounds—no substantial evidence exists that these requirements have either reduced prospective patients' willingness to seek treatment and to cooperate with physicians or significantly impaired the physician–patient relationship.[54]

In a consequentialist account, then, *nonabsolute* rules of confidentiality are attractive and acceptable as long as it is understood that when physicians breach medical confidentiality, they infringe their patients' rights. Such an infringement clearly has negative effects for confiders. A physician who breaks confidence cannot ignore the potential for eroding the system of medical confidentiality, trust, and fidelity. A consequentialist justification for breaching confidentiality can thus meet its own high standards only if *all* probable consequences are taken into account.

Arguments from autonomy and privacy rights. A second set of arguments to justify rules and rights of confidentiality derives from the principle of respect for autonomy and rules of privacy. The claim is that values of the exercise of autonomy and the right to control one's privacy support rules of confidentiality. Like the first argument, this second argument does not support absolute rules of confidentiality. When rules of confidentiality are used as absolute shields, they can eventuate in outrageous and preventable injuries and harms.[55]

Justified Infringements of Rules of Confidentiality

Infringements of prima facie rules of confidentiality are often justified when third parties face serious dangers. We concentrate on such situations, while recognizing that paternalistic breaches of confidentiality are also sometimes ethically justifiable.

Assessing and reducing risks to others. In assessing which risks to others outweigh rights of confidentiality, we must balance both the probability that harm will materialize and the magnitude of that harm against the obligation of confidentiality. The chart of risk assessment introduced on pp. 224 supplies the basic categories:

		Major	Minor
		Magnitude of Harm	
	High	1	2
Probability of Harm			
	Low	3	4

As health professionals' assessments of a situation approach a high probability of a major harm (category 1) to a third party, the weight of the obligation to breach confidentiality increases. As the situation approaches category 4, it is more likely that breaching confidentiality will be wrong. Many particularities of the case will determine whether the professional is justified in breaching confidentiality in categories 2 and 3. These particularities include the foreseeability of a harm's occurrence, the preventability of that harm through a health professional's intervention, and the potential impact of disclosure on policies and laws regarding confidentiality. However, these abstractions are often difficult to put into practice, and measurements of probability and magnitude of harm are often imprecise. Accordingly, we move now to problems of practice.

Disclosure of HIV infection to third parties. Controversy surrounds the question whether physicians and other health care professionals should notify at-risk persons that a patient has tested positive for HIV infection and therefore has the potential to infect others through sexual intercourse or other exchanges of bodily fluids. In one case, after several weeks of dry, persistent coughing and night sweats, a bisexual man visited his family physician, who arranged for a test to determine whether he had antibodies to HIV. The physician informed the patient of a positive test, of the risk of infection for his wife, and of the risk that their children might lose both parents. The patient refused to tell his wife and insisted that the physician maintain strict confidentiality. The physician reluctantly yielded to this demand. Only in the last few weeks of his life did the patient allow the physician to inform his wife of the nature of her husband's illness, and a test then showed that she too was antibody-positive for HIV. When symptoms appeared a year later, she angrily—and we think appropriately—accused the physician of violating his moral responsibilities to her and to her children.[56] This case presents a high probability (if we assume unprotected sexual intercourse) of a major harm to an identifiable individual, which is the paradigm case of a justified breach of confidentiality.

Many well-grounded reasons support informing spouses and sexual partners that a person has tested positive for exposure to the AIDS virus. For example, if people are at risk of serious harms, and the disclosure is necessary to prevent and probably would prevent the harms (to their spouses or lovers), then disclosure that breaks confidentiality is virtually always justified. Variations on these conditions appear in several statements of professional ethics by medical associations, but ambiguities and gaps in their statements point to the difficulties of fully specifying the nature, scope, and strength of the clinician's ethical obligation to protect third parties. For example, which actions will discharge the physician's moral obligation to protect third parties? Guidelines often do not oblige the physician to determine whether the patient has, in fact, carried out a promise to terminate risky conduct or to warn those endangered, and it is not clear how far the physician should go in monitoring compliance, particularly without the patient's consent. One study concludes that it is very ineffective to leave partner notification to patients.[57] The most responsible, although demanding, strategy is one proposed by the AMA's Council on Ethical and Judicial Affairs: A physician who "knows that a seropositive individual is endangering a third party...should, within the constraints of the law, (1) attempt to persuade the infected patient to cease endangering the third party; (2) if persuasion fails, notify authorities; and (3) if the authorities take no action, notify the endangered third party."[58]

There are also questions about how far the patient must go to reduce the risk of HIV transmission. Suppose the patient refuses to notify his or her sexual partner and refuses to abstain completely from sexual intercourse, but indicates that he or she will insist on the use of a condom. This promise is usually not sufficient to release the physician from an obligation of disclosure.

Prior notification by a physician to a patient of the limits of confidentiality regarding HIV status is an important practice, but its omission does not preclude the possibility of a justified disclosure to an endangered third party. Without prior notification, the physician breaches confidentiality but may be justified in doing so; with prior notification, the physician breaches privacy but not confidentiality. In either case, the physician should seek the patient's permission to warn a third party if the patient is unwilling to do so, but the patient's permission is not a necessary condition for warning an endangered third party.

Some guidelines stress the ethical *permissibility* of the physician's disclosure, rather than its *obligatoriness,* whereas the AMA's Council on Ethical and Judicial Affairs rightly focuses on the physician's obligation. The primary justification for disclosure is that health professionals are obligated to reduce the risk of death in particular cases under their control. Public officials, however, need to consider not only endangered third parties, but also which societal rule of confidentiality would save more lives in the long run. Solutions to this problem hinge, in part, on disputed claims about the role of voluntary testing in reducing risky conduct over time. One consequentialist argument is that people who have been exposed to the AIDS virus but do not yet have symptoms will be reluctant to seek testing unless confidentiality is protected. As a result, they will fail to obtain valuable information that could lead them to reduce risks to others. A counterargument holds that carefully limited breaches of confidentiality—namely, disclosure only to sexual partners or needle-sharing partners who are at risk of harm—would not deter people from seeking testing and medical attention, especially now that HIV infection and AIDS have been increasingly defined as chronic diseases. According to this argument, people would still seek testing if they were informed that confidentiality would be breached only under strictly limited conditions and, even then, only to parties at risk of harm.[59] (This debate parallels in some respects the debate about the *Tarasoff* case; see earlier pp. 305–06.)

Solid evidence regarding the effects of breaches of confidentiality on individuals' willingness to be tested is difficult to obtain. Robert Klitzman and Ronald Bayer have found available empirical studies too narrowly focused on the potential benefits and costs of disclosure for HIV-infected persons themselves, rather than on the moral issues regarding their sexual partners. Hence, they sought to determine how persons with HIV/AIDS understand the moral complexities and challenges of disclosure to sexual partners and others in their lives.[60] Their research indicates that many HIV-infected persons prefer to see confidentiality breached to prevent another person's infection. They often disclose to a doctor that "they are troubled about or seeking help in informing their partners."[61] Nevertheless, successful notification of partners, whether by physicians or by public health officials, depends largely on patients' cooperation in providing relevant information. Any policy should be carefully constructed to elicit such cooperation.

Disclosure of genetic information to third parties. Another problem about notification of at-risk parties arises from genetic information about a particular individual, which may also reveal information about particular family members. Those who learn that they have a serious genetic condition may have a moral obligation to share that information with at-risk relatives who may then be able to take actions to reduce risks to themselves or their offspring or to seek treatment. Health care providers should underline this obligation to their patients or clients. Genetic counselors, in particular, may have to overcome their proclivity for nondirective counseling and seek to persuade counselees to disclose this information. It would be preferable for the counselors to make the disclosure to ensure that adequate information is transmitted about risks and preventive or therapeutic options. However, directive counseling is different from disclosing the information to relatives against the counselee's explicit directives.

We concur with the recommendation of the Institute of Medicine Committee on Assessing Genetic Risks that "confidentiality should be breached and relatives informed about genetic risks only when (1) attempts to elicit voluntary disclosure fail, (2) there is a high probability of irreversible or fatal harm to the relative, (3) the disclosure of the information will prevent the harm, (4) the disclosure is limited to the information necessary for diagnosis or treatment of the relative, and (5) there is no other reasonable way to avert the harm."[62]

In this approach, health care professionals should respect the confidentiality of an individual's personal genetic information but may have a right or obligation, under some circumstances, to disclose that information to protect others from harm even if the individual objects. The default is nondisclosure to family members at risk, unless the individual consents. Some critics of this approach propose that we take more seriously the familial nature of genetic information.[63] By analogy with a bank account, they recommend a model of genetic information as a joint account, whereas our approach views it as a personal account. The personal account model fits well with respect for autonomy, confidentiality, maintenance of trust in health care relationships, and good practice in most of health care. In the joint account model, the default is the availability of genetic information to all on the joint familial account unless there are good reasons not to do so, such as serious harm to the individual from whom the information was generated. This is based on considerations of justice, or possibly, in the language of Chapter 6, reciprocity-based beneficence. Given the essentially and unavoidably familial nature of genetic information, one family member should not be able to benefit from this joint information while excluding others from those benefits.

However, in any transition to this joint account model, it would be morally obligatory to inform those using genetic services, at the point of entry, about the nature and limits of confidentiality, so they can choose whether to proceed. In this regard, the principle of respect for autonomy remains essential to an ethically justified use of the joint account model. Each participant has to understand at the outset that the information will be available to all. In our judgment, rather than changing the default regarding the sharing of information with family members, it would be better to educate individuals about their responsibilities to family members who could benefit or avoid harm by access to the genetic information.

FIDELITY

Paul Ramsey argued that the fundamental ethical question in research, medicine, and health care is, "What is the meaning of the faithfulness of one human being to another?"[64] Few today would agree that fidelity is the fundamental moral norm in health care and research, but it is clearly a central norm.

The Nature and Place of Fidelity

Obligations of fidelity arise whenever a physician or other health care professional establishes a significant relationship with a patient. Abandonment of a patient is thus a breach of fidelity, amounting to disloyalty. Conflicts of fidelity also create significant problems of divided loyalties, and we begin with these conflicts.

Conflicts of fidelity and divided loyalties. Professional fidelity, or loyalty, has been traditionally conceived as giving the patient's interests priority in two respects: (1) the professional effaces self-interest in any situation that may conflict with the patient's interests, and (2) the professional favors the patient's interests over others' interests. In practice, fidelity has never been so pristine. To take one example, caring for patients in epidemics has often been considered praiseworthy and virtuous rather than an obligatory instance of fidelity, and physicians have never been expected to care for a great many patients without compensation. In addition, health care professionals regularly use their clinical skills to serve social purposes beyond the individual patient's interests, such as public health concerns. They may, for instance, recommend vaccination when, in a context of high rates of immunization, its risks would outweigh its benefits to certain patients. Or physicians may select particular antibiotics in light of a concern about the development of antibiotic-resistant bacteria. Clinical skills also sometimes serve various non-health-related social activities, such as criminal justice and war, as well as religious and cultural practices, such as male circumcision. Finally, physicians serve as gatekeepers in society's assignment of certain goods and burdens. Examples include providing psychiatric evaluation as part of a criminal trial and conducting a medical review of a person's disability insurance claims.[65]

Divided loyalties typically occur when fidelity to patients, subjects, or clients conflicts with allegiance to colleagues, institutions, funding agencies, corporations, or the state. In such cases, two or more roles and their associated loyalties and obligations become incompatible and irreconcilable, forcing a moral choice. This choice, as we will see, may alter the landscape of one's commitments.[66]

Third-party interests. Physicians, nurses, and hospital administrators sometimes find aspects of their role obligations in conflict with obligations to patients.

In some cases, they may have a therapeutic contract with a party other than the patient. When parents bring a child to a physician for treatment, for instance, the physician's primary responsibility is to serve the child's interests, although the parents made the contract and the physician has obligations of fidelity to the parents. The latter obligations are sometimes easily and validly overridden, as occurs when physicians go to court to oppose parents' decisions that seriously threaten their children. Courts have often allowed adult Jehovah's Witnesses, for example, to reject blood transfusions for themselves, while rightly overriding their rejections of medically necessary blood transfusions for their children. Parents are also sometimes charged with child neglect when they fail to seek or permit potentially beneficial medical treatment recommended by physicians.[67]

Maternal–fetal relations have likewise become more complex and open to conflicts.[68] The fetus typically becomes a patient because of the pregnant woman's decision to enter the health care system. Once both patients (the pregnant woman and the fetus) are under care, conflicting obligations of fidelity and divided loyalties may develop. For example, the possibility of a cesarean section late in pregnancy sometimes presents a conflict between the survival and health of the fetus and the wishes of the pregnant woman.

Institutional interests. In some types of conflict, it is unclear what the health care professional owes the "patient." Often the institutions involved are not health care institutions, but, in discharging their functions, they may need medical information about individuals and may even provide some care for those individuals. Examples include a physician's contract to provide medical examinations of applicants for positions in a company or to determine whether applicants for insurance policies are safe risks. In some circumstances the health care professional may rightly not regard the person examined as his or her patient, but, even so, the professional still has certain responsibilities of due care.

In some jurisdictions, the health care professional does not have a legal obligation to disclose the discovery of a disease to the examinee. However, nondisclosure is a morally dubious practice. At a minimum, health care professionals have a moral responsibility to oppose, avoid, and withdraw from contracts that would require them to withhold information of significant potential benefit to examinees. Physicians similarly owe "due care" to individuals who become their patients under a third-party contract in an institutional arrangement. Examples include health care professionals in industries, prisons, and the armed services.

When care of an individual conflicts with institutional objectives and policies, the individual's needs may not take precedence. For example, the military physician must accept a different set of obligations than the nonmilitary physician—in particular, to place the military's interests above both the patient's and the physician's interests. However, some actions so grossly violate canons of medical ethics that they warrant disobedience of orders and defiance of superiors, rather than loyalty and compliance. An example is a commander's order for a physician to help torture a prisoner of war.[69]

Medical assistance in prisons also presents moral problems, in part because of the institutional mandate to punish the criminal, which limits the obligations of fidelity to the criminal as patient. Medical values are sometimes subordinated to the correctional institution's functions, and yet the physician is expected to be loyal to both. The correctional institution may expect physicians and other health care professionals to participate in the administration of justice and punishment. Examples include surgical removal of a bullet for evidence when the bullet is not a hazard to the inmate and can be safely left in place, forced examinations of inmates' body cavities for evidence of contraband drugs, and participation in corporal or capital punishment—for instance, by administering a lethal injection.[70]

Moral questions arise about medical assessments of prisoners' physical conditions to determine whether they can endure punishments, and about medical monitoring of prisoners during punishment. Medical supervision can prevent extreme or unintended injury or harm, but participation in the administration of punishment, whether corporal or capital, represents a compromise of fidelity.[71] For similar reasons, the AMA's Council on Ethical and Judicial Affairs has held for several years that physician participation in capital punishment through administration of a lethal injection is unethical. Over time it defined unethical participation to include administering tranquilizers or other medications as part of an execution, monitoring a condemned prisoner's vital signs, witnessing an execution in a professional capacity, or rendering technical advice for an execution.[72] The reason, we suggest, is that in these acts a physician's conflicts of fidelity are unjustifiably resolved in favor of institutional needs that could be satisfied without the participation of physicians.

Nursing. Nursing may be the area of health care with the most pervasive conflicts among obligations of fidelity. Codes of nursing ethics in the latter part of the twentieth century began to frame the moral responsibility of nurses in different ways than some earlier codes that had discouraged nurses from making their own moral judgments. In 1950, the first code of the American Nurses' Association stressed the nurse's obligation to carry out the physician's orders, whereas the 1976 revision and subsequent revisions stress the nurse's obligation to the client and the obligation to safeguard both the client and the public from the "incompetent, unethical or illegal" practices of any person.

Moral problems can be expected wherever one group of professionals makes the decisions and orders their implementation by other professionals who have not participated in the decision making. In one study of relationships in health care, investigators examined different perceptions of ethical problems by nurses and doctors in acute care units. In structured interviews, both nurses and physicians said they frequently encountered ethical problems. Most physicians (twenty-one of twenty-four) and most nurses (twenty-five of twenty-six) recognized ethical conflicts within the health care team. However, in twenty-one of the twenty-five cases reported by nurses, the ethical conflict was between a nurse and a physician, whereas only one physician reported a conflict with a nurse rather than with another physician. The authors of the study conclude that it is likely that conflicts with nurses occurred, but that the physicians "were not aware of them, or did not see conflict with a nurse as forming an *ethical* problem."[73] Several features of the working relationship between physicians and nurses may explain these findings. Physicians write orders and nurses carry them out. By virtue of their close relationships with patients, nurses often experience the problems that arise from medical decisions more immediately and fully than physicians. These features of nursing roles heighten obligations of fidelity to patients but also open avenues of conflict with colleagues.

Conflicts of Interest

Over the last several years, conflicts that have weakened or threatened traditional rules of fidelity have often involved conflicts of interest, a topic of fairly recent origin.[74] A conflict of interest exists when an individual's personal interests would lead an impartial observer to question whether the individual's professional actions or decisions are unduly influenced by considerations of significant personal interest. Such personal interests create temptations or biases that may lead to a breach of role responsibilities through judgments, decisions, and recommendations other than those reasonably expected in the role. Even if a potential conflict is not a real conflict (i.e., does not in fact bias the individual's judgment), and even if no wrong has been committed, it is reasonable to anticipate possibly tainted judgments and to require that they be avoided. High moral standards of probity and impartiality require avoidance of even the appearance of conflict.

Although discussion of conflict of interest has centered on personal financial interests, other interests, such as professional advancement or standing and friendships, are no less important. Any personal interest in an outcome, institution, or entity that is at odds with the person's professional obligations should be avoided. The professional's personal interest may be perfectly legitimate (e.g., an interest in promoting a favored charitable cause) but conflicts of interest threaten to destroy professionals' primary commitments and loyalties and are not to be tolerated except in the most restricted circumstances in which a compelling moral justification can be given.

Conflicts of interest occur in medicine, health care, biomedical research, and the review of grant proposals and articles submitted for publication in all of these fields. The medical profession has seen a concerted attempt to address numerous financial conflicts of interest, including fee splitting, self-referring, accepting gifts, accepting fees for recruiting patients for a research protocol, outside consulting with a regulated industry by government-employed physicians, appointing industry-based physicians to government regulatory agencies, industry-paid lecturing on an industry product, and author disclosures of funding sources when publishing journal articles.[75]

Consider the problem of self-referral, the referral of patients to medical facilities or services physicians own or in which they have a financial investment. Such referral threatens fidelity to patients' interests by extending the temptation inherent in fee-for-service to provide unnecessary or excessively expensive care. Physicians create these financial conflicts of interest by owning or investing in medical facilities or services, such as diagnostic imaging centers, laboratories, or physical therapy services, to which they refer patients. Physician ownership of radiation therapy and physical therapy services, for instance, can substantially increase use and costs, without compensatory benefits such as increased access.[76] Self-referral is generally more problematic than fee-for-service because the patient cannot as easily identify the physician's potential economic gain—unless it is explicitly disclosed—in ordering additional procedures and thus cannot proceed cautiously, perhaps by seeking a second opinion.

Although disclosure is not a common practice, physicians have an ethical obligation to disclose these economic conflicts of interest. Fidelity and honesty require such disclosure as an ethical minimum. However, often disclosure is not sufficient. For example, a legal or professional prohibition of self-referral should be adopted in many cases.[77] In other cases—such as voting as a trustee when one has a conflict of interest and serving on a review committee that is assessing a friend's or colleague's grant proposal(s)—recusal is the only satisfactory remedy.

In recent decades, third-party payers and institutional providers have increasingly imposed constraints on medical decisions about diagnostic and therapeutic procedures through mechanisms designed to control costs. These mechanisms sometimes limit and constrict the physician's fidelity to the patient through incentives and disincentives that can place the physician's self-interest in conflict with the patient's best medical interest. For example, health maintenance organizations (HMOs) often withhold a substantial part of the primary physician's income. They return part or all at the end of the year, depending on the overall financial condition of the HMO and, in some cases, the physician's productivity and frugality. This arrangement creates an incentive for physicians to severely limit expensive procedures—a worrisome conflict of interest. The patient is in a different position when the physician has incentives to *restrict* needed treatment than when the physician has incentives to provide *unnecessary* treatment. In the latter situation, patients can obtain another opinion. In the former situation, patients may not be aware of a needed treatment.[78]

Financial incentive structures such as those used in many diagnostic laboratories also create a powerful motive for physicians to limit both their time and expensive procedures. Physicians are there paid by output—for example, how many slides they read. Annual payments are tied to productivity (e.g., number of slides read), but a rapid reading of data adds risk of error, substantially increasing risks of false negative results and misdiagnosis. Pathologists who read many hundreds of slides per day looking for the presence of carcinoma will substantially increase their salary, but also will substantially increase the likelihood of failing to detect a carcinoma. Every physician will occasionally make some mistake or follow an incorrect, yet excusable, strategy, but it is not excusable to make mistakes where there is an inherent conflict of interest encouraging behavior that falls below an appropriate standard of due care.

Difficult judgments need to be made regarding the best way to address particular conflicts of interest, whether by *eliminating* them, *managing* or *mitigating* them, or requiring *disclosure* of conflicts to alert parties at risk. Each of these is justifiable in some contexts, and each is preferable to the traditional convention of relying on professional or personal character to determine whether a conflict is actual or merely potential. Worthy of strong condemnation and legislation (buttressed by professional sanctions) are so-called "gag clauses," which in some contracts for services prohibit clinicians from disclosing conflicts of interest (e.g., economic incentives for physicians to provide fewer or less expensive diagnostic and therapeutic procedures) and conflicts of obligations (e.g., a managed care organization's rationing strategy or clinical guidelines).

Another set of conflicts of interest is subtle and ambiguous. Several training programs, institutions, and professional organizations—as well as individual physicians—have wrestled with conflicts of interest created by gifts from pharmaceutical and medical device manufacturers. Financial support by these companies provides for continuing medical education and supplies free, sponsored lunches and free product samples.[79]

Some efforts at industry, professional, and institutional self-regulation have distinguished gifts according to amount and purpose. For instance, the PhRMA (Pharmaceutical Research and Manufacturers of America) Code of Interaction with Healthcare Professionals allows companies to offer physicians certain items that are primarily for the benefit of patients and that do not have substantial value ($100 or less).[80] Many professional medical associations, including the AMA, also allow their members to accept such gifts. The assumption is that physicians' judgments about medical products will not be affected by temptations and biases created by such relatively small gifts and the relationships they support. However, there is good evidence that even small gifts intended as ways to build and maintain relationships influence physicians' prescribing behavior.[81] Moreover, gift relationships, however small, create a variety of temptations, dependencies, friendships, and forms of indebtedness—all of which may create conflicts of interest with the physician's primary obligation to act in the best interest of the patients.[82]

Although disclosure to patients helps to reduce the negative impact of many forms of conflict of interest, it appears to be relatively useless for conflicts of interest created by industry gifts. More stringent institutional regulations, including for academic medical centers, is needed to eliminate or greatly modify common practices in the interactions between for-profit industries and physicians. Examples include banning gifts, limiting reimbursement, and reducing the practice of supplying free samples.[83]

Conflicts of interest reach beyond practice to research. For instance, clinical trials of pharmaceutical products are financially supported by companies willing to assume the financial risk because the returns from a successful trial are the life-blood of the company. The financial advantages for physician-investigators and corporations promote a relationship with a steady and reliable flow of funding. This relationship risks creating a motive to find positive results, thereby compromising scientific objectivity. Data always must be interpreted for significance or insignificance. It is vital to control the process of interpretation and assessment through objective procedures and independent controls such as data safety and monitoring committees. The personal financial interests of physician-investigators and management should be strictly controlled.[84]

In addition, conflicts of interest may arise for members of institutional review boards and of data and safety monitoring boards as well as for advisory committees to governmental agencies, such as the Food and Drug Administration. Mitigation of such conflicts of interest is vital, even if they cannot be avoided altogether. At a minimum, public disclosure of conflicts of interest should be a basic moral norm governing these practices.

THE DUAL ROLES OF CLINICIAN AND INVESTIGATOR

The Physician's Oath of the World Medical Association affirms that "the health of my patient will be my first consideration." But can research involving patients and other subjects or participants consistently honor this obligation? The dual roles of research scientist and clinical practitioner pull in different directions. As an investigator, the physician acts to generate scientific knowledge to benefit individual patients and populations in the future. As a clinician, he or she has the responsibility to act in the best interests of present patients. Both roles are intended to benefit the sick, but the scientific enterprise is directed at unknown, future patients, whereas the clinical role is aimed at known, current patients. Accordingly, responsibilities to future generations may conflict with due care for current patients who become research subjects.

Research involving human subjects is socially important, but morally troublesome, because it exposes subjects to risk for the advancement of science.

Ethically justified research must satisfy several conditions, including (1) a goal of valuable knowledge, (2) a reasonable prospect that the research will generate the knowledge that is sought, (3) the necessity of using human subjects, (4) a favorable balance of potential benefits over risks to the subjects, (5) fair selection of subjects, and (6) protection of privacy and confidentiality.[85] (In addition, some conditions of nonexploitation must be satisfied, as discussed in Chapter 7.) It is appropriate to ask potential subjects to participate only if these conditions have been met.

Because society encourages and supports extensive research and because investigators and subjects are unequal in knowledge and vulnerability, public policy and review committees are responsible for ensuring that the research meets these ethical conditions. Some cases warrant a straightforward paternalistic decision.[86] For example, if healthy persons free of heart disease volunteer to participate in a research protocol to test an artificial heart, as once happened,[87] an IRB should declare that the risk relative to benefit for a healthy subject is too substantial to permit the research. Of course, the risk relative to benefit for a patient with a seriously diseased heart may be acceptable.

These considerations apply to both research that offers no prospect of medical benefit to the subject and research that offers some prospect of medical benefit to the patient-subject and that may be conducted as a part of the care of the patient. The term "therapeutic research" should be avoided, because it can draw attention away from the fact that *research* is being conducted. Scientific research is distinguishable from both routine therapy and experimental or innovative therapy, which are directed at particular patients. Attaching the positive term "therapeutic" to research suggests "justified intervention" in the care of particular patients and may create a "therapeutic misconception," in which participants construe the protocol as therapy rather than as research designed to generate generalizable knowledge.

Conflicts in Clinical Trials

Controlled clinical trials are needed to establish or confirm that an observed effect, such as reduced mortality from a disease, results from a particular intervention rather than from an unknown variable in the patient population. The evidence supporting many available treatments is tenuous, and some procedures have never been adequately tested for either safety or efficacy. If doubt surrounds the efficacy or safety of a treatment, or its relative merits in comparison to another treatment, scientific research aimed at resolving the doubt is in order. Controlled trials are scientific instruments intended to protect current and future patients against medical enthusiasm and hunches. In this research, one group receives the experimental therapy, while a "control group" receives either a standard therapy or a placebo so that investigators can determine whether an experimental therapy is more effective and safer than a standard therapy or a placebo. Commonly, subjects are randomly assigned to control and experimental groups to avoid intentional or unintentional bias. Randomization is designed to keep variables other than the treatments under examination from distorting study results. Blinding certain persons to some information about the randomized controlled trial (RCT) provides additional protection against bias. An RCT may be single-blind (the subject does not know whether he or she is in the control group or the experimental group), double-blind (neither the subject nor the investigator knows), or unblinded (all parties know). Double-blind studies are designed specifically to reduce bias in observations and interpretations by subjects, physicians, and investigators. Blinding the physician-investigator also serves an ethical function, because it obviates the conflict of interest for those who both provide therapy and conduct research.

Problems of consent. Subjects in RCTs usually do not know which treatment or placebo they will receive. However, no justification exists for not disclosing to potential subjects the full set of methods, treatments, and placebos (if any) that will be used, their known risks and probable benefits, and any uncertainties. Likewise, no justification exists for failing to disclose the fact of randomization and the rationale for it. Any physician-researcher with dual responsibilities has a fiduciary obligation to inform patient-subjects of matters directly relevant to their decisions, including any conflicts of interest.[88] If this information is supplied, potential subjects should have an adequate informational base for deciding whether to participate. In conventional RCTs, investigators screen patients for eligibility and then inform them about the study, its different arms, the risks and benefits, and the use of randomization for assignment to the different arms. If a patient consents to participate, he or she is then randomized to one arm of the study. Even in the face of scientific evidence that two proposed treatments are roughly equal in safety and efficacy, patients may have strong subjective preferences for one treatment over another. Suppose two surgical procedures for treating the same disease appear to have the same survival rate (say, an average of fifteen years), and suppose we want to test their effectiveness by an RCT. A patient might have a preference if treatment A has little risk of death during the operation but a high rate of death after ten years, and treatment B has a high risk of death during the operation or postoperative recovery but a low rate of death after recovery (say, for thirty years). A patient's age, family responsibilities, and other circumstances might be other factors leading to a preference for one over the other. Accordingly, some patients may choose not to enter a particular RCT even though, from the standpoint of safety and efficacy, the different arms are in equipoise.

The problem of clinical equipoise. Serving the patient's best interests intuitively seems inconsistent with assigning a treatment randomly to promote social goals of accumulating knowledge and benefiting future patients. No two patients are alike, and a physician should be able to select and modify the course of therapy, as required by the patient's best interests. But is this axiom of medical ethics consistent with RCTs?

Proponents argue that RCTs do not violate moral obligations to patients because they are used only in circumstances in which justifiable doubt exists about the relative merits of existing, standard, and new therapies. No one knows, prior to conducting the research, whether it is more advantageous to be in the control group or in the experimental group. The community of reasonable physicians is therefore in a state of "clinical equipoise":[89] On the basis of the available evidence, members of the relevant expert medical community are equally poised between the treatment strategies being tested in the RCT, because they are equally uncertain about, and equally comfortable with, the known advantages and disadvantages of the treatments to be tested (or the placebo being used). No patient, then, will receive a treatment known to be less effective or more dangerous than an available alternative. Because current patients are not asked to forgo a superior treatment, the use of RCTs seems justifiable, especially in light of the promise of benefit to future patients. No one has scientific grounds before the trial for preferring to be in one group rather than another, although he or she may prefer one over the other on the basis of hunches or intuitions about effectiveness and safety or on the basis of factors not being studied in the trial. If two treatments for breast cancer are in veritable clinical equipoise from the standpoint of survival, a woman still may prefer the less disfiguring treatment.

Some critics suppose that proponents of clinical equipoise as a condition for ethically justified RCTs hold that it is the only condition or a sufficient condition for ethically justified RCTs.[90] However, we take the view that clinical equipoise is simply an important threshold condition. Whether particular RCTs satisfy this threshold condition is frequently debated.[91] If a cooperating physician strongly believes prior to a trial that one therapy is more beneficial or safer, he or she will have to decide whether to suspend this belief in the interests of scientific objectivity and in deference to the views of the community of experts, who find themselves in clinical equipoise. The physician is obligated to indicate both his or her own viewpoint and that of the relevant community of experts to patients who are potential candidates for the RCT. The obligation to obtain the patient's informed consent prior to the initiation of treatment, or research, entails the disclosure of the risks and benefits of all reasonable alternatives.[92]

The problem of placebo controls. Some examples illustrate problems with RCTs, particularly the use of placebo controls when no effective treatments exist and the condition is fatal. In a classic case, a conflict erupted over placebo-controlled trials of AZT (azidothymidine) in the treatment of AIDS. Promising laboratory tests led to a trial (phase I) to determine the safety of AZT among patients with AIDS. Several patients showed clinical improvement. Because AIDS was then considered invariably fatal, many people argued that compassion dictated making it immediately available to all patients with AIDS and, perhaps, to those who were antibody-positive to the AIDS virus. However, the pharmaceutical company (Burroughs Wellcome Company, later GlaxoSmithKline) did not have an adequate supply of the drug to satisfy this plan, and, as required by federal regulations, it used a placebo-controlled trial of AZT to determine its effectiveness for certain groups of patients with AIDS. A computer randomly assigned some patients to AZT and others to a placebo. For several months, no major differences emerged in effectiveness, but then patients receiving the placebo began to die at a significantly higher rate. Of the 137 patients on the placebo, 16 died. Of the 145 patients on AZT, only one died.[93] Many moral problems surround starting a placebo controlled trial when a disease appears to be universally fatal and no promising alternative to the new treatment exists. There are related questions about when to stop a trial, as well as how to distribute a new treatment.

Consider a second example. Although commonly used in the investigation of pharmaceutical agents, RCTs (particularly placebo-controlled) are rare in surgery. Some worry that surgical procedures are too easily introduced without sufficiently rigorous evidence of their efficacy or safety. In one case, surgical researchers sought a clinical trial to determine whether transplanting fetal neural tissue into the brains of patients with Parkinson's disease (a disorder of motor function, marked by tremor, rigidity, unsteady walking, and unstable posture) would be safe and effective. Standard medical treatment consisted of levodopa, which may not restore lost motor function, may have adverse effects over a long period, and may not adequately control new manifestations of the disease. Researchers contended that surgical therapy using cells is more like the administration of pharmaceutical agents than conventional surgical procedures. They proposed a randomized, double-blind, placebo-controlled trial. Because surgery itself may have some effects, such as evoking patients' favorable subjective responses, researchers maintained that a placebo control was preferable to the use of standard medical treatment as the control. The placebo consisted of sham surgery, that is, the administration of general anesthesia followed by bilateral surgery, a skin incision with a partial burr hole that does not penetrate the skull's inner cortex. This sham surgery was to be compared to two other procedures that differ from each other only in the amount of fetal tissue transplanted. The thirty-six subjects in this study all knew that twelve of them would undergo sham surgery, and researchers promised all of them free access to the real surgery if the trial demonstrated its net benefits.

The basic moral argument against the use of sham surgery as a placebo control in this research is that risks from the procedure and the anesthesia are substantial. In this trial, the best research design, from the standpoints of both the researchers involved and future patients, conflicted with researchers' obligations of beneficence and nonmaleficence to current patients invited to serve as research subjects. The ethical question that arises is whether the patient-subjects' consent was sufficient to justify proceeding with the research.[94] In our view, consent is not sufficient, and must be considered in the context of the risk involved, the necessity of reducing bias by blinding participants, the alternatives that might obviate the need for sham surgery, and so forth.

Early Termination of and Withdrawal from Clinical Trials

Physician-researchers can face difficult questions about whether to stop an experiment before its planned completion—particularly whether to withdraw patient-subjects from the trial before sufficient scientific data are available to support conclusions. Access to data is limited during clinical trials to protect the integrity of the research. Consequently, physicians may be excluded from access to critical information about trends. If they were aware of trends prior to the point of statistical significance, they might pull their patients from the trial, but this might invalidate the research.

However, if a physician determines that a particular patient's condition is deteriorating and that this patient's interests dictate withdrawal from the research, the physician should be free to act on behalf of the patient, assuming the patient concurs. In an RCT, it may be very difficult to determine whether the experiment should be stopped, even if some physician-researchers are satisfied by what they have observed. One procedural solution is to differentiate roles, distinguishing between the responsibilities of individual physicians who must make decisions regarding their own patients and those of a data and safety monitoring committee established to determine whether to continue or stop a trial. Unlike the physicians, this committee is charged to consider the impact of its decision on future patients, as well as on current patient-subjects. One function of such committees is to stop a trial if accumulated data indicate that the circumstance of equipoise has shifted and uncertainty no longer prevails.

This differentiation of roles by using a monitoring committee, particularly in a double-blind RCT, is procedurally sound, but it relocates, rather than resolves, some ethical questions. The committee must determine if it is legitimate to impose, or to continue to impose, risks on current patients, to benefit future patients, by establishing with a higher degree of probability the superiority of one treatment over another. A committee will likely decide that clinical equipoise must have been eliminated from the perspective of the expert medical community.[95] However, the individual physician and his or her patient may be concerned primarily with whether clinical uncertainty has been eliminated *for them*.

Many questions are relevant to a patient-subject's decision to withdraw from an RCT, including questions about interim data and early trends. Trends are often misleading and sometimes prove to be temporary aberrations. However, they might be relevant at a given point to a patient-subject's decision about whether to continue to participate, despite the fact that the evidence would not satisfy statisticians or the expert medical community. If information about trends is not to be released prior to the completion or early termination of the RCT, potential subjects need to understand this rule and accept it as a condition of participation.[96]

Justifying Conditions for Randomized Clinical Trials

Despite several problems, RCTs can be justified if they satisfy the following specific substantive and procedural conditions (in addition to the broad conditions identified earlier):

1. True clinical equipoise exists in the community of relevant medical experts.
2. The trial is designed as a crucial experiment to determine which therapeutic alternative is superior and shows scientific promise of achieving this result.
3. An IRB or its functional equivalent has approved the protocol and certified that no physician has a conflict of interest or incentive that would threaten the patient–physician relationship.
4. Patient-subjects give comprehensive informed consent (as specified in Chapter 4).
5. Placebos cannot be used if an effective treatment exists for the condition being studied, if that condition involves death or serious morbidity, and if a new treatment is promising.
6. A data and safety monitoring committee will either end the trial when statistically significant data displace clinical equipoise or will supply physicians and patients with significant safety and therapeutic information that is relevant to a reasonable person's decision to remain in or to withdraw from the trial.
7. Physicians have the right to recommend withdrawal and patients have the right to withdraw at any time.

Medical knowledge and scientific progress are vital societal goals, but particular research protocols are often optional, and some are ethically unacceptable. Some research can generate knowledge only by violating the rights and interests of current patients. As important as they are, RCTs should not become necessary canons of valid research. Historical controls may be sufficient, and some prospective studies can be conducted without randomization.

CONCLUSION

In this chapter we have further interpreted and specified principles of respect for autonomy, nonmaleficence, beneficence, and justice. We have concentrated on obligations of veracity, privacy, confidentiality, and fidelity. We have explored the basis, meaning, limits, and stringency of these obligations in the context of professional–patient or professional–subject relationships. At this point we have concluded our discussion of the four principles of biomedical ethics and their implications. In the remaining two chapters, we turn to a closer examination of ethical theory as it is pertinent to biomedical ethics.

NOTES

1. *Current Opinions of the Judicial Council of the American Medical Association* (Chicago: AMA, 1981), p. ix; *Code of Medical Ethics of the American Medical Association, 2006–2007 Edition* (Chicago: AMA, 2006), p. xv.

2. Henry Sidgwick, *The Methods of Ethics,* 7th ed. (Indianapolis, IN: Hackett, 1907), pp. 315–16.

3. G. J. Warnock, *The Object of Morality* (London: Methuen, 1971), p. 85.

4. See W. D. Ross, *The Right and the Good* (Oxford: Clarendon, 1930), chap. 2.

5. See Daniel K. Sokol, "Dissecting 'Deception,'" *Cambridge Quarterly of Healthcare Ethics* 15 (2006): 457–64 (although the definition of "deception" is problematic).

6. In *Truth, Trust, and Medicine* (London: Routledge, 2001), Jennifer Jackson too sharply distinguishes truthfulness and disclosure.

7. On sociocultural contexts of physician–patient communication about cancer and nondisclosure, see Antonella Surbone and Matjaz Zwitter, eds., "Communication with the Cancer Patient: Information and Truth," in *Annals of the New York Academy of Sciences* 809 (February 20, 1997); and Loretta M. Kopelman, "Multiculturalism and Truthfulness: Negotiating Difference by Finding Similarities," *South African Journal of Philosophy* 19 (2000): 51–55.

8. Bettina Schöne-Seifert and James F. Childress, "How Much Should the Cancer Patient Know and Decide?" *CA-A Cancer Journal for Physicians* 36 (1986): 85–94.

9. See Donald Oken, "What to Tell Cancer Patients: A Study of Medical Attitudes," *Journal of the American Medical Association* 175 (1961): 1120–28; Dennis H. Novack et al., "Changes in Physicians' Attitudes Toward Telling the Cancer Patient," *Journal of the American Medical Association* 241 (March 2, 1979): 897–900.

10. Elisa J. Gordon and Christopher K. Daugherty, "'Hitting You over the Head': Oncologists' Disclosure of Prognosis to Advanced Cancer Patients," *Bioethics* 17 (2003): 142–68.

11. James Boswell, *Life of Johnson,* as quoted in Alan Donagan, *The Theory of Morality* (Chicago: University of Chicago Press, 1997), p. 89.

12. Leo Tolstoy, in Aylmer Maude, trans., *The Death of Ivan Ilyich and Other Stories* (New York: The New American Library, 1960), p. 137.

13. Nicholas A. Christakis, *Death Foretold: Prophecy and Prognosis in Medical Care* (Chicago: University of Chicago Press, 1999), esp. chap. 5. See also Afaf Girgis and Rob Sanson-Fisher,

"Breaking Bad News: Consensus Guidelines for Medical Practitioners," *Journal of Clinical Oncology* 13 (1995): 2449–56.

14. Joel Stein, "A Fragile Commodity," *Journal of the American Medical Association* 283 (January 19, 2000): 305–06.

15. Thurstan B. Brewin, "Telling the Truth" (Letter), *The Lancet* 343 (June 11, 1994): 1512. Several subsequent letters to the editor support the physician's response; see *The Lancet* 344 (July 16, 1994): 196.

16. Antonella Surbone, "Truth Telling to the Patient," *Journal of the American Medical Association* 268 (October 7, 1992): 1661–62; and Surbone, "Truth-Telling, Risk, and Hope," in *Communication with the Cancer Patient: Information and Truth, Annals of the New York Academy of Sciences* 809 (February 20, 1997): 72–79.

17. Daniel Rayson, "Lisa's Stories," *Journal of the American Medical Association* 282 (November 3, 1999): 1605–06.

18. K. T. Kohn, J. M. Corrigan, and M. S. Donaldson, *To Err Is Human: Building a Safer Health System* (Washington, D.C.: National Academy Press, 1999).

19. See Troyen A. Brennan, "The Institute of Medicine Report on Medical Errors—Could It Do Harm?" *New England Journal of Medicine* 342 (April 13, 2000): 1123–25; and Clement J. McDonald et al., "Deaths Due to Medical Errors Are Exaggerated in Institute of Medicine Report," *Journal of the American Medical Association* 264 (July 5, 2000): 93–97.

20. See Rae M. Lamb et al., "Hospital Disclosure Practices: Results of a National Survey," *Health Affairs* 22 (2003): 73–83; Lamb, "Open Disclosure: The Only Approach to Medical Error," *Quality and Safety in Health Care* 13 (2004): 3–5; Lisa Lehmann et al., "Iatrogenic Events Resulting in Intensive Care Admission: Frequency, Cause, and Disclosure to Patients and Institutions," *The American Journal of Medicine* 118 (2005): 409–13.

21. See Thomas H. Gallagher et al., "Choosing Your Words Carefully: How Physicians Would Disclose Harmful Medical Errors to Patients," *Archives of Internal Medicine* 166 (August 14–28, 2006): 1585–93. See also David K. Chan et al., "How Surgeons Disclose Medical Errors to Patients: A Study Using Standardized Patients," *Surgery* 138 (November 2005): 851–58.

22. See, for example, *Code of Medical Ethics of the American Medical Association, 2006–2007 Edition* 8.12 and 8.121 (pp. 240–43); and Joint Commission on Accreditation of Healthcare Organizations, Standard R11.2.2, July 1, 2001.

23. See Steve S. Kraman and Ginny Hamm, "Risk Management: Extreme Honesty May Be the Best Policy," *Annals of Internal Medicine* 131 (December 21, 1999): 963–67; and A. Kachalia et al., "Does Full Disclosure of Medical Errors Affect Malpractice Liability? The Jury Is Still Out," *Joint Commission Journal on Quality and Patient Safety* 29 (October 2003): 503–11. See also Nancy Berlinger, *After Harm: Medical Error and the Ethics of Forgiveness* (Baltimore: Johns Hopkins University Press, 2005).

24. Joanna M. Cain, "Is Deception for Reimbursement in Obstetrics and Gynecology Justified?" *Obstetrics & Gynecology* 82 (September 1993): 475–78.

25. Kaiser Family Foundation, "Survey of Physicians and Nurses," http://www.kff.org/1999/1503 (accessed August 20, 2007).

26. M. K. Wynia, D. S. Cummins, J. B. VanGeest, and I. B. Wilson, "Physician Manipulation of Reimbursement Rules for Patient: Between a Rock and a Hard Place," *Journal of the American Medical Association* 283 (April 12, 2000): 1858–65; and the Commentary by M. Gregg Bloche, "Fidelity and Deceit at the Bedside" in the same issue, 1881–84. Contrast James L. Bernat et al., "Attitudes of U.S. Neurologists Concerning the Ethical Dimensions of Managed Care," *Neurology* 49 (1997): 4–13.

27. Victor G. Freeman et al., "Lying for Patients: Physician Deception of Third-Party Payers," *Archives of Internal Medicine* 159 (October 25, 1999): 2263–70.

28. Rachel M. Werner et al., "Lying to Insurance Companies: The Desire to Deceive among Physicians and the Public," *The American Journal of Bioethics* 4 (Fall 2004): 53–59, with eleven commentaries on pp. 60–80.

29. *Griswold v. Connecticut,* 381 U.S. 479 (1965), at 486.

30. Anita L. Allen, "Genetic Privacy: Emerging Concepts and Values," in *Genetic Secrets: Protecting Privacy and Confidentiality in the Genetic Era,* ed. Mark A. Rothstein (New Haven, CT: Yale University Press, 1997), pp. 31–59. Proprietary privacy merits more attention in biomedical ethics than it has received. The law extends propertylike notions to individuals' interests in possessing and controlling aspects of their person. For example, stored tissue samples may involve this privacy interest. See *Research Involving Human Biological Materials: Ethical Issues and Policy Guidance,* vol. I: Report and Recommendations of the National Bioethics Advisory Commission (Rockville, MD: NBAC, August 1999).

31. Ruth Gavison, "Privacy and the Limits of Law," *The Yale Law Journal* 89 (1980): 428.

32. Charles Fried, "Privacy: A Rational Context," *The Yale Law Journal* 77 (1968): 475–93.

33. Warren and Brandeis, "The Right to Privacy," *Harvard Law Review* 4 (1890): 193–220.

34. Thomson, "The Right to Privacy," *Philosophy and Public Affairs* 4 (Summer 1975): 295–314, as reprinted in Schoeman, ed., *Philosophical Dimensions of Privacy* (New York: Cambridge University Press, 1984). pp. 272–89; esp. 280–87.

35. James Rachels, "Why Privacy Is Important," p. 292; and Edward Bloustein, "Privacy as an Aspect of Human Dignity," both as reprinted in Schoeman, ed., *Philosophical Dimensions of Privacy.*

36. Fried, "Privacy: A Rational Context."

37. Joel Feinberg, *Harm to Self,* vol. III in *The Moral Limits of the Criminal Law* (New York: Oxford University Press, 1986), chap. 19.

38. Public health ethics has recently received considerable attention. See James F. Childress, Ruth R. Faden, Ruth D. Gaare, et al., "Public Health Ethics: Mapping the Terrain," *Journal of Law, Medicine & Ethics* 30 (2002): 170–78; Angus Dawson and Marcel Verweij, eds., *Ethics, Prevention, and Public Health* (Oxford: Oxford University Press, 2007); Madison Powers and Ruth Faden, *Social Justice: The Moral Foundations of Public Health and Health Policy* (New York: Oxford University Press, 2006); and Ronald Bayer, Lawrence O. Gostin, Bruce Jennings, and Bonnie Steinbock, eds. *Public Health Ethics: Theory, Policy, and Practice* (New York: Oxford University Press, 2006).

39. See Lawrence O. Gostin, *The AIDS Pandemic: Complacency, Injustice, and Unfulfilled Expectations* (Chapel Hill, NC: The University of North Carolina Press, 2004).

40. George J. Annas, "Control of Tuberculosis—The Law and the Public's Health," *New England Journal of Medicine* 328 (February 25, 1993): 585–88; Ronald Bayer and Laurence Dupuis, "Tuberculosis, Public Health, and Civil Liberties," *Annual Review of Public Health* 16 (1995): 307–26; Michael D. Iseman, David L. Cohn, and John A. Sbarbaro, "Directly Observed Treatment of Tuberculosis: We Can't Afford Not to Try It," *New England Journal of Medicine* 328 (February 25, 1993): 576–78; Tom Oscherwitz et al., "Detention of Persistently Nonadherent Patients with Tuberculosis," *Journal of the American Medical Association* 278 (September 10, 1997): 843–46.

41. See Richard Coker, "Public Health, Civil Liberties, and Tuberculosis: How Society Encourages Compliance Reflects Society's Approach to the Vulnerable," *British Medical Journal* 318 (May 29, 1999), esp. 1434–35; and Coker, *From Chaos to Coercion: Detention and the Control of Tuberculosis* (London: Palgrave Macmillan, 2000).

42. See Allen, "Genetic Privacy: Emerging Concepts and Values." In addition, as we emphasize in our discussion of confidentiality, genetic information also implicates what we have called relational privacy because an individual's genetic information is also familial information.

43. See George J. Annas, "Privacy Rules for DNA Databanks: Protecting Coded 'Future Diaries,'" *Journal of the American Medical Association* 270 (1993): 2346–50; contrast Thomas H. Murray, "Genetic Exceptionalism and 'Future Diaries': Is Genetic Information Different from Other Medical Information?" in *Genetic Secrets,* ed. Rothstein, chap. 3.

44. Neil C. Manson and Onora O'Neill, *Rethinking Informed Consent in Bioethics* (Cambridge: Cambridge University Press, 2007), pp. 104ff.

45. See Lawrence O. Gostin, "Genetic Privacy," *Journal of Law, Medicine & Ethics* 23 (1995): 320–30 and "Health Information Privacy," *Cornell Law Review* 80 (1995): 101–84.

46. Mark A. Rothstein, "Genetic Exceptionalism and Legislative Pragmatism," *The Journal of Law, Medicine & Ethics* 35, Special Supplement (Summer, 2007): 59–65, reprinted from *Hastings Center Report* 35, no. 4 (2005): 27–44.

47. Mark A. Rothstein, "Genetic Secrets: A Policy Framework," in *Genetic Secrets,* ed. Rothstein, chap. 23; and Rothstein, "Genetic Privacy and Confidentiality: Why They Are so Hard to Protect," *Journal of Law, Medicine and Ethics* 26 (1998): 198–204.

48. Mark A. Rothstein, "Genetic Secrets: A Policy Framework," p. 453.

49. Mark Siegler, "Confidentiality in Medicine—A Decrepit Concept," *New England Journal of Medicine* 307 (1982): 1518–21; and see Bernard Friedland, "Physician–Patient Confidentiality: Time to Re-examine a Venerable Concept in Light of Contemporary Society and Advances in Medicine," *Journal of Legal Medicine* 15 (1994): 249–77.

50. Superior Court of New Jersey, Law Division, Mercer County, Docket No. L88–2550 (April 25, 1991).

51. Barry D. Weiss, "Confidentiality Expectations of Patients, Physicians, and Medical Students," *Journal of the American Medical Association* 247 (1982): 2695–97.

52. *Bratt v. IBM,* 467 N.E.2d 126 (1984).

53. *Tarasoff v. Regents of the University of California,* 17 Cal. 3d 425 (1976); 131 California Reporter 14 (1976). The majority opinion was written by Justice Tobriner; the dissenting opinion was written by Justice Clark.

54. See Kenneth Appelbaum and Paul S. Appelbaum, "The HIV Antibody-Positive Patient," in *Confidentiality Versus the Duty to Protect: Foreseeable Harm in the Practice of Psychiatry,* ed. James C. Beck (Washington, D.C.: American Psychiatry Press, 1990), pp. 127–28.

55. For views to the contrary, see Michael H. Kottow, "Medical Confidentiality: An Intransigent and Absolute Obligation," *Journal of Medical Ethics* 12 (1986): 117–22; and Kenneth Kipnis, "A Defense of Unqualified Medical Confidentiality," *The American Journal of Bioethics* 6, No. 2 (2006): 7–18 (followed by critical commentaries, pp. 19–41).

56. Grant Gillett, "AIDS and Confidentiality," *Journal of Applied Philosophy* 4 (1987): 15–20, from which this case study has been adapted.

57. See Susanne E. Landis, Victor J. Schoenbach, David J. Weber, et al., "Results of a Randomized Trial of Partner Notification in Cases of HIV Infection in North Carolina," *New England Journal of Medicine* 326 (January 9, 1992): 101–06. See also Michael D. Stein et al., "Sexual Ethics: Disclosure of HIV-Positive Status to Partners," *Archives of Internal Medicine* 158 (February 1998): 253–57.

58. *Code of Medical Ethics of the American Medical Association,* 2006–2007 Edition, 2.23, p. 109.

59. See Gillett, "AIDS and Confidentiality"; and Case Studies, "AIDS and a Duty to Protect," *Hastings Center Report* 17 (February 1987): 22–23. Two decades later, Kenneth Kipnis argued for a virtually absolute duty of confidentiality in such cases: "A Defense of Unqualified Medical Confidentiality," pp. 7–18. For analysis of dilemmas of confidentiality in the context of the HIV/AIDS epidemic, see Robert L. Barret, "Confidentiality and HIV/AIDS: Professional Challenges," in *Privacy and Confidentiality in Mental Health Care,* ed. John J. Gates and Bernard S. Arons (Baltimore: Paul H. Brookes, 2000), pp. 157–71.

60. Robert Klitzman and Ronald Bayer, *Mortal Secrets: Truth and Lies in the Age of AIDS* (Baltimore: Johns Hopkins University Press, 2003), p. 11, et passim.

61. Robert Klitzman, "Qualifying Confidentiality: Historical and Empirical Issues and Facts," *The American Journal of Bioethics* 6 (March–April 2006): 36; and Klitzman et al., "Naming Names: Perceptions of Name-Based HIV Reporting, Partner Notification, and Criminalization of Non-Disclosure among Persons Living with HIV," *Sexuality Research and Social Policy* 1 (2004): 38–57.

62. Lori B. Andrews et al., eds. (for the Committee on Assessing Genetic Risks, Institute of Medicine), *Assessing Genetic Risks: Implications for Health and Social Policy* (Washington, D.C.: National Academy Press, 1994), p. 278, see also pp. 264–73; and David H. Smith et al., *Early Warning: Cases and Ethical Guidance for Presymptomatic Testing in Genetic Diseases* (Bloomington, IN: Indiana University Press, 1998).

63. Michael Parker and Anneke Lucassen, "Genetic Information: A Joint Account?" *British Medical Journal* 329 (July 17, 2004): 165–67; and Parker and Lucassen, "Concern for Individuals and Families in Clinical Genetics," *Journal of Medical Ethics* 29 (2003): 70–74. See also Lucassen's case of intrafamilial conflict about genetic information, discussed from the standpoint of several different approaches to ethics, in Richard Ashcroft et al., *Case Analysis in Clinical Ethics* (Cambridge: Cambridge University Press, 2005).

64. Paul Ramsey, *The Patient as Person* (New Haven, CT: Yale University Press, 1970), p. xii.

65. See M. Gregg Bloche, "Clinical Loyalties and the Social Purposes of Medicine," *Journal of the American Medical Association* 281 (January 20, 1999): 268–74.

66. Our formulation is indebted to Stephen Toulmin, "Divided Loyalties and Ambiguous Relationships," *Social Science and Medicine* 23 (1986): 784.

67. *In re Sampson,* 317 N.Y.S.2d (1970).

68. See Donna L. Dickenson, ed., *Ethical Issues in Maternal-Fetal Medicine* (Cambridge: Cambridge University Press, 2002).

69. In *Oath Betrayed: Torture, Medical Complicity, and the War on Terror* (New York: Random House, 2006), Steven H. Miles asks, "Where were the doctors and nurses at Abu Ghraib?" and challenges medical and health professionals to recognize their responsibilities to disarmed captives. See also M. Gregg Bloche and Jonathan H. Marks, "When Doctors Go to War," *New England Journal of Medicine* 352, no. 1 (2005): 3–6; and Michael L. Gross, *Bioethics and Armed Conflict: Moral Dilemmas of Medicine and War* (Cambridge, MA: MIT Press, 2006).

70. See Curtis Prout and Robert N. Ross, *Care and Punishment: The Dilemmas of Prison Medicine* (Pittsburgh, PA: University of Pittsburgh Press, 1988); and Kenneth Kipnis, "Ethical Conflict in Correctional Health Services," in *Conflict of Interest in the Professions,* ed. Michael Davis and Andrew Stark (Oxford: Oxford University Press, 2001), pp. 302–15.

71. Richard J. Bonnie, "The Death Penalty: When Doctors Must Say No," *British Medical Journal* 305 (August 15, 1992): 381–82; and A. Sikora and Alan R. Fleischman, "Physician Participation in Capital Punishment: A Question of Professional Integrity," *Journal of Urban Health* 76 (1999): 400–08.

72. See *Code of Medical Ethics of the American Medical Association,* 2006–2007 Edition, 2.06, pp. 19–20, and the discussion in Robert D. Truog and Troyen Brennan, "Participation of Physicians in Capital Punishment," *New England Journal of Medicine* 329 (October 28, 1993): 1346–50.

73. Gregory F. Gramelspacher, Joel D. Howell, and Mark J. Young, "Perceptions of Ethical Problems by Nurses and Doctors," *Archives of Internal Medicine* 146 (March 1986): 577–78. For various ethical problems in nursing, see Sara T. Fry and Robert M. Veatch, *Case Studies in Nursing Ethics,* 3rd ed. (Boston: Jones & Bartlett, 2005).

74. See Michael Davis and Andrew Stark, eds., *Conflict of Interest in the Professions* (New York: Oxford University Press, 2001); Marc A. Rodwin, *Medicine, Money, and Morals: Physicians' Conflicts of Interest* (New York: Oxford University Press, 1993); and Edmund Erde et al., eds., *Conflicts of Interest in Clinical Practice and Research* (New York: Oxford University Press, 1996).

75. See Teddy D. Warner and John P. Gluck, "What Do We Really Know about Conflicts of Interest in Biomedical Research?" *Psychopharmocology* 171 (2003): 36–46. On the subject of disclosures of funding sources when publishing, see Sheldon Krimsky and L. S. Rothenberg, "Conflict of Interest Policies in Science and Medical Journals: Editorial Practices and Author Disclosures," *Science and Engineering Ethics* 7 (2001): 205–18.

76. See, among other studies, Jean M. Mitchell and Jonathan Sunshine, "Consequences of Physicians' Ownership of Health Care Facilities—Joint Ventures in Radiation Therapy," *New England Journal of Medicine* 327 (November 19, 1992): 1497–1501; Jean M. Mitchell and T. R. Sass, "Physician Ownership of Ancillary Services: Indirect Demand Inducement or Quality Assurance?" *Journal of Health Economics* 14 (August 1995): 263–89.

77. Several empirical studies in the late 1980s and early 1990s led to a federal prohibition of physician self-referral for Medicare or Medicaid patients, and to state laws prohibiting physician self-referral for privately insured patients. The federal legislation has several loopholes allowing opportunities for self-referral to return. See Jean M. Mitchell, "The Prevalence of Physician Self-Referral Arrangements after Stark II: Evidence from Advanced Diagnostic Imaging," *Health Affairs* Web Exclusive, April 17, 2007, W415–W424; Bruce J. Hillman, "Trying to Regulate Imaging Self-Referral Is Like Playing Whack-A-Mole," *American Journal of Roentgenology* 189 (2007): 267–68. The Council on Ethical and Judicial Affairs of the AMA has a general ban on self-referral, with exceptions; *Code of Medical Ethics of the American Medical Association,* 2006–2007 Edition, 8.032, pp. 188–90, passim.

78. See E. Haavi Morreim, *Balancing Act: The New Medical Ethics of Medicine's New Economics* (Boston: Kluwer Academic, 1991), which has influenced this discussion.

79. See Eric C. Campbell et al., "A National Survey of Physician-Industry Relationships," *New England Journal of Medicine* 356 (April 26, 2007): 1742–50; and Ashley Wazana, "Physicians and the Pharmaceutical Industry," *Journal of the American Medical Association* 283 (January 19, 2000): 373–80.

80. Pharmaceutical Research and Manufacturers of America, *Code on Interaction with Healthcare Professionals* (2002). Available from http://www.phrma.org/code_on_interactions_with_healthcare_professionals/ (accessed June 21, 2007).

81. Adriane Fugh-Berman and Shahram Ahiri, "Following the Script: How Drug Reps Make Friends and Influence Doctors," *PloS Medicine* 4 (April 2007): 621–25; Jason Dana and George Loewenstein, "A Social Science Perspective on Gifts to Physicians from Industry," *Journal of the American Medical Association* 290 (July 9, 2003): 252–55; R. B. Cialdini and M. R. Trost, "Influence, Social Norms, Conformity, and Compliance," in *The Handbook of Social Psychology,* 4th ed., ed. D. T. Gilbert et al. (New York: Oxford University Press, 1998); and Richard F. Adair and Leah R. Holmgren, "Do Drug Samples Influence Resident Prescribing Behavior? A Randomized Trial," *The American Journal of Medicine* 118 (2005): 881–84.

82. Dana Katz et al., "All Gifts Large and Small: Toward an Understanding of the Ethics of Pharmaceutical Industry Gift-Giving," *American Journal of Bioethics* 3 (Summer 2003): 39–45, accompanied by commentaries.

83. For these and other proposals, see Troyen A. Brennan et al., "Health Industry Practices that Create Conflicts of Interest: A Policy Proposal for Academic Medical Centers," *Journal of the American Medical Association* 295 (January 25, 2006): 429–33.

84. See several chapters in Part IV, "Clinical Research," in *Conflicts of Interest in Clinical Practice and Research*, ed. Erde et al.

85. Versions of several of these conditions appear in the Nuremberg Code and U.S. Department of Health and Human Services, Protections of Human Subjects, 45 CFR 46 (1991). See also Ezekiel J. Emanuel et al., "What Makes Clinical Research Ethical?" *Journal of the American Medical Association* 283 (May 24, 2000): 2701–11.

86. For analysis and criticism of pervasive paternalism in research ethics, see Franklin G. Miller and Alan Wertheimer, "Facing Up to Paternalism in Research Ethics," *Hastings Center Report* 37, No. 3 (2007): 24–34.

87. Disclosed by surgeon William DeVries at the University of Utah, as reported in Denise Grady, "Summary of Discussion on Ethical Perspectives," in *After Barney Clark: Reflections on the Utah Artificial Heart Program,* ed. Margery W. Shaw (Austin, TX: University of Texas Press, 1984), p. 49.

88. See Gunnel Elander and Goran Hermeren, "Placebo Effect and Randomized Clinical Trials," *Theoretical Medicine* 16 (1995): 171–82; B. P. Minogue et al., "Individual Autonomy and the Double-Blind Controlled Experiment: The Case of Desperate Volunteers"; and Gerald Logue and Stephen Wear, "A Desperate Solution: Autonomy and the Double-Blind Controlled Experiment," both in *Journal of Medicine and Philosophy* (1995): 43–64.

89. See Benjamin Freedman, "Equipoise and the Ethics of Clinical Research," *New England Journal of Medicine* 317 (July 16, 1987): 141–45; and Eugene Passamani, "Clinical Trials—Are They Ethical?," *New England Journal of Medicine* 324 (May 30, 1991): 1590–91.

90. See Franklin G. Miller and Howard Brody, "Clinical Equipoise and the Incoherence of Research Ethics," *Journal of Medicine and Philosophy* 32 (2007): 161. In a series of singly and jointly authored articles, Miller has sharply criticized appeals to clinical equipoise in research ethics. See also Miller and Brody, "A Critique of Clinical Equipoise: Therapeutic Misconception in the Ethics of Clinical Trials," *Hastings Center Report* 33, No. 3 (2003): 19–28.

91. Fred Gifford, "So-Called 'Clinical Equipoise' and the Argument from Design," *Journal of Medicine and Philosophy* 32 (2007): 135–50; and Ezekiel Emanuel, W. Bradford Patterson, and Samuel Hellman, "Ethics of Randomized Clinical Trials," *Journal of Clinical Oncology* 16 (1998): 365–71.

92. Don Marquis, "How to Resolve an Ethical Dilemma Concerning Randomized Clinical Trials," *New England Journal of Medicine* 341 (August 26, 1999): 691–93.

93. See M. A. Fischl et al., "The Efficacy of Azidothymidine (AZT) in the Treatment of Patients with AIDS-Related Complex: A Double-Blind, Placebo-Controlled Trial," *New England Journal of Medicine* 317 (1987): 185–91; and D. D. Richman et al., "The Toxicity of Azidothymidine (AZT) in the Treatment of Patients with AIDS and AIDS-Related Complex: A Double-Blind, Placebo-Controlled Trial," *New England Journal of Medicine* 317 (1987): 192–97.

94. For contrasting views, see Thomas B. Freeman et al., "Use of Placebo Surgery in Controlled Trials of a Cellular-Based Therapy for Parkinson's Disease," *New England Journal of Medicine* 341 (September 23, 1999): 988–92; Ruth Macklin, "The Ethical Problems with Sham Surgery in Clinical Research," *New England Journal of Medicine* 341 (September 23, 1999): 992–96; and Franklin G. Miller, "Sham Surgery: An Ethical Analysis," *The American Journal of Bioethics* 3 (2003): 41–48, with several commentaries (pp. 50–71).

95. This was Freedman's proposal in "Equipoise and the Ethics of Clinical Research."

96. See treatments of consent, data monitoring, and the control of information in Robert J. Levine and David K. Dennison, "Randomized Clinical Trials in Periodontology: Ethical Considerations," *Annals of Periodontology* 2 (1997): 83–94; and Valery M. Gordon, Jeremy Sugarman, and Nancy Kass, "Toward a More Comprehensive Approach to Protecting Human Subjects: The Interface of Data Safety Monitoring Boards and Institutional Review Boards in Randomized Clinical Trials," *IRB: A Review of Human Subjects Research* 20 (1998): 1–5.

PART III

THEORY AND METHOD

9

Moral Theories

In this chapter we examine the moral theories that we have mentioned in earlier chapters but did not pursue in detail. We examine four types of moral theory: utilitarianism, Kantianism, rights theory, and communitarianism.[1] Knowledge of these theories is indispensable for reflective study in biomedical ethics, because much of the field's literature discusses, and often relies on, these theories.

A so-called "textbook approach" to moral theory presents several competing theories and then proceeds to criticize each one. Often the criticisms are so harsh that each type of theory seems irreparably wounded, and readers become skeptical about the value of ethical theory in general. This skepticism is unfortunate. Defects and excesses appear in all major theories, but the theories discussed in this chapter all contain insights and arguments that deserve careful study. Our goal is to eliminate what is unacceptable in each type of theory and to appropriate what is relevant and acceptable for biomedical ethics.

Here and in the next chapter we refer to our own account of ethics as a "theory," but a word of caution is in order regarding this term. "Ethical theory" and "moral theory" are commonly used to refer to each of the following: (1) abstract moral reflection and argument, (2) systematic presentation of the basic components of ethics, (3) an integrated body of moral principles, and (4) a systematic justification of moral principles. We have attempted in this book to construct a coherent body of virtues, principles, and rules for *biomedical ethics only*. We do not claim to have developed a comprehensive ethical theory in ways suggested by the combination of (3) and (4). We engage *in theory* (e.g., in evaluating other ethical theories), and in doing so we engage in abstract reflection and argument (1). We also present an organized system of principles (3) and engage in systematic reflection and argument (2). But, at most, we present only elements of a comprehensive *general* theory. Our views on theory, method, and justification appear in Chapter 10.

Each section of this chapter, except the first and the last, is divided into subsections structured as follows: (1) an overview of the characteristic features of the theory being considered (introduced by examining how its proponents might approach a case); (2) an outline of the salient features of the theory; (3) an examination of criticisms regarding the theory's limitations and problems; and (4) an assessment of the theory's potential or actual contribution. This structure may suggest that we accept several moral theories, but this is not the best way to frame our conclusions. We accept as legitimate various *aspects* of many theories advanced in the history of ethics.[2] However, we reject both the hypothesis that all leading principles of the major moral theories can be assimilated into a coherent whole and the hypothesis that each of the theories offers an equally tenable moral framework.

CRITERIA FOR THEORY CONSTRUCTION

We begin with eight conditions of adequacy for an ethical theory. These criteria for theory construction set forth exemplary conditions for theories, but not so exemplary that no theory could satisfy them. The fact that all available theories only partially satisfy these conditions is not our concern here. Our objective is to provide a basis from which to assess theories.

Some philosophers reject the criteria that we propose on grounds that they present a distorted view of ethics. We cannot fully engage this controversy, but we offer two observations: First, we believe that these criteria are useful tools for assessing theories in ethics, including our own. Second, we believe that careful attention to actual moral practices often yields more insight into the moral life than general theories. Even illuminating theories are not the only source of moral insight. These theories are more plausible if they are applied only to some *limited range* of morality, rather than to all of it. For example, we suggest that utilitarianism is a better theoretical model for public policy than for clinical medical ethics.

There is a conflict between a once-popular conception of ethical theory and a newer and less settled account. In the older conception, popular from the late eighteenth century to the late twentieth century, the task of moral theory is to locate and justify general norms as a system. In the newer and less settled conception, the task of ethics is to reflect critically on actual and proposed moral norms and practices. In this chapter we discuss both conceptions, but our sympathies are decidedly with the latter.

Eight conditions express a more or less traditional understanding of criteria for ethical theories:[3]

1. *Clarity.* Taken as a whole or in its parts, a theory should be as clear as possible. Although, as Aristotle suggested, we can expect only as much clarity and precision of language as is appropriate for the subject matter, more obscurity and vagueness exist in the literature of ethical theory and biomedical ethics than is warranted by the subject matter.
2. *Coherence.* An ethical theory should be internally coherent. There should be neither conceptual inconsistencies (e.g., "hard medical paternalism

is justified only by consent of the patient") nor apparently contradictory statements (e.g., "to be virtuous is a moral obligation, but virtuous conduct is not obligatory"). If an account contains implications that are incoherent with other parts of that account, some aspect of the theory must be changed in a way that does not produce further incoherence. As we argue in Chapters 1 and 10, a major goal of a theory is to bring into coherence all of its normative elements (principles, virtues, rights, considered judgments, and the like).

3. *Comprehensiveness.* A theory should be as comprehensive as possible. A theory would be fully comprehensive if it could account for all justifiable moral norms and judgments. Any theory that includes fewer moral norms (e.g., one that includes only respect for autonomy) will range from partially complete to empty of important norms. Although the principles presented in this book under the headings of respect for autonomy, nonmaleficence, beneficence, and justice are far from a complete system for general normative ethics, they do provide a comprehensive general framework for the specific practical domain of *biomedical ethics.* We do not need additional general principles, but we do specify these four principles to generate such rules as promise-keeping, truthfulness, privacy, and confidentiality (see especially Chapter 7). These rules increase the comprehensiveness of the account.

4. *Simplicity.* A theory that distills the demands of morality to a few basic norms is preferable to a theory with more norms but no additional content. A theory should have no more norms than are necessary (simplicity in the sense of theoretical parsimony), and also no more than people can use without confusion (a practical simplicity). However, morality is complicated both theoretically and practically, and any comprehensive moral theory is certain to be complex. If the inherent complexity of morality demands a theory too difficult for practical use, the theory cannot be faulted for this reason alone. Developing a theory is a different enterprise than fashioning practical action guides.

5. *Explanatory power.* A theory has explanatory power when it provides enough insight to help us understand morality: its purpose, its objective or subjective status, how rights are related to obligations, and the like. For the sake of clarity, we should distinguish between normative theories and the theories we described in Chapter 1 as metaethical theories. While a general normative theory should not be held to the task of shedding light on metaethical questions, the ideal theory is one that seamlessly constructs a normative system while addressing the relevant metaethical questions. (We do not here distinguish between theory and method; our assumption is that theory and method go hand in hand.)

6. *Justificatory power.* A theory should also give us grounds for *justified* belief, not merely a reformulation or repackaging of beliefs we already

possess. For example, the distinction between acts and omissions under-lies many traditional beliefs in biomedical ethics, such as the belief that killing is impermissible and allowing to die permissible. But a moral theory would be impoverished if it only incorporated this distinction without determining whether the distinction is justifiable. A good theory also should have the power to criticize defective beliefs, no matter how widely accepted those beliefs may be.

7. *Output power.* A theory has output power when it produces judgments that were not in the original database of considered moral judgments on which the theory was constructed. If a normative theory did no more than repeat the list of judgments thought to be sound prior to the construction of the theory, it would have accomplished nothing. For example, if the parts of a theory pertaining to obligations of beneficence do not yield new judgments about role obligations of care in medicine beyond those assumed in constructing the theory, the theory will amount to no more than a classification scheme. A theory, then, must generate more than a list of axioms already present in pretheoretic belief.

8. *Practicability.* A proposed moral theory is unacceptable if its require-ments are so demanding that they cannot be satisfied or could be satisfied by only a few extraordinary persons or communities. A moral theory that presents utopian ideals or unfeasible recommendations fails the criterion of practicability. For example, if a theory proposed such high require-ments for personal autonomy (see Chapter 4) or such lofty standards of social justice (see Chapter 7) that no person could be autonomous and no society just, the proposed theory would be deeply problematic. (We are making certain assumptions about human nature and what is socially possible, but these assumptions will not be analyzed here.)

We could formulate other general criteria, but the eight we have identified are the most important for our purposes. A theory can receive a high score on the basis of one or more criteria and a low score on the basis of other criteria. For example, utilitarianism is arguably an internally coherent, simple, and compre-hensive theory with exceptional output power, but it is not coherent with some of our vital considered judgments, especially with certain judgments about justice, human rights, and the importance of personal projects. By contrast, Kantian theories are consistent with many of our considered judgments, but their clarity, simplicity, and output power are limited.

UTILITARIANISM

Consequentialism is a label affixed to theories holding that actions are right or wrong according to the balance of their good and bad consequences. It is a general term denoting theories that take the promotion of value to determine the rightness or wrongness of actions. The right act in any circumstance is the act that produces the best overall result as determined by the relevant theory of value. As the most prominent consequentialist theory, utilitarianism concentrates on the value of well-being, which may be analyzed in terms of pleasure, happiness, welfare, preference satisfaction, or the like. Utilitarianism accepts one and only one basic principle of ethics: the principle of utility. This principle asserts that we ought always to produce the maximal balance of positive value over disvalue (or the least possible disvalue, if only undesirable results can be achieved). It is often formulated as a requirement to do the greatest good for the greatest number, as determined from an impersonal perspective that gives equal weight to the legitimate interests of each affected party. The classical origins of this theory are found in the writings of Jeremy Bentham (1748–1832) and John Stuart Mill (1806–1873).

The Concept of Utility

Although utilitarians share the conviction that we should morally assess human actions in terms of their production of maximal value, they often disagree concerning which values should be maximized. Many utilitarians maintain that we ought to produce *agent-neutral* or *intrinsic* goods; that is, goods such as happiness, freedom, and health that every rational person values.[4] These goods are valuable in themselves, without reference to their further consequences or to the particular values held by individuals.

Bentham and Mill are *hedonistic* utilitarians because they conceive utility entirely in terms of happiness or pleasure, two broad terms that they treat as synonymous.[5] They acknowledge that many human actions do not appear to be performed for the sake of happiness. For example, when highly motivated professionals, such as research scientists, work themselves to the point of exhaustion in search of new knowledge, they do not appear to be seeking personal happiness. Mill proposes that such persons are initially motivated by success, recognition, or money, which all promise happiness. Along the way, either the pursuit of knowledge provides happiness or such persons never stop associating their hard work with the success, recognition, or money that they hope to gain.

However, many recent utilitarian philosophers have argued that a diverse set of values other than happiness contribute to well-being. Examples are knowledge, health, success, understanding, enjoyment, and deep personal relationships.[6] Even when their lists differ, these utilitarians concur that we should assess the greatest good in terms of the total intrinsic value produced by an action. Still other utilitarians hold that the concept of utility does not refer to *intrinsic goods,* but to an individual's *preferences;* that is, we are to maximize the overall satisfaction of the preferences of the greatest number of individuals.

A Case of Risk and Truthfulness

To distinguish the major themes of each theory treated in this chapter, each of the four sections devoted to a theory explicates how its proponents might approach the same case. This case centers on a five-year-old girl who has progressive renal failure and is not responding well on chronic renal dialysis. The medical staff is considering a renal transplant, but its effectiveness is "questionable" in her case. Nevertheless, a "clear possibility" exists that the transplanted kidney will not be affected by the disease process. The parents concur with the plan to try a transplant, but an additional obstacle emerges. The tissue typing indicates that it would be difficult to find a match for the girl. The staff excludes her two siblings, ages two and four, as too young to provide a kidney. The mother is not histocompatible, but the father is compatible and has "anatomically favorable circulation for transplantation."

Meeting alone with the father, the nephrologist gives him the results and indicates that the prognosis for his daughter is "quite uncertain." After reflection, the father decides that he will not donate a kidney to his daughter. His several reasons include his fear of the surgery, the uncertain prognosis for his daughter even with a transplant, the slight prospect of a cadaver kidney, and the suffering his daughter has already sustained. The father then requests that the physician "tell everyone else in the family that he is not histocompatible." He is afraid that if family members know the truth, they will accuse him of failing to save his daughter when he could have. He maintains that truth-telling would have the effect of "wrecking the family." The physician is uncomfortable with this request, but after further discussion he agrees to tell the man's wife that the father should not donate a kidney "for medical reasons."[7]

Utilitarians evaluate this case in terms of the probable consequences of the different courses of action open to the father and the physician. The goal is to realize the greatest good by balancing the interests of all affected persons. This evaluation depends on judgments concerning probable outcomes. Whether the father ought to donate his kidney depends on the probability of successful transplantation as well as the risks and other costs to him (and indirectly to other dependent members of the family). The potential effectiveness is questionable and the prognosis uncertain, although a possibility exists that a transplanted kidney would not undergo the same disease process. There is a slight possibility that a cadaver kidney could be obtained.

The girl will probably die without a transplant from either a cadaveric or a living source, but the transplant also offers only a small chance of survival. The risk of death to the father from anesthesia during kidney removal is 1 in 10,000 to 15,000 (at the time of this case). It is difficult to put an estimate on other possible long-term health effects. Nevertheless, because the chance of success is likely greater than the probability that the father will be harmed, many utilitarians would hold that the father or anyone else similarly situated is *obligated* to undertake what others would consider a heroic act that surpasses obligation (see chap. 9, pp. 336ff, 341–42). On one balance of probable benefits and risks, an uncompromising utilitarian would suggest tissue typing the patient's two siblings and then removing a kidney from one if there were a good match and parental approval. However, utilitarians disagree among themselves in these various judgments because of their different theories of value and their different predictions and assessments of probable outcomes.

Probabilistic judgments would likewise play a role in the physician's utilitarian calculation of the right action in response to the father's request. The physician would need to bear in mind a variety of sociological and psychological considerations, including whether a full disclosure would wreck the family, whether lying to the family would have serious negative effects, and whether the father would subsequently experience serious guilt from his refusal to donate. A utilitarian would argue that the physician is obligated to consider the whole range of facts and possible consequences in light of the best available information.

Act and Rule Utilitarianism

The principle of utility is the ultimate standard of right and wrong for all utilitarians. Controversy has arisen, however, over whether this principle pertains to particular acts in particular circumstances or instead to general rules that themselves determine which acts are right and wrong. Whereas the *rule utilitarian* considers the consequences of adopting certain rules, the *act utilitarian* disregards the level of rules and justifies actions by direct appeal to the principle of utility, as the following chart indicates:

Rule Utilitarianism	*Act Utilitarianism*
Principle of Utility	Principle of Utility
↑	
Moral Rules	↑
↑	
Particular Judgments	Particular Judgments

The act utilitarian asks, "What good and bad consequences will probably result from *this action in this circumstance?*" Although moral rules are useful in guiding human actions, they are also expendable if they do not promote utility in a particular context. For the rule utilitarian, by contrast, an act's conformity to a rule that is justified by utility makes the act right, and the rule is not expendable in a particular context, even if following the rule does not maximize utility in that context.[8]

Physician Worthington Hooker, a prominent nineteenth-century figure in academic medicine and medical ethics, was a rule utilitarian who attended to rules of truth-telling in medicine as follows:

> The good, which may be done by deception in a *few* cases, is almost as nothing, compared with the evil which it does in *many,* when the prospect of its doing good was just as promising as it was in those in which it succeeded. And when we add to this the evil which would result from a *general* adoption of a system of deception, the importance of a strict adherence to the truth in our intercourse with the sick, even on the ground of expediency, becomes incalculably great.[9]

Hooker argued that widespread deception in medicine will have an increasingly negative effect over time and will eventually produce more harm than good.

Act utilitarians, by contrast, argue that observing a rule such as truth-telling does not always maximize the general good, and that such rules are properly understood as rough guidelines. They regard rule utilitarians as unfaithful to the fundamental demand of the principle of utility, which is to "Maximize value." In some circumstances, they argue, abiding by a generally beneficial rule will not prove most beneficial to the persons affected by the action, even in the long run. According to one act utilitarian, a third possibility exists between never adopting any rules and always obeying rules—namely, *sometimes* obeying rules.[10] From this perspective, physicians do not and should not always tell the truth to their patients or their families. Sometimes physicians should even lie to give hope. According to this account, selective obedience does not erode either moral rules or general respect for morality.

Because of the benefits to society of the general observance of moral rules, the rule utilitarian does not abandon rules, even in difficult situations. Abandonment threatens the integrity and existence of both the particular rules and the whole system of rules.[11] The act utilitarian's reply is that although promises usually should be kept to maintain trust, they may be set aside when doing so would maximize overall good.

An Absolute Principle with Derivative Contingent Rules

From the utilitarian's perspective, the principle of utility is the sole and absolute principle of ethics. No derivative rule is absolute, and no rule is unrevisable. For example, rules in medicine against actively ending a patient's life may be overturned or substantially revised. In Chapter 5 we assessed current debates about whether seriously suffering patients should, at their request, be actively assisted in dying rather than merely being "allowed to die." The rule utilitarian argues that we should support rules that permit physicians to hasten death if and only if those rules would produce the most utility. Likewise, there should be rules against physician-assisted death if and only if those rules would maximize utility. Utilitarians often point out that we do not currently permit physicians to actively bring about a patient's death because of the adverse social consequences that are believed to follow for those directly and indirectly affected. If, however, under a different set of social conditions, legalization of physician-assisted death would maximize overall social welfare, the utilitarian would see no reason to prohibit it. Utilitarians thus regard their theory as responsive in constructive ways to changing social practices.

A Critical Evaluation of Utilitarianism

Utilitarianism is not a fully adequate moral theory for several reasons.

Problems with immoral preferences and actions. Problems arise for utilitarians who are concerned about the maximization of individual preferences when some of these individuals have what considered judgments tell us are morally unacceptable preferences. For example, if a researcher derived supreme satisfaction from inflicting pain on animals or on human subjects in experiments, we would condemn this preference and would seek to prevent it from being satisfied. A theory based on subjective preferences is a plausible theory only if we can formulate a range of *acceptable* preferences and determine "acceptability" independently of agents' preferences. This task seems inconsistent with a pure preference approach to utility.[12]

There is an additional problem concerned with immoral actions. Suppose the only way to achieve the maximal utilitarian outcome is to perform an immoral act (as judged by the standards of the common morality) such as killing one person to distribute his organs to several others who will die without them. Utilitarianism seems to say not only that such killing is permissible, but that it is morally obligatory. This requirement seems blatantly immoral.

Does utilitarianism demand too much? Some forms of utilitarianism seem to demand too much in the moral life, because the principle of utility requires *maximizing* value. Utilitarians have a difficult time maintaining the crucial distinction (see in Chapter 2) between *morally obligatory actions* and *supererogatory actions* (those above the call of moral obligation and performed for the sake of personal ideals). Alan Donagan has described a variety of situations in which utilitarian theory regards an action as obligatory even though our firm moral conviction is that the action is ideal and praiseworthy rather than obligatory.[13] For example, Donagan would regard the "voluntary" suicide of frail elderly persons who suffer from severe disabilities who are no longer useful to society as an example of acts that could never rightly be considered obligatory, regardless of the consequences. The same holds for heroic donation of bodily parts, such as kidneys and even hearts, to save another person's life. If utilitarianism makes such actions obligatory, then it is a defective theory. Donagan argues, and we agree, that all utilitarians face these problems, because none can rule out the ever-present possibility that what is today praiseworthy (but optional) will, through altered social circumstances, become obligatory by utilitarian standards.

Bernard Williams and John Mackie offer extensions of the thesis that utilitarianism demands too much. Williams argues that utilitarianism abrades personal integrity by making persons as morally responsible for consequences that they *fail to prevent* as for those outcomes they *directly cause,* even when the consequences are not of their doing. Mackie argues that a utilitarian "test of right actions" is so distant from our moral experience that it becomes "the ethics of fantasy," because it demands that people strip themselves of many goals and relationships they value in life to maximize outcomes for others. From this perspective, the utilitarian demands that we act like saints without personal interests and goals.[14]

Problems of unjust distribution. A third problem is that utilitarianism, in principle, permits the interests of the majority to override the rights of minorities, and does not have the resources to adequately guard against unjust social distributions. The charge is that utilitarians assign no independent weight to justice and are indifferent to unjust distributions because they distribute value according to net aggregate satisfaction.[15] If an already prosperous group of persons could have more value added to their lives than could be added to the lives of the indigent in society, the utilitarian must recommend that the added value go to the prosperous group.

An example of problematic (although not necessarily unjust) distribution appears in the following case. Two researchers wanted to determine the most cost-effective way to control hypertension in the American population. As they developed their research, they discovered that it is more cost-effective to target patients already being treated for hypertension than to identify new cases of hypertension among persons without regular access to medical care. They concluded that "a community with limited resources would probably do better to concentrate its efforts on improving adherence of known hypertensives (that is, those already identified as sufferers of hypertension), even at a sacrifice in terms of the numbers screened." If accepted by the government, this recommendation would exclude the poorest sector, which has the most pressing need for medical attention, from the benefits of publicly funded high blood pressure education and management. The investigators were concerned because of the apparent injustice in excluding the poor and minorities. Yet their statistics were compelling. No matter how carefully planned the efforts, nothing worked efficiently (i.e., nothing produced utilitarian results), except programs directed at known hypertensives already in contact with physicians. The investigators therefore recommended what they explicitly referred to as a utilitarian allocation scheme.[16]

Medical research since this study has continued to support its findings. Society could probably achieve a greater net improvement in overall public health by targeting patients who have primary-care physicians, yet such a strategy is likely to underserve poor and minority populations who already suffer disproportionately from health problems.[17]

A Constructive Evaluation of Utilitarianism

Despite these criticisms, utilitarianism has many strengths, two of which we have appropriated in other chapters. The first is the acceptance of a significant role for the principle of utility in formulating public policy. The utilitarian's requirements for an objective assessment of everyone's interests and of an impartial choice to maximize good outcomes for all affected parties are acceptable norms of public policy, except insofar as they lead to unjust distributions and the like. Second, when we formulated principles of beneficence in Chapter 5, utility played an important role. We have characterized utilitarianism as primarily a *consequence*-based theory, but it is also *beneficence*-based. That is, the theory sees morality primarily in terms of the goal of promoting welfare.

A theory that balances the principle of beneficence with other principles should eliminate the several problems with an unqualified use of the principle of utility previously discussed. We agree with Amartya Sen that "Consequentialist reasoning may be fruitfully used even when consequentialism as such is not accepted. To ignore consequences is to leave an ethical story half told."[18]

KANTIANISM

A second type of theory denies much that utilitarian theories affirm. Often called *deontological*[19] or *nonconsequentialist*[20] (i.e., a theory of duty holding that some features of actions other than or in addition to consequences make actions right or wrong), this type of theory is now frequently called *Kantian*, because the ethical thought of Immanuel Kant (1724–1804) has most deeply shaped its formulations.

Consider how a Kantian might approach the previously mentioned case of the five-year-old in need of a kidney. A Kantian would insist that we should rest our moral judgments on reasons that also apply to all other persons who are similarly situated. If the father has no generalizable moral obligation to his daughter, then no basis is available for morally criticizing him. The strict Kantian maintains that if the father chooses to donate out of affection, compassion, or concern for his dying daughter, his act would lack moral worth, because it would not be based on a generalizable obligation; but the donation would have moral worth if done from the duty of beneficence. Using one of the girl's younger siblings as a source of a kidney would be illegitimate because this recourse to children who are too young to consent to donation would involve using persons merely as means to others' ends. This principle would also exclude coercing the father to donate against his will.

Regarding the physician's options after the father requests to deceive the family, a strict Kantian views lying as an act that cannot consistently be universalized as a norm of conduct. The physician should not lie to the man's wife or to other members of the family, even if it would help keep the family intact (a consequentialist appeal). Although the physician's statement is not, strictly speaking, a lie, he still intentionally uses this formulation to conceal relevant facts from the wife, an act Kantians typically view as morally unacceptable.

A Kantian will also consider whether the rule of confidentiality has independent moral weight, whether the tests the father underwent with the nephrologist established a relationship of confidentiality, and whether the rule of confidentiality protects information about the father's histocompatibility and his reasons for not donating. If confidentiality prohibits the nephrologist from letting the family know that the father is histocompatible, then the Kantian must face an apparent conflict of obligations: truthfulness in conflict with confidentiality. Before we can address such conflict, however, we need to understand Kantian theory better.

Obligation from Categorical Rules

Kant argued that morality is grounded in reason, rather than in tradition, intuition, or attitudes such as sympathy. He saw human beings as creatures with rational powers that motivate them morally, that resist tempting desire, and that allow humans to prescribe moral rules to themselves.

One of Kant's most important claims is that the moral worth of an individual's action depends exclusively on the moral acceptability of the rule (an objective "maxim") on which the person acts. As Kant puts it, moral obligation depends on an objective rule determining the individual's will; the rule provides a moral reason that justifies the action.[21] For Kant, one must act not only *in accordance with* but *for the sake of* obligation. That is, to have moral worth, a person's motive for acting must come from a recognition that he or she intends that which is known to be morally required. For example, if an employer discloses a health hazard to an employee only because the employer fears a lawsuit, and not because of the importance of truth-telling, then the employer has performed the right action but deserves no moral credit for the action. If agents do what is morally right simply because they are scared, because they derive pleasure from doing that kind of act, or because they seek recognition, they lack the requisite goodwill that derives from acting for the sake of obligation.

To see how a Kantian would judge the moral worth of a proposed course of action, imagine a man who desperately needs money and knows that he will not be able to borrow it unless he promises repayment in a definite time, but who also knows that he will not be able to repay it within this period. He decides to make a promise that he knows he will break. Kant asks us to examine the man's reason, that is, his maxim: "When I think myself in want of money, I will borrow money and promise to pay it back, although I know that I cannot do so." This maxim, Kant says, cannot pass a test that he calls the *categorical imperative*. This imperative tells us what must be done irrespective of our desires. In its major formulation, Kant states the categorical imperative as follows: "I ought never to act except in such a way that I can also will that my maxim become a universal law." Kant says that this one principle justifies all particular impera- tives of obligation (all "ought" statements that morally obligate).[22]

The categorical imperative is a canon of the acceptability of moral rules; that is, a criterion for judging the acceptability of the maxims that direct actions. This imperative adds nothing to a maxim's content. Rather, it determines which maxims are objective and valid. The categorical imperative functions by testing what Kant calls the "consistency of maxims": A maxim must be capable of being conceived and willed without contradiction. When we examine the maxim of the person who deceitfully promises, we discover, Kant seems to say, that this maxim is incapable of being conceived and willed universally without yielding a contradiction. It is inconsistent with what it presupposes and is like saying, "Though promising is not deceitful, this promise of mine is deceitful." The uni- versalized maxim is inconsistent with the very point of the proposed maxim of action—a maxim that would be undermined if everyone acted on it. Lying, too, works only if the person lied to expects or presupposes that people are truthful, but in a world in which everyone lied, a maxim approving lying would make the purpose of truth-telling impossible, and no one would believe the person who told a lie. Many examples from everyday life illustrate this thesis. For instance, maxims permitting cheating on tests are inconsistent with the practices of hon- esty on tests that they presuppose.[23]

Kant appears to have more than one version of what he calls the categorical imperative, because his several formulations are notably different. His second formulation is widely cited in biomedical ethics and, more generally, is at least as influential as the first: "One must act to treat every person as an end and never as a means only."[24] It has often been said that this principle categori- cally requires that we should never treat another as a means to our ends, but this interpretation misrepresents Kant's views. He argues only that we must not treat another *merely* or *exclusively* as a means to our ends. When human research subjects volunteer to test new drugs, they are treated as a means to others' ends, but they have a choice in the matter and retain control over their lives. Kant does not prohibit such uses of consenting persons. He insists only that they be treated with the respect and moral dignity to which every person is entitled.

Autonomy and Heteronomy

We saw in Chapter 4 that the word *autonomy* typically refers to that which makes judgments and actions one's own. The concept of autonomy is more restricted for Kant. Persons have "autonomy of the will" if and only if they knowingly act in accordance with the universally valid moral principles that pass the requirements of the categorical imperative. He contrasts this *moral* autonomy with "heteronomy," which refers to any determinative influence over the will other than motivation by moral principles.[25] If, for example, people act from passion, ambition, or self-interest, they act heteronomously. Only a rational will acting morally chooses autonomously. Kant regards acting from desire, fear, impulse, personal projects, and habit as no less heteronomous than actions manipulated or coerced by others.

To say that an individual must "accept" a moral principle to be autonomous does not mean that the principle is subjective or that each individual must create (author or originate) his or her moral principles. Kant requires only that each individual *will the acceptance* of moral principles. If a person freely accepts objective moral principles, that person is a lawgiver unto himself or herself. For Kant this account extends beyond the *nature* of autonomy to its *value*. "The principle of autonomy," he contends, is "the sole principle of morals," and it is autonomy that gives people respect, value, and proper motivation. A person's dignity—indeed, "sublimity"—comes from being morally autonomous.[26]

Although Kant's theory of respect is grounded in his conception of autonomy, his theory of autonomy differs considerably from the theory of autonomy we presented in Chapter 4 when developing the principle of respect for autonomy. Kant's theory of autonomy is not about respect for self-determination in general (as ours is); it is exclusively about *moral* self-determination. However, Kant's second formulation of the categorical imperative is reasonably close to the normative commitments in the principle of respect for autonomy that we developed in Chapter 4.

Contemporary Kantian Ethics

Several writers in contemporary ethical theory have accepted and developed Kantian moral theories, broadly construed.

An example is *The Theory of Morality* by Alan Donagan. He seeks the "philosophical core" of the morality expressed in the Hebrew-Christian tradition (which he interprets in secular rather than religious terms). Donagan's philosophical elaboration of this point of view relies heavily on Kant's theory of persons as ends in themselves, especially the imperative that one must treat humanity as an end and never as a means only. Donagan expresses the fundamental principle of the Hebrew-Christian tradition as a Kantian principle grounded in rationality: "It is impermissible not to respect every human being, oneself or any other, as a rational creature."[27]

A second Kantian theory derives from the work of John Rawls. Rawls challenged utilitarian theories while developing Kantian themes of reason, autonomy, individual worth, self-respect, and equality.[28] His *A Theory of Justice* builds on and reconstructs Kant's moral theory as the foundation of a theory of justice (a theory we briefly treated in Chapter 7). The theory appeals to Kant's conception of deriving principles of ethics (principles of justice, in Rawls's case) from a circumstance of pure rationality. In selecting the basic moral principles, agents implement the Kantian idea of autonomy. Rawls insists, as Kant did, that autonomous derivation of basic principles is independent of the historical features of any given society. The principles of justice in some societies can be shown to be rationally better than the principles of justice adopted in other societies. For Rawls, the right to individual autonomy (as we discussed in Chapter 4)— of an agent or of a political state—does not outweigh what rational moral principles determine to be morally right. Even conscientious acts of individual autonomy do not merit respect unless they are in accord with moral principles derived from moral autonomy.[29]

Several philosophers, including Bernard Williams and Thomas Nagel, have developed a doctrine of "deontological constraints" that is related to Kant's injunction never to use another person merely as a means.[30] These philosophers argue that Kant was correct to maintain that certain actions are impermissible regardless of the consequences. For example, in research involving human subjects, even if achieving certain results would have good consequences for millions of people, researchers would be treating their subjects unethically if they violated fundamental constraints on behavior. These constraints limit actions even if they will bring about the overall best state of affairs. Such constraints are essentially negative duties. That is, they specify what we may not justifiably do to others even in the pursuit of worthy goals. However, they do not specify any actions that we should perform for the sake of others. For example, stealing a sibling's share of the family inheritance would violate deontological constraints, but those constraints do not tell us how to divide wealth among siblings.

This conception of deontological constraints highlights an obvious difference between Kantian and utilitarian theories. The latter require us to seek the best possible state of affairs, irrespective of the position of particular agents who act in those states of affairs. Utilitarians demand an external, impartial view to weigh each person's interests equally, but a person's role and sense of integrity have no independent force. They are only important insofar as they are factors in the calculus of utilities. Kantian thought firmly resists these utilitarian conclusions.

A number of writers have reinvigorated Kant scholarship and infused it with innovative moral theories. Three such writers are Christine Korsgaard, Barbara

Herman, and Onora O'Neill, who have offered stimulating interpretations of Kant, constructive extensions of his moral philosophy, and responses to many objections that other philosophers make to Kant. Kant, at their hands, is rather different from the rigid, rule-bound Kant of traditional interpretation. Herman argues that Kant's categorical imperative is a sensitive and practical moral tool, not merely a rigid element in a rationalistic theory of duty. Korsgaard uses various Kantian themes to justify moral normativity. She also develops interpretations of the several different formulations that Kant provides of the categorical imperative. O'Neill has extended her work into several areas of biomedical ethics and global justice. Her Kantian themes focus heavily on "principled autonomy," public reason, a robust interpretation of universalizability, and the importance of creating conditions of trust.[31]

A Critical Evaluation of Kantianism

Like utilitarianism, Kant's theory fails to provide a comprehensive and adequate theory of the moral life.

The problem of conflicting obligations. Kant construes moral requirements as categorical imperatives, but this produces a severe problem with conflicting obligations. Suppose we have promised to take our children on a long-anticipated trip, but now find that if we do so, we cannot assist our sick mother in the hospital. A rule of promise-keeping and a rule of assistance or obligation of care generate this conflict. Conflict can also arise from a single moral rule rather than from two different rules, as, for example, when two promises come into conflict, although the promisor could not have anticipated the conflict when making the promises. Because moral rules are *categorical* for Kant, he seems to say that we are obligated to do the impossible and perform both actions. Any ethical theory that leads to this conclusion is incoherent, yet no clear way out exists for Kant or for any theory with truly categorical or absolutist rules.[32] (Our own solution to the general problem of moral conflicts is found on pp. 15–26).

Overemphasizing law, underemphasizing relationships. Kant's arguments concentrate on lawful obligations, and some recent Kantian theories feature a contractual basis for obligations. But whether equality, contract, law, and other staples of Kantianism deserve to occupy such a central position in a moral theory is questionable. (They are, we can readily agree, central ingredients in legal and political theories.) These visions of the moral life fail to capture much in personal relationships that generate moral responsibilities. For example, we rarely think or act in terms of law, contract, or absolute rules in relationships among friends and family.[33] This suggests that Kant's theory (like utilitarianism) is better suited for relationships among strangers than for relationships among friends or other intimates.

Virtue, emotion, and the theory of moral worth. Kant maintains that actions done from sympathy, emotion, and the like have no moral worth; only actions done from duty (i.e., the motive of duty) have moral worth. Kant does not disallow or even discourage sympathies and emotions, but these motives count for nothing morally. Yet, we argued in Chapter 2 that actions done from sympathy, emotion, and the like can have moral worth. Persons with appropriate feelings and concern about their friends, for example, are morally worthier than persons who discharge obligations of friendship entirely from a sense of duty. A "friend," or a physician or a nurse, who is lacking in appropriate attitudes of care is morally deficient. Kant's theory seems defective not because we want people to act from feelings rather than from a sense of obligation. Of course we want people to be attentive to and discharge their obligations, and there is nothing wrong with a motive of duty. At the same time, there is also something meritorious about motivation from deep care and concern. The goodness of the action seems intimately connected, in many cases, with the feelings of the actor. Duty is a meritorious motive, but so is caring feeling, and actions can derive from both.[34]

A Constructive Evaluation of Kantianism

Kant argued that when good reasons support a moral judgment, those reasons are good for all relevantly similar circumstances. Most moral theories now accept this claim, and Kant must be given credit for a compelling theoretical account of the claim. It is a far-reaching claim. For example, if we are required to obtain valid consent for all subjects of biomedical research, we cannot make exceptions of certain persons merely because we could advance science by doing so. We cannot use institutionalized populations without consent any more than we can use people who are not in institutions without their consent. Kant and many Kantians have driven home the point that persons cannot privilege or exempt themselves or their favored group and still act morally.

Kant and contemporary Kantians have worked diligently on perhaps the single most important issue in modern moral philosophy: Are some actions wrong not because of their good or bad effects, but rather for a reason pertaining to the inherent wrongness of either the actions or the rules from which the action is performed? Also, as we touched on earlier, Kant's second formulation of the categorical imperative—that persons must be treated as ends and not as means only—can be, and often has been, interpreted as the substantive basis of what, in Chapter 4 and throughout this book, we refer to as the principle of respect for autonomy. Kant's second formulation has been enormously, and justifiably, influential on contemporary biomedical ethics.

RIGHTS THEORY

The language of *rights* is as important as that of obligation. Statements of rights provide vital protections of life, liberty, expression, and property. They protect against oppression, unequal treatment, intolerance, arbitrary invasion of privacy, and the like. Some philosophers, political activists, lawyers, and framers of political declarations regard rights as the single most important category for expressing the moral point of view.

An ethical analysis of the case of the five-year-old in need of a transplant would, from the perspective of rights theories, focus on the rights of all the parties, in an effort to determine their meaning and scope as well as their weight and strength. The father could be considered to have rights of autonomy, privacy, and confidentiality that protect his bodily integrity and sphere of decision making from interference by others. In addition, he has a right to information, which he apparently received, about the risks, benefits, and alternatives of living kidney donation. The father's decision not to donate is within his rights, as long as it does not violate another's rights. No apparent grounds support a general right to assistance that could permit anyone, including his daughter, to demand a kidney. However, there are various specific rights to assistance, and it might be argued that the daughter has a right to receive a kidney from her family on the basis of either parental obligations or medical need. But even if such a right exists, which is doubtful, it would be circumscribed. For example, it is implausible to suppose that such a right could be enforced against the interests of the girl's two young siblings. Their right to noninterference, when the procedure is not for their direct benefit, carries risks, and they lack the capacity to consent, precludes their use as sources of a kidney.

Analysis of this case in terms of rights would note that the father has exercised his rights of autonomy and privacy in allowing the physician to run some tests. He then seeks protection under his right of confidentiality, which he believes allows him to control access to any information generated in his relationship with the physician. However, the precise scope and limits of his rights and competing rights need to be approached cautiously. For example, does the mother herself have a right to the information generated in the relationship between the father and the nephrologist, particularly information bearing on the fate of the daughter?

An analysis using rights would also consider whether the physician has a right of conscientious refusal. The physician might resist becoming an instrument of the father's desire to keep others from knowing why he is not donating a kidney. But even if the physician does have a right to protect his personal integrity, does this right trump the rights of others?

Liberal Individualism as Rights Theory

Rights are *justified claims* that individuals and groups can make on other individuals or on society; to have a right is to be in a position to determine, by one's choices, what others should or should not do.[35] All rights exist or fail to exist because of a normative structure that either allows or disallows the claim in question. *Legal* rights are justified by normative structures in law, and *moral* rights are justified by normative structures in morality. It is arguably the case that claiming a right is a rule-governed activity, where the rules may be legal rules, moral rules, institutional rules, or rules of games. However, there is a priority problem here: It is not always clear that the right is derived from a rule. Perhaps rules are derived from rights. For example, perhaps the right to free speech is the basis of various rules of freedom of expression, rather than the converse. Accordingly, we leave the precise basis of rights an open question.[36]

We analyze rights theory in this section in terms of what has often been called *liberal individualism*. Rights could rest on other bases, but liberal individualism is an important theory, and, historically, it has been intertwined with rights theory. Liberal individualism starts with the basic presumption that a just political system must carve out a certain space within which the individual may pursue personal projects. Liberal individualism has, in recent years, challenged the reigning utilitarian and Kantian moral theories. H. L. A. Hart once described this challenge as a switch from an "old faith that some form of utilitarianism...*must* capture the essence of political morality" to a new faith in "a doctrine of basic human rights, protecting specific basic liberties and interests of individuals."[37]

This faith may be new, but liberal individualism is not a new development in moral and political theory. At least since Thomas Hobbes, liberal individualists have employed the language of rights to buttress moral and political arguments, and the Anglo-American legal tradition has relied heavily on this language. The language of rights has served, on occasion, as a means to oppose the status quo, to demand recognition and respect, and to promote social reforms that aim to secure legal protections for individuals. Historically, this language has been instrumental in wresting certain freedoms—such as freedom of the press and freedom of religious expression—from established orders of religion, society, and state.

The legitimate role of civil, political, and legal rights in protecting the individual from societal intrusions seems undeniable, but the proposition that individual rights provide the fountainhead for moral and political theory has been strongly resisted—for example, by many utilitarians and communitarians. They note that individual interests said to be protected by rights are often at odds with communal and institutional interests. In discussions of health care delivery, for example, proponents of a broad availability of medical services often appeal to the "right to health care," whereas opponents sometimes appeal to the "rights of the medical profession." Many participants in these moral, political, and legal discussions presuppose that arguments cannot be persuasive unless stated in the language of rights, although other participants find this language too confrontational and adversarial.

Absolute and Prima Facie Rights

Perhaps rights are neither as strong nor as confrontational as they first appear. Some rights may be absolute (e.g., the right to choose one's religion or to reject all religion), but, typically, rights are not absolute claims. Like principles of obligation, rights assert only prima facie claims (in the sense of "prima facie" introduced in Chapter 1).

Some writers seem to suggest that rights are absolute, or at least absolute in some restricted contexts. Ronald Dworkin has argued the well-known thesis that some political rights are so basic that ordinary justifications for interference with rights by the state, such as reducing inconvenience or promoting utility, have no warrant. The stakes must be far more significant to justify such invasions, he argues, because rights are "trumps" held by an individual against general plans and background justifications in the political state.[38] Democratic governments typically frame their policies to promote the general welfare and to conform to majority decisions, but rights are instruments that function to *guarantee* that individuals cannot be sacrificed to these government or majority interests.

However, as Dworkin recognizes, if the claims of public utility are highly significant, the individual cannot actually claim to have a trump card.[39] Rights are not so strong that they may never be overridden. If the state needs to protect the rights of others (e.g., the state needs to prevent the spread of a catastrophic disease), then it may legitimately override some individual rights (e.g., the right to refuse vaccination). What we cannot do, Dworkin insists, is to act as if the right did not exist and so make decisions based entirely on net social utility. Mere benefit to the community is not of itself sufficient to override rights, which is the fundamental point of rights guarantees.

We believe that all rights, like all principles and rules of obligation, are prima facie (i.e., presumptively) valid claims that sometimes must yield to other claims. Even the right to life is not absolute, irrespective of competing claims or social conditions, as evidenced by common moral judgments about killing in war and killing in self-defense. In light of this need to balance claims, we should distinguish a *violation* of a right from an *infringement* of a right.[40] Violation refers to an unjustified action *against* a right, whereas infringement refers to a justified action *overriding* a right.

Positive Rights and Negative Rights

A *positive* right is a right to receive a particular good or service from others, whereas a *negative* right is a right to be free from some action by others. A person's positive right entails another's obligation to do something for that person; a negative right entails another's obligation to refrain from doing something.[41] Examples of both sorts of rights appear in biomedical practice, research, and policy. If a right to health care exists, for example, it is a positive right to goods and services grounded in a claim of justice (see Chapter 7). The right to forgo a recommended surgical procedure, by contrast, is a negative right grounded in the principle of respect for autonomy. The liberal individualist tradition generally has found it easier to justify negative rights, but the recognition of welfare rights in modern societies has led to an extension of the scope of positive rights.

The Correlativity of Rights and Obligations

How, then, are rights connected to obligations? To answer this question, consider the meaning of "X has a right to do or have Y." X's right entails that some party has an obligation either not to interfere if X does Y or to provide X with Y. Suppose, for example, that a physician agrees to take John Doe as a patient and commences treatment. The physician incurs an obligation to Doe, and Doe gains correlative rights. Likewise, if a state has an obligation to provide goods such as food or health care to needy citizens, then any citizen who meets the relevant criteria of need can claim an entitlement to food or health care.

This analysis suggests a firm but untidy *correlativity* between obligations and rights.[42] It is untidy because at least one use of the words *requirement, obligation,* and *duty* indicates that not all obligations imply corresponding rights. For example, although we sometimes refer to requirements or obligations of charity, no person can claim another person's charity as a matter of right. If such norms of charity express what we "ought to do," they do so not from moral obligation but from personal ideals that exceed obligation (see Chapter 2). We can best construe these commitments as self-imposed "oughts" that are not required by morality and that do not generate rights claims for other persons. Thus, rights language is correlative to obligation language, but in a way that requires careful attention to particular contexts and often entails further specification of both rights and their correlative obligations.

Some writers use the language of rights in a more robust way, so that certain particularly critical interests of persons are firmly protected by rights. These rights protect persons against having their interests balanced or traded off to serve the public interest or the interests of others. In particular, rights offer special protection against public utility being used to override rights.[43] Although we appreciate the moral importance of this point, we do not think that this robust sense of rights undercuts either the claim that rights are prima facie or that they are not strictly correlative to obligations.

The Primacy of Rights

The correlativity thesis does not determine whether rights or obligations, if either, is the more fundamental or primary category in moral theory. The proposal made by some philosophers that moral theory should be "rights-based"[44] springs from a particular conception of the function and justification of morality.

If the function of morality is to protect individuals' interests (rather than communal interests), and if rights (rather than obligations) are our primary instruments to this end, then moral action guides seem to be fundamentally rights based. Rights, on this account, precede obligations.

A theory we encountered in Chapter 7 illustrates this position: the libertarian theory of justice. One representative, Robert Nozick, maintains that "Individuals have rights, and there are things no person or group may do to them [without violating their rights]."[45] He takes the following rule to be basic in the moral life: All persons have a right to be left free to do as they choose. The obligation not to interfere with this right follows from the right itself. That it "follows" indicates the priority of a rule of right over a rule of obligation. That is, an obligation is derived from a right.

Alan Gewirth has proposed another rights-based argument that recognizes *positive* or *benefit* rights:

> Rights are to obligations as benefits are to burdens. For rights are justified claims to certain benefits, the support of certain interests of the subject or right-holder. Obligations, on the other hand, are justified burdens on the part of the respondent or duty-bearer; they restrict his freedom by requiring that he conduct himself in ways that directly benefit not himself but rather the right-holder. But burdens are for the sake of benefits, and not vice versa. Hence obligations, which are burdens, are for the sake of rights, whose objects are benefits. Rights, then, are prior to obligations in the order of justifying purpose...in that respondents have correlative obligations *because* subjects have certain rights.[46]

These rights-based accounts accept *correlativity* of rights and obligations, but they also accept a *priority* thesis that obligations follow from rights, rather than the converse. Rights form the justificatory basis of obligations, they maintain, because they best capture the purpose of morality, which is to secure liberties or other benefits for a rights-holder.

A Critical Evaluation of Rights Theory and Liberal Individualism

Problems with rights-based theories. One problem with basing ethics on rights is that rights are only a piece of a more general account that identifies what makes a claim valid. Justification of the system of rules within which valid claiming occurs does not itself seem to be rights-based. (See Chapters 1, 10, pp. 381–87, 392–96.) Pure rights-based accounts run the risk of truncating or impoverishing our understanding of morality, because rights cannot account for the moral significance of motives, supererogatory actions, virtues, and the like. Such a limited theory would fare poorly under the criteria of comprehensiveness and explanatory and justificatory power proposed at the beginning of this chapter. Accordingly, we should not force a rights-based theory into the model of a comprehensive or complete moral theory. This type of theory is best understood as a statement of minimal and enforceable rules that communities and individuals must observe in their treatment of all persons.

Normative questions about the exercise of rights. Often the question is not whether someone has a right, but whether rights-holders should or should not *exercise* their rights. If a person says, "I know you have the right to do X, but you should not do it," this moral claim goes beyond a statement of a right. One's obligation or character, not one's right, is in question.

The neglect of communal goods. Liberal individualists sometimes write as if social morality's major concern is to protect individual rights against government intrusion. This vision is too limited, because it excludes not only group interests, but also communal values, such as public health, biomedical research, and the protection of animals. The better perspective is that social ideals and principles of obligation are as critical to social morality as are rights, and that none is dispensable.

A Constructive Evaluation of Liberal Individualism

In recent ethical theory, some writers have sought to eliminate the language of rights. They suggest either that rights language can be replaced by another vocabulary (e.g., obligations or virtues) or that the assertion of valid individual claims against society has risky implications. We reject such views, and we accept both the correlativity thesis and the moral and social purposes served by traditional interpretations of basic human rights, in their positive as well as their negative forms.[47]

No part of the moral vocabulary has done more to protect the legitimate interests of citizens in political states than the language of rights. Predictably, injustice and inhumane treatment occur most frequently in states that fail to recognize human rights in their political rhetoric and documents, as well as their actions. As much as any part of moral discourse, rights language crosses international boundaries and enters into treaties, international law, and statements by international agencies and associations. Rights thereby become acknowledged as international standards for the treatment of persons. The language of "human rights" has understandably come, in much of today's moral discourse, to refer to individual entitlements that political states, military forces, and the global order must observe. It is appropriate that these entitlements have become the substantive basis of cross-cultural moral evaluation as well as international law.

Being a rights-bearer in a society that enforces rights is both a source of personal protection and a source of dignity and self-respect. By contrast, to maintain that someone has an *obligation* to protect another's interest may leave the beneficiary in a passive position, dependent on the other's good will in fulfilling the obligation. When persons possess enforceable rights correlative to obligations, they are enabled to be independent agents, pursuing their projects and making legitimate claims. What we often cherish most is not that someone is obligated to us, but that we have a right that secures for us the opportunity to pursue and claim as our own the benefit or liberty that we value.

COMMUNITARIANISM

Several approaches in contemporary philosophy and political theory have little sympathy with rights theory in the form of liberal individualism. In these theories, communal values, the common good, social goals, traditional practices, and cooperative virtues are fundamental in ethics. Communitarianism is such a theory. Conventions, traditions, loyalties, and the social nature of life and institutions figure more prominently in communitarianism than in the types of theory discussed to this point.

In the case of the potential kidney transplantation discussed in introducing the previous three theories, communitarians ask not which rights are at stake, but whether communal values and relationships are recognized. They focus on the family as a small community intermediate between the individual and the state. They ask which acts, rules, and policies (e.g., those governing organ donation, privacy, and confidentiality) best express, reinforce, and promote communal values, including family values.

Communitarian critics of the father's behavior, which reduces his daughter's chances of survival, would maintain that he is insufficiently committed to the good of the family and that he asserts the values of liberal individualism (in standing on his rights) without adequately attending to his responsibilities. The father contends that if the physician tells other members of the family the true reasons for his decision not to donate, it would wreck the family. The father's prediction about this negative impact may or may not be correct, but what his actions express about his own lack of commitment to the family's welfare is notable. Communitarians might also view the physician as focused unduly on protecting rights of the father, such as autonomy and privacy. From the communitarian perspective, the physician would be expected to consider whether his actions conform to traditions of medicine, with its communal goods, codes, and virtues. These traditions have often defended the use of deception in treating patients, but in this case the father asks the physician to deceive *others,* a relatively rare request and one with less clear historical precedent in medical practice. Nondisclosure to others because of confidentiality does have clear historical precedent in medicine, but rules of confidentiality are not absolute and have often been justifiably overridden by the interests of others. (See our discussion of veracity and confidentiality in Chapter 8.)

The Repudiation of Liberalism

Unfortunately, no systematic and classic account of communitarianism exists that rivals the systematic theories in Mill, Kant, and philosophers of rights such as Locke and Hobbes. Contemporary communitarianism is usually analyzed in terms of a few key themes that emerge from a few leading writers. The most prominent themes are the influence of society on individuals and the roots of values in communal history, traditions, and practices, as well as the value of community.

Contemporary communitarians repudiate central tenets in what is often called *liberalism,* a term that is defined through premises in all three of the types of theory discussed in the three previous sections: utilitarian, Kantian, and rights theories (especially liberal individualism). What cements them jointly as "liberal" is their commitment to what Mill defended as *individuality,* what Kant called *autonomy,* and what liberal individualists protect as *rights.* Each type of theory protects the individual against the state, and, according to the communitarian interpretation, each also asserts that the state should neither reward nor penalize different conceptions of the good life held by individuals. Postulates of individual autonomy, rights against the state, and community neutrality toward conflicting values, then, are the central liberal tenets that communitarians oppose. [48]

Contemporary communitarians both repudiate liberal theory and question societies established on liberal premises. According to communitarians, these societies lack a commitment to the general welfare, to common purposes, and to education in citizenship, while expecting and even encouraging social and geographic mobility, distanced personal relations, welfare dependence, breakdowns in family life and marital fidelity, political fragmentation, and the like. The number of abandoned children and elderly parents, social and familial disintegration, and the lack of effective communal programs are, according to communitarians, the disastrous products of liberalism.

The meaning of *community* and its synonyms varies in these theories. Some communitarians refer to the political state as the community, whereas others refer to smaller communities and institutions with defined goals and role obligations. Some include the family as a basic communal unit, within which being a parent and being a child involve specific roles and responsibilities. Much of what a person ought to do in communitarian theories is determined by the social roles assigned to or acquired by this person as a member of the community. Understanding a particular system of moral rules requires understanding the community's history, sense of cooperative life, and conception of social welfare.

Communitarian criticisms of liberal theories center on ideas that liberalism (1) fails to appreciate the constructive role of the cooperative virtues and the political state in promoting values and creating the conditions of the good life, (2) fails to acknowledge shared goals and obligations that come not from freely made contracts among individuals, but from communal ideals and responsibilities, and (3) fails to understand the human person as historically constituted by and embedded in communal life and social roles.[49]

Every major communitarian thinker has contested the thesis of the priority of individual rights over the common good. Charles Taylor's challenge is perhaps the most straightforward, even though Taylor does not seem to entirely repudiate liberalism, the liberal state, or autonomy rights. He argues that all conceptions of the rights of individuals already contain within their fabric some conception of the individual and social good. The liberal's claim of the priority of right is itself, from this perspective, premised on a conception of the human good (e.g., the good of autonomous moral agency). Furthermore, Taylor argues, the type of autonomy suggested by individualism cannot be developed in the absence of the family and other community structures. Liberalism's emphasis on individual rights therefore needs to make provision for the development and maintenance of the necessary communities. It is a mistake to view individuals as isolated atoms existing independently of one another.[50]

Communitarianism can be distinguished into *militant* and *moderate* forms. Militants firmly support community control and reject liberal theories, whereas moderates emphasize the importance of various forms of community—including the family and the political state—while attempting to accommodate strands in liberal theories. Militant communitarianism sees liberalism as antagonistic to all tradition and as opposed to rights and rights language. These communitarians aim to perpetuate and even impose on individuals conceptions of virtue and the good life that limit the rights conferred by liberal societies. Militant communitarians see persons as intrinsically *constituted* by communal values and as best suited to achieve personal goods through communal life.[51] The moderate communitarian takes a stance far less opposed to autonomy and individual rights.

The Primacy of Social Practices

Alasdair MacIntyre and other communitarians have traced to Aristotle the thesis that local community practices and their corresponding virtues have a moral priority. MacIntyre uses "practice" to designate a cooperative arrangement in pursuit of goods that are internal to a structured communal life. Social roles of parenting, teaching, governing, healing, and the like involve practices. "Goods internal to a practice" are achievable, according to MacIntyre, only by engaging in the practice and conforming to its constraints and standards of excellence. In the practice of medicine, for example, goods internal to the profession exist, and these determine what it means to be a good physician. The virtues of physicians flow from communal and institutional practices of care, practical wisdom, and education. Medicine, like other professions and political institutions, has a history that sustains a tradition requiring participants in the practice to cultivate certain virtues.[52]

As an example of communitarians' promotion of the common good in biomedical ethics, consider their debate with liberal individualists over policies of obtaining cadaveric organs for transplantation. Based on principles of individual rights, all states in the United States adopted the Uniform Anatomical Gift Act in the late 1960s and early 1970s. This act gives individuals the right to donate their organs after death and to express their decisions through a donor card or other gift documents. If the individual has not made a decision prior to death, the law authorizes the family to decide whether to donate the decedent's organs. Opinion polls had suggested that many individuals would sign donor cards and provide a sufficient supply of organs, thereby avoiding the need to search for living donors as in the case we have been investigating of the five-year-old girl needing a kidney transplant.

In practice, however, few individuals sign donor cards, the cards are rarely available at the time of death, and procurement teams routinely seek authorization from the family, even if the decedent left a valid donor card. As a result, a communitarian focus has emerged.[53] The family has become the primary donor (i.e., the decision maker about donation) rather than the individual, and because the supply of organs has remained severely limited, various policies have been considered and some adopted that aim to promote the common good more vigorously. Even approaches that protect individual rights attempt to educate people about the need for organs, and some writers propose *requiring* people to make a decision about donation—for instance, when obtaining a driver's license. Laws and regulations also require hospitals to ask families whether they know the wishes of the decedent and want to donate the decedent's organs.

Some communitarians now recommend still stronger laws and policies to make organ procurement a community project rather than a matter of individual or even family decisions. Some communitarians defend so-called *presumed consent* laws, which have been adopted in several European countries. These laws presume that individuals are willing to donate if they have not registered a dissent. They operate with an assumption of individuals' dispositional authority over organs after death, but the absence of dissent is interpreted as tacit consent. Such a policy of organ procurement would be difficult to adopt in the United States, and it might prove counterproductive. Many individuals would opt out because of distrust of the system, which would block familial donation and decrease the overall supply of transplantable organs.

An even stronger communitarian policy would involve the *routine salvaging* of organs in the absence of registered objections. Arguments for such a policy stress either the individual's obligation to donate to help others or the society's ownership of cadaveric organs. Some communitarians argue for such a policy on grounds that members of a community should be willing to provide others objects of lifesaving value when they can do so at no cost to themselves.[54] Others recommend policies of routine salvaging that assume communal, rather than individual or familial ownership of cadaveric body parts (even if they would also allow for conscientious refusals). Routine organ salvaging, especially if based on communal ownership of cadaveric organs, conflicts so deeply with individualistic values and rights that it has not received, and is not likely soon to receive, sympathetic consideration in the United States.[55]

An emphasis on the community and the common good also appears in issues about the allocation of health care, as we observed in Chapter 7. According to Daniel Callahan's communitarian account, we should enact public policy from a shared consensus about the good society rather than on the basis of individual rights. We should relax liberal assumptions about government neutrality, and society should be free to implement a substantive concept of the good. Biomedical ethics should use communitarian values to implement or revise social laws and regulations governing the promotion of health, the use of genetic knowledge, the use of advances in medical technology, responsibilities to future generations, and the limits of health care for the elderly. In each case, Callahan would have us ask, "What is most conducive to a good society?" rather than simply, "Is it harmful, or does it violate autonomy?"[56]

A Critical Evaluation of Communitarian Ethics

Several claims made by militant communitarians rely on questionable accusations and arguments, and we now concentrate on problems in these theories.

An unfair account of liberal theories. Militant communitarians suggest that liberal theorists defend atomistic, isolated individuals and leave a trail of skepticism about communal goods. This characterization is unwarranted. Mill and Rawls, the figures most frequently attacked by communitarians, never depict either individuals or the communal good in these terms, and both philosophers develop a theory of the common good, as well as an account of social traditions and political community.[57] Mill thought he had captured how historical traditions converge to the principle of utility, which he construed as a principle of communal welfare. Liberty functions in his arguments to protect individuals against mistakes in planning communal pursuits of the good, and he defends individuality *because* it conduces to a constantly readjusted and improved community. Similarly, Rawls defends rights and liberties, in part, because an open society can correct and revise social ends better than a society controlled by tradition.[58]

A false dichotomy: Community or autonomy. Communitarians present us with misleading dichotomies: (1) either liberal accounts of rights and justice have priority or the communal good has priority,[59] and (2) either we protect autonomy in public decision making or we protect communal decision making in setting social goals. A more accurate picture is available: We inherit social roles and goals. We then critique, adjust, and attempt to improve our beliefs over time through discussion and collective arrangements. Individuals and groups alike progressively interpret, revise, and sometimes even replace traditions with new conceptions that adjust for and foster community values. This liberal outlook is, as Joel Feinberg has argued, entirely compatible with communal interests: "It is impossible to think of human beings except as part of ongoing communities, defined by reciprocal bonds of obligation, common traditions, and institutions.... The ideal [in liberal accounts] of the autonomous person is that of an authentic individual whose self-determination is as complete as is consistent with the requirement that he is, of course, a member of a community."[60]

A failed challenge to rights. Communitarians sometimes argue against rights on grounds that rights function to give individuals too much power, thereby stalling communal organization and activities and dulling our sense of social union. This claim misses the value of rights for communities. We value rights because, when enforced, they provide protections against unscrupulous behavior, promote orderly change and cohesiveness in communities, and allow diverse communities to coexist peacefully within a single political state.[61] Rights are necessary both to enable individuals to live safely and to protect them from oppressive communities. Even if we grant communitarian arguments that the best life is communal life, it would not follow that communities should determine the individual's goals or truncate individual rights. The major reason for giving prominence to rights in moral and political theory is that they stand as a shield against communal intrusion and control.

A Constructive Evaluation of Communitarianism

By emphasizing historical traditions and institutional practices, communitarian theories have redirected ethical theory in recent years and have helped us rediscover the importance of community, even if we accept liberal values. For instance, communitarians rightly emphasize the need to foster neighborhood associations, create communal ties, promote public health, and develop national goals.

CONVERGENCE OF THEORIES

Whenever several competing theories, systems, or general depictions of some phenomenon are available, we tend to seek out the best account and affirm it. However, affiliation with a single type of ethical theory is precarious in general ethics as well as biomedical ethics. If the two authors of this book were forced to rank the types of theory examined in this chapter, we would differ. However, for both of us, the most satisfactory theory—if we could find only *one* to be most satisfactory—would be only slightly preferable, and no theory would fully satisfy all relevant criteria.

It would exaggerate differences among types of theory if they were presented as warring armies locked in combat. Many and perhaps most theories lead to similar action guides and to similar virtues. This is less true of act-based theories (e.g., act utilitarianism), but it is generally true of theories committed to rules. These theories defend roughly the same principles, obligations, rights, responsibilities, and the like. For example, although rule utilitarianism often appears both starkly different from and hostile to nonconsequentialist theories, utilitarian Richard Brandt rightly notes that his theory is similar, at the level of principle and obligation, to W. D. Ross's deontological theory (which is itself sharply critical of utilitarianism):

> [The best code] would contain rules giving directions for recurrent situations which involve conflicts of human interests. Presumably, then, it would contain rules rather similar to W. D. Ross's list of prima facie obligations: rules about the keeping of promises and contracts, rules about debts of gratitude such as we may owe to our parents, and, of course, rules about not injuring other persons and about promoting the welfare of others where this does not work a comparable hardship on us.[62]

That Brandt appeals to utility and Ross to intuitive induction to justify similar sets of rules is a significant difference at the level of moral justification, and the two authors might interpret, specify, and balance their rules differently. Yet, their lists of primary obligations display only trivial differences. This convergence is not restricted to Brandt and Ross. Most of the theories this chapter addresses accept similar general principles or values, including respect for autonomy, nonmaleficence, and the like. Such agreement springs from an initial shared database, namely, the norms of the common morality. We can say without undue paradox that the proponents of these theories all accept these principles of common morality before they devise their theory, and that when they attend to practical problems they often rely as much on the principles they share with others as on their own unique theory.

Convergence as well as consensus about principles among a group of persons is common in assessing *cases* and framing *policies,* even when deep theoretical differences divide the group. Agreement may similarly emerge about precedent cases. In the real world of practical judgments and public policies, we often need no more agreement than an agreement of principle—not an agreement regarding the foundation of the principle. At the same time, we should not confuse convergence to principles with whether or not a theory adequately justifies its principles. Theoretical inquiry is appropriate even if practical agreement has been achieved.

Reasons exist, then, for holding that moral theory is an important enterprise, but that distinctions among types of theory are not as significant for *practical* ethics as some seem to think. It is a mistake to suppose that a series of continental divides separates moral theorists into distinct and hostile groups who reach different practical conclusions and fail to converge on principles. Many theories are closer in substantive principles and rules to allegedly rival theories than they are to some theories of their own "type."

CONCLUSION

Contemporary biomedical ethics reflects theoretical differences of considerable complexity, and the diverse theories explored in this chapter help us see why. Competition exists among the various normative theories, and competing conceptions exist about how such theories relate to biomedical practice. Nonetheless, we stand to learn from all of these theories. Where one theory is weak in accounting for some part of the moral life, another is strong. Although every general theory clashes at some point with our considered moral convictions, each articulates some point of view that we should be reluctant to relinquish. This approach to theories allows us to focus on acceptable features in theories without having to choose one theory to the exclusion of the others.

NOTES

1. We do not examine a theory, or perspective, that we included as a section in this chapter in the fifth edition: "Ethics of Care: Relationship-Based Accounts." In this edition, we have modified that material and placed it as a section on the ethics of care in Chapter 2.

2. Our views on pluralism are influenced by Thomas Nagel, "The Fragmentation of Value," in *Mortal Questions* (Cambridge: Cambridge University Press, 1979), pp. 128–37; and Baruch Brody's treatment in *Life and Death Decision Making* (New York: Oxford University Press, 1988), p. 9.

3. Our discussion has profited from Shelly Kagan, *The Limits of Morality* (Oxford: Clarendon, 1989), esp. pp. 11 15, and from criticisms of our views privately presented by David DeGrazia and Avi Craimer.

4. For analysis of this utilitarian thesis, see Samuel Scheffler, *Consequentialism and Its Critics* (Oxford: Clarendon, 1988).

5. Jeremy Bentham, *An Introduction to the Principles of Morals and Legislation,* ed. J. H. Burns and H. L. A. Hart (Oxford: Clarendon, 1970), pp. 11–14, 31, 34. John Stuart Mill, *Utilitarianism,* in vol. 10 of the *Collected Works of John Stuart Mill* (Toronto: University of Toronto Press, 1969), chap. 1, p. 207; chap. 2, pp. 210, 214; chap. 4, pp. 234–35.

6. See a representative theory in James Griffin, *Well-Being: Its Meaning, Measurement and Moral Importance* (Oxford: Clarendon, 1986), especially p. 67.

7. This case is based on Melvin D. Levine, Lee Scott, and William J. Curran, "Ethics Rounds in a Children's Medical Center: Evaluation of a Hospital-Based Program for Continuing Education in Medical Ethics," *Pediatrics* 60 (August 1977): 205.

8. Among writers in bioethics, Joseph Fletcher and Peter Singer are examples of act utilitarians, and R. M. Hare is (at what he calls level 2) an example of a rule utilitarian. See Joseph Fletcher, *Humanhood: Essays in Biomedical Ethics* (Buffalo, NY: Prometheus Books, 1979); Peter Singer, *Practical Ethics,* 2nd ed. (Cambridge: Cambridge University Press, 1993); R. M. Hare, *Essays on Bioethics* (Oxford: Oxford University Press, 1993); and Hare, "A Utilitarian Approach to Ethics," in *A Companion to Bioethics,* ed. Helga Kuhse and Peter Singer (Oxford: Blackwell, 1998), pp. 80–85. For a full rule-utilitarian view, see Brad Hooker, *Ideal Code, Real World: A Rule-Consequentialist Theory of Morality* (Oxford: Oxford University Press, 2000).

9. Worthington Hooker, *Physician and Patient* (New York: Baker & Scribner, 1849), pp. 357ff, 375–81.

10. J. J. C. Smart, *An Outline of a System of Utilitarian Ethics* (Melbourne: University Press, 1961); and "Extreme and Restricted Utilitarianism," in *Contemporary Utilitarianism,* ed. Michael Bayles (Garden City, NY: Doubleday, 1968), esp. pp. 104–07, 113–15.

11. Richard B. Brandt, "Toward a Credible Form of Utilitarianism," in *Contemporary Utilitarianism,* ed. Bayles, pp. 143–86, and in Brandt's *Morality, Utilitarianism, and Rights* (Cambridge: Cambridge University Press, 1992). For a rule-utilitarian alternative to Brandt's rule-utilitarian formulation, see Hooker, *Ideal World, Real World.*

12. This question is discussed in Madison Powers, "Repugnant Desires and the Two-Tier Conception of Utility," *Utilitas* 6 (1994): 171–76.

13. Alan Donagan, "Is There a Credible Form of Utilitarianism?" in *Contemporary Utilitarianism,* ed. Bayles, pp. 187–202.

14. Williams, "A Critique of Utilitarianism," in *Utilitarianism: For and Against,* J. J. C. Smart and Bernard Williams (Cambridge: Cambridge University Press, 1973), pp. 116–17; and J. L. Mackie, *Ethics: Inventing Right and Wrong* (New York: Penguin, 1977), pp. 129, 133. For an extension, see Edward Harcourt, "Integrity, Practical Deliberation and Utilitarianism," *Philosophical Quarterly* 48 (1998): 189–98; for critical commentary, see Alastair Norcross, "Consequentialism and Commitment," *Pacific Philosophical Quarterly* 78 (1997): 380–403. Recent efforts to develop consequentialist theories that reduce or eliminate the "demandingness" problem include Tim Mulgan, *The Demands of Consequentialism* (Oxford: Clarendon, 2005), which offers a "moderately demanding" theory of mixed consequentialism.

15. For a defense of utilitarianism (set against egalitarianism) in forming just policies toward people with disabilities, see Mark S. Stein, *Distributive Justice and Disability: Utilitarianism against Egalitarianism* (New Haven, CT: Yale University Press, 2006).

16. Milton Weinstein and William B. Stason, *Hypertension* (Cambridge, MA: Harvard University Press, 1977); "Public Health Rounds at the Harvard School of Public Health: Allocating of Resources to Manage Hypertension," *New England Journal of Medicine* 296 (1977): 732–39; and "Allocation Resources: The Case of Hypertension," *Hastings Center Report* 7 (October 1977): 24–29.

17. Jane Morley et al., "Hypertension Control and Access to Medical Care in the Inner City," *American Journal of Public Health* 88 (November 1998): 1696–99; Steven Shea et al., "Correlates of Nonadherence to Hypertension Treatment in an Inner-City Minority Population," *American Journal of Public Health* 82 (December 1992): 1607–12.

18. Amartya Sen, *On Ethics and Economics* (Oxford: Basil Blackwell, 1987), p. 75.

19. See Stephen Darwall, ed., *Deontology* (Oxford: Blackwell, 2002), for a representative collection of classic and recent works.

20. See, for example, the writings of F. M. Kamm, including *Intricate Ethics: Rights, Responsibilities, and Permissible Harm* (New York: Oxford University Press, 2007).

21. Kant sought to show that unaided reason can and should be a proper motive to action. What we should do morally is determined by what we would do "if reason completely determined the will." *The Critique of Practical Reason,* trans. Lewis White Beck (New York: Macmillan, 1985), pp. 18–19. Ak. 20. "Ak." designates the page-reference system of the 22-volume Preussische Akademie edition conventionally cited in Kant scholarship.

22. Kant, *Foundations of the Metaphysics of Morals,* trans. Lewis White Beck (Indianapolis, IN: Bobbs-Merrill, 1959), pp. 37–42; Ak. 421–24.

23. There are competitive interpretations of Kant's idea of contradiction in conception. See Christine Korsgaard, "Kant's Formula of Universal Law," *Pacific Philosophical Quarterly* 66 (1985): 24–47; "Kant's Formula of Humanity," *Kant-Studien* 77 (1986): 183–202, both reprinted with other essays in her *Creating the Kingdom of Ends* (Cambridge: Cambridge University Press, 1996); and Barbara Herman, *The Practice of Moral Judgment* (Cambridge, MA: Harvard University Press, 1993), pp. 132–58.

24. *Foundations,* p. 47; Ak. 429.

25. *Foundations,* pp. 51, 58–63; Ak. 432, 439–44.

26. *Foundations,* p. 58; Ak. 439–40.

27. Alan Donagan, *The Theory of Morality* (Chicago: University of Chicago Press, 1977), pp. 63–66.

28. See *A Theory of Justice* (Cambridge, MA: Harvard University Press, 1971; rev. ed., 1999), pp. 3–4, 27–31 (1999: pp. 3–4, 24–28). For an approach to Kant influenced by Rawls, see Thomas Hill, Jr., *Human Welfare and Moral Worth: Kantian Perspectives* (Oxford: Clarendon, 2002).

29. Rawls, *A Theory of Justice,* pp. 252, 256, 515–20 (1999: pp. 221–22, 226–27, 452–56). See also "A Kantian Conception of Equality," *Cambridge Review* (February 1975): 97ff.

30. See, for example, Thomas Nagel, "Personal Rights and Public Space," *Philosophy and Public Affairs* 24 (1995): 83–107, and his *The View from Nowhere* (New York: Oxford University Press, 1986); Bernard Williams, *Ethics and the Limits of Philosophy* (Cambridge, MA: Harvard University Press, 1985), and his *Moral Luck: Philosophical Papers, 1973–1980* (Cambridge: Cambridge University Press, 1981).

31. Onora O'Neill, *Toward Justice and Virtue: A Constructive Account of Practical Reasoning* (Cambridge: Cambridge University Press, 1996), pp. 5–6. See also *Constructions of Reason: Explorations of Kant's Practical Philosophy* (Cambridge: Cambridge University Press, 1989). Her important work in bioethics includes *Autonomy and Trust in Bioethics* (Cambridge: Cambridge University Press, 2002) and, with Neil C. Manson, *Rethinking Informed Consent in Bioethics* (Cambridge: Cambridge University Press, 2007).

32. For innovative interpretations that respond to such an objection by giving more flexibility to Kant, see Barbara Herman, *The Practice of Moral Judgment,* pp. 132–58; Nancy Sherman, *Making a Necessity of Virtue* (Cambridge: Cambridge University Press, 1997); and Tamar Schapiro, "Kantian Rigorism and Mitigating Circumstances," *Ethics* 117 (2006): 32–57. These writings supply responses to forms of the third objection we mention in this section, especially regarding the place of virtue in Kant's theory.

33. Cf. Annette Baier, "The Need for More than Justice," in her *Moral Prejudices* (Cambridge, MA: Harvard University Press, 1994).

34. We are indebted to the analysis in Karen Stohr, "Virtue Ethics and Kant's Cold-Hearted Benefactor," *Journal of Value Inquiry* 36 (2002): 187–204.

35. Compare H. L. A. Hart, "Bentham on Legal Rights," in *Oxford Essays in Jurisprudence,* 2nd series, ed. A. W. B. Simpson (Oxford: Oxford University Press, 1973), pp. 171–98.

36. Cf. Joel Feinberg, *Social Philosophy* (Englewood Cliffs, NJ: Prentice Hall, 1973), p. 67.

37. H. L. A. Hart, "Between Utility and Rights," in *Jurisprudence and Philosophy* (Oxford: Clarendon, 1983), p. 198. For debates about liberalism, see Nancy L. Rosenblum, ed. *Liberalism and the Moral Life* (Cambridge, MA: Harvard University Press, 1989).

38. Ronald Dworkin, *Taking Rights Seriously* (Cambridge, MA: Harvard University Press, 1977), p. xi; and *Law's Empire* (Cambridge, MA: Harvard University Press, 1986), p. 223.

39. Ronald Dworkin, *Taking Rights Seriously*, pp. xi, 92, 191, and "Is There a Right to Pornography?" *Oxford Journal of Legal Studies* 1 (1981): 177–212.

40. See Judith Jarvis Thomson, *The Realm of Rights* (Cambridge, MA: Harvard University Press, 1990), pp. 122ff.

41. See Feinberg, *Social Philosophy*, p. 59; and Eric Mack, ed., *Positive and Negative Duties* (New Orleans, LA: Tulane University Press, 1985).

42. See David Braybrooke, "The Firm but Untidy Correlativity of Rights and Obligations," *Canadian Journal of Philosophy* 1 (1972): 351–63; and Carl P. Wellman, *Real Rights* (New York: Oxford University Press, 1995).

43. See Hart, "Between Utility and Rights."

44. Ronald Dworkin argues that political morality is rights based in *Taking Rights Seriously*, pp. 169–77, esp. p. 171. John Mackie has applied this thesis to morality generally in "Can There Be a Right-Based Moral Theory?," *Midwest Studies in Philosophy* 3 (1978), esp. p. 350. For a view that the ancients had a theory of rights in place, but not a theory of the primacy of rights, see Myles Burnyeat, "Did the Ancient Greeks Have the Concept of Human Rights?" *Polis* 13 (1994): 1–11.

45. Robert Nozick, *Anarchy, State, and Utopia* (New York: Basic Books, 1974), pp. ix, 149–82. See also Jan Narveson, *The Libertarian Idea* (Philadelphia, PA: Temple University Press, 1988) and *Respecting Persons in Theory and Practice* (Lanham, MD: Rowman & Littlefield, 2002).

46. Alan Gewirth, "Why Rights Are Indispensable," *Mind* 95 (1986): 333. See Gewirth's later book, *The Community of Rights* (Chicago: University of Chicago Press, 1996); and a partial challenge to his theses that connects the theory to positive and negative rights in Jan Narveson, "Alan Gewirth's Foundationalism and the Well-Being State," *Journal of Value Inquiry* 31 (1997): 485–502.

47. For discussions of bioethical issues in the framework of human rights, see Lawrence O. Gostin and Zita Lazzarini, *Human Rights and Public Health in the AIDS Pandemic* (New York: Oxford University Press, 1997); and George J. Annas, *American Bioethics: Crossing Human Rights and Health Law Boundaries* (New York: Oxford University Press, 2004).

48. See Daniel Callahan, "Individual Good and Common Good: A Communitarian Approach to Bioethics," *Perspectives in Biology and Medicine* 46 (2003): 496–507, esp. 500ff; Callahan, "Principlism and Communitarianism," *Journal of Medical Ethics* 29 (2003): 287–91; Michael Sandel, *Democracy's Discontent: America in Search of a Public Philosophy* (Cambridge, MA: Harvard University Press, 1996); Sandel, *Public Philosophy: Essays on Morality in Politics* (Cambridge, MA: Harvard University Press, 2005); Alasdair MacIntyre, *After Virtue,* 3rd ed. (Notre Dame, IN: University of Notre Dame Press, 2007); and Michael Walzer, "The Communitarian Critique of Liberalism," *Political Theory* 18 (1990): 6–23.

49. Sandel, "Introduction," in *Liberalism and Its Critics,* ed. Sandel (New York: New York University Press, 1984), p. 6, and "Morality and the Liberal Ideal," *The New Republic* (May 7, 1984): 15–17; MacIntyre, *After Virtue,* chap. 1. For a balanced assessment of these theses, see Alisa L. Carse, "The Liberal Individual: A Metaphysical or Moral Embarrassment?" *Nous* 28 (1994): 184–209.

50. Charles Taylor, "Atomism," in *Powers, Possessions, and Freedom*, ed. Alkis Kontos (Toronto: University of Toronto Press, 1979): 39–62.

51. Sandel, *Liberalism and the Limits of Justice*, pp. 15–23, 84–87, 92–94, 139–51; Alasdair MacIntyre, *Whose Justice? Which Rationality?* (Notre Dame, IN: University of Notre Dame Press, 1988), p. 10.

52. MacIntyre, *After Virtue*.

53. Some states have now passed laws that give clear priority to the decedent's previously articulated wish to donate over the family's objection, thereby restoring the individualistic orientation.

54. See James L. Nelson, "The Rights and Responsibilities of Potential Organ Donors: A Communitarian Approach," *Communitarian Position Paper* (Washington, DC: The Communitarian Network, 1992); James Muyskens, "Procurement and Allocation Policies," *The Mount Sinai Journal of Medicine* 56 (1989): 202–06.

55. See James F. Childress and Catharyn T. Liverman, eds., *Organ Donation: Opportunities for Action*, A report of an Institute of Medicine Committee on Increasing Rates of Organ Donation (Washington, DC: National Academies Press, 2006), esp. chap. 7, "Presumed Consent." For the range of issues and positions in organ procurement, see James F. Childress, *Practical Reasoning in Bioethics* (Bloomington and Indianapolis, IN: Indiana University Press, 1997), chaps. 14–16.

56. Callahan, *What Kind of Life* (New York: Simon & Schuster, 1990), chap. 4, esp. pp. 105–13, and *Setting Limits* (New York: Simon & Schuster, 1987), esp. pp. 106–14.

57. See arguments to this conclusion in Will Kymlicka, "Communitarianism, Liberalism, and Superliberalism," *Critical Review* 8 (1994): 263–84; "Liberalism and Communitarianism," *Canadian Journal of Philosophy* 18 (June 1988): 181–204; and "Liberal Individualism and Liberal Neutrality," *Ethics* 99 (July 1989): 883–905. Even John Locke and Thomas Hobbes—the communitarians' arch-enemies—emphasize promoting the commonweal. Locke gives an elegant statement in *Two Treatises of Civil Government, Works* (London: C. and J. Rivington, 1824), 12th ed., bk. 2, note 8, p. 357.

58. See Amy Gutmann, "Communitarian Critics of Liberalism," *Philosophy and Public Affairs* 14 (Summer 1985): 308–22; Andrew Jason Cohen, "A Defense of Strong Voluntarism," *American Philosophical Quarterly* 35 (1998): 251–65.

59. Sandel interprets Rawls as creating this dilemma by his account of the alleged priority of the right over the good. See *Liberalism and the Limits of Justice*, pp. 1–10, 17–24, 168–72, and "Morality and the Liberal Ideal," pp. 16–17.

60. Joel Feinberg, *Harm to Self*, vol. 3 in *The Moral Limits of the Criminal Law* (New York: Oxford University Press, 1986), p. 47.

61. See William R. Lund, "Politics, Virtue, and the Right to Do Wrong: Assessing the Communitarian Critique of Rights," *Journal of Social Philosophy* 28 (1997): 101–22; Allen Buchanan, "Assessing the Communitarian Critique of Liberalism," *Ethics* 99 (July 1989): 852–82, esp. 862–65; and William A. Galston, *Liberal Purposes* (Cambridge: Cambridge University Press, 1991).

62. Brandt, "Toward a Credible Form of Utilitarianism," p. 166.

10
Method and
Moral Justification

Wide agreement exists that we can teach, practice, and do research in biomedical ethics, but little agreement exists about the methods for achieving these goals. Related disagreement exists about how to justify moral conclusions. In this chapter we step back from the first-order problems of normative ethics that have preoccupied us to this point and reflect on second-order problems of whether there is method and justification in bioethics, and, if so, which methods and forms of justification are preferable.

Questions about method are intimately connected to questions about justification. The first three major sections of this chapter explicate three models of method and justification and evaluate the arguments of several critics of our methods and principles. Later in the chapter, we connect our (second-order) account of method and justification to the (first-order) common-morality theory introduced in Chapter 1 and also to the account of moral character developed in Chapter 2.

JUSTIFICATION IN ETHICS

What is justification in ethics, and by what method(s) of reasoning do we achieve it?

Justification has several meanings, some specific to disciplines. In law, for example, justification is a demonstration in court that one has a sufficient reason and evidence for one's claim or for what one has been called to answer. In ethical discourse, the objective is to establish one's case by presenting sufficient reasons for it. A mere listing of reasons will not suffice, because those reasons may not adequately support the conclusion. Not all reasons are good reasons, and not all good reasons are sufficient for justification. We therefore need to distinguish a reason's *relevance* to a moral judgment from its *sufficiency* to support that judgment, and we need to distinguish an *attempted* justification from a *successful* justification. For example, chemical companies in the United States at one time took the presence of toxic chemicals in a work environment to provide a legally and morally sound reason to exclude women of childbearing age from a hazardous workplace, but the U.S. Supreme Court overturned these policies on grounds that they discriminate against women.[1] The dangers to health and life presented by hazardous chemicals constitute a *good* reason for protecting employees from a workplace, but this reason is not a *sufficient* reason for a ban that impacts women alone.

Several models of method and justification operate in ethical theory and contemporary biomedical ethics. We analyze and evaluate three influential models. The first model approaches justification and method from a top-down perspective that emphasizes moral norms (as discussed in Chapter 1) and ethical theory (as discussed in Chapter 9). The second approaches justification and method from a bottom-up perspective that emphasizes precedent cases in moral tradition, experience, and particular circumstances. The third refuses to assign priority to either a top-down or a bottom-up strategy. We adopt a version of the third.

Top-Down Models: Theory and Application

A top-down model holds that we reach justified moral judgments through a structure of normative precepts that cover the judgments. This model is inspired by disciplines such as mathematics, in which a claim follows logically (deductively) from a credible set of premises. The idea is that justification occurs if and only if general principles and rules, together with the relevant facts of a situation, support an inference to the correct or justified judgment(s). This model is simple and conforms to the way many people have been raised to learn to think morally: Its method involves applying a general norm (principle, rule, ideal, right, etc.) to a clear case falling under the norms. The deductive form is sometimes considered an "application" of general precepts, a conception that motivated use of the term *applied ethics*.

The following is the deductive form involved in "applying" a norm (here using what is *obligatory,* rather than what is *permitted* or *prohibited,* although the deductive model is the same for all three):

1. Every act of description A is obligatory.
2. Act b is of description A.
    Therefore,
3. Act b is obligatory.

A simple example is:

1x. Every act in a patient's overall best interest is obligatory for the patient's doctor.

2x. Act of resuscitation b is in this patient's overall best interest. Therefore,

3x. Act of resuscitation b is obligatory for this patient's doctor.

Covering precepts, such as 1 and 1x, occur at various levels of generality, and they are always universal in their logical form. The level of generality varies according to the specificity of the description A, while the statement's universality is ensured by the claim that "every act" of such a description is obligatory. We may justify a particular judgment, belief, or hypothesis by bringing it under the scope of one or more moral rules; or justify the rules by bringing them under general principles; or defend both rules and principles by appeal to a full ethical theory. Consider the example of a nurse who refuses to assist in an abortion procedure. The nurse might attempt to justify the act of refusal by the rule that it is wrong to kill an innocent human being intentionally. If pressed further, the nurse may justify this moral rule by reference to a principle of the sanctity of human life. Finally, the particular judgment, rule, and principle might all find support in an ethical theory (as such theory is discussed in Chapters 1 and 9) and in a theory of moral status (as discussed in Chapter 3) that is only implicit and inchoate in the nurse's original judgment.

This deductivist model functions smoothly in the simple case of a judgment brought directly and unambiguously under a rule or a principle. Consider the following justification: "You must tell Mr. Sanford that he has cancer and will probably die soon, because a clinician must observe rules of truthfulness to properly respect the autonomy of patients." The top-down model suggests that the judgment, "You should not lie to Mr. Sanford," descends in its moral content directly from the covering principle, "You should respect autonomy," from which we derive and justify the covering rule, "You should not lie to patients."

Problems in the Model

This model is overrated if presented as the only correct account of moral thinking and method in ethics. It suggests an ordering in which theories, principles, and rules enjoy priority over traditional practices, institutional rules, and case judgments. Although much in the moral life conforms roughly to this conception, much does not. Particular moral judgments in hard cases almost always require that we specify and balance norms (see Chapter 1), not merely that we bring a particular instance under a preexisting covering rule or principle. The abstract rules and principles in moral theories are extensively indeterminate. That is, the content of these rules and principles is too abstract to determine the acts that we should perform. In the process of specifying and balancing norms and in making particular judgments, we often must take into account factual beliefs about the world, cultural expectations, judgments of likely outcome, and precedents to help assign relative weights to rules, principles, and theories.

The moral life often requires even more than *specified* general norms. A situation may be such that no general norm (principle or rule) clearly applies. The facts of cases are usually complex, and the different moral norms that can be brought to bear on the facts may yield inconclusive, or even contradictory, results. For example, in the controversy over whether it is permissible to destroy a human embryo for purposes of scientific research, embryo destruction does not clearly violate rules against killing or murder, nor does the rule that a person has a right to protect his or her bodily integrity and property clearly apply to the destruction of human embryos. Even if we have all of the facts straight, our selection of pertinent facts and pertinent rules will generate a judgment that may be incompatible with another person's selection of facts and rules. Selecting the right set of facts and bringing the right set of rules to bear on these facts are not reducible to a deductive form of judgment. Therefore, general ethical theory, absent the necessary specification, is inadequate by itself to address such cases.

The top-down model also creates a potentially infinite regress of justification—a never-ending demand for final justification—because each level of appeal to a covering precept requires some further general level to justify that precept. Theoretically, we could handle this problem by presenting a principle that is self-justifying or one that it is irrational not to hold, but proof that some principles occupy this status and that they justify all other principles or rules is an arduous demand that current ethical theory cannot meet. Yet, if all standards are unjustified until brought under a justified covering precept, it would appear, on the assumptions of this approach, that there are no justified principles or judgments.

Finally, the appeal to theory in the covering-precept model suggests that only one normative theory has a sufficiently attractive defense to warrant its use. Yet many distinct theories have attractive defenses (as we saw in Chapter 9). There is no authoritative or even dominant theory. As a practical matter, in the absence of general agreement about the adequacy of theories, we cannot rely on any given theory as an adequate basis for moral justification.

Impartial-Rule Theory

One important version of top-down theory in general philosophy and in biomedical ethics (although not a pure deductivism) has been developed over the last four decades by Bernard Gert and his coauthors H. Danner Clouser and Charles Culver. When challenges arose to our framework of principles in the late 1980s, these authors emerged as our most unsparing critics. Clouser and Gert wrote several articles and part of a book to express concerns about prima facie principles. They coined the label "principlism" to refer to all accounts of ethics comprised of a plurality of potentially conflicting prima facie principles. They directed their criticism primarily at our framework of four principles and offered, as a substitute, a framework centered on less abstract rules. This impartial-rule theory, as we will call it, allegedly provides an alternative body of general norms and framework of decision making in biomedical ethics.[2]

Clouser and Gert bring several accusations against our proposed use of principles.[3] First, they charge that principles function like names, checklists, or headings for values worth remembering, but lack deep moral substance and capacity to guide action. That is, principles point to moral themes that merit consideration by grouping those themes under broad headings, but do little more. A second and related criticism is that, because moral agents confronted with bioethical problems receive no specific, directive guidance from principles, they are left free to deal with the problems in their own way. They may give a principle whatever weight they wish, or even no weight at all. From this perspective, our account is insubstantial and permissive, in part because it lacks a controlling theory. A third criticism is that the prima facie principles (and other action guides in our framework) often conflict, and our account is too indeterminate to provide a decision procedure to adjudicate the conflicts.

Clouser and Gert are particularly fond of pointing to these deficiencies in the principles of justice discussed in Chapter 7 of this book. There is, they say, no specific guide to action that derives from these principles. All principles of justice mentioned in this chapter instruct persons to attend to matters of justice and think about justice, but they give no specific normative guidance. Because such vagueness and generality underdetermine solutions to problems of justice, agents are free to decide what is just and unjust as they see fit.

Gert and Clouser also criticize principlism for giving status to *both* nonmaleficence *and* beneficence as principles of obligation. They maintain that there are no moral rules of beneficence (although they agree that we should encourage *moral ideals* of beneficence). The only obligations in the moral life, apart from duties encountered in professional roles and other specific stations of duty, are captured by moral rules that prohibit causing harm or evil. For Gert and colleagues, the general goal of morality is to minimize evil or harm, not to promote good (a basic thesis that they judge obvious, but do little to justify). Rational persons can act impartially at all times in regard to all persons with the aim of not causing evil, they say, but rational persons cannot impartially promote the good for all persons at all times.[4]

The Limitations of Impartial-Rule Theory

We agree that the problems Gert, Clouser, and Culver present deserve sustained reflection. We reject, however, their requirement that there be "a single, clear, coherent, and comprehensive decision procedure for arriving at answers."[5] We are skeptical of this enterprise, even as a model for ethical theory, for reasons we have presented in Chapters 1 and 9.

Moreover, we believe that the very same criticisms they direct at our account affect their impartial-rule theory. In particular, their criticism that our principles lack directive moral substance (being unspecified principles) applies to their rules in a near-identical way, one level down in the order of abstraction. Any norm, principle, or rule will have this problem if it is underspecified for the task at hand. A basic norm of any sort is intrinsically general, designed to cover a broad range of circumstances.[6] If general rules are not specified in biomedical ethics, they are almost always too general and will fail to provide adequate normative guidance. Clouser and Gert's rules (e.g., "Don't cheat," "Don't deceive," and "Do your duty") are comparable to our principles in just this way: They lack specificity in their original general form. One tier less abstract than principles, their rules constitute a first level of *specified* principles, which explains why their rules do, we agree, have a more directive and specific content than our abstract principles. Our full account of principles and rules, however, already includes a set of rules that is effectively identical to the rules embraced by Gert and his colleagues.[7]

Regarding their criticism that our principles are checklists or headings without deep moral substance, we agree that principles order, classify, and group moral norms that require additional content and specificity. However, until we analyze and interpret the principles (as we do in every first section of Chapters 4–7) and then specify and connect them to other norms (as we do in later sections of each of these chapters), it is unreasonable to expect much more than a classification scheme that organizes the normative content and provides very general moral guidance.[8]

Regarding the criticism that principles compete with other principles in ways that our account cannot handle, we acknowledge that moral frameworks of principles do not themselves resolve conflicts among principles and derivative rules. No framework of guidelines could reasonably anticipate the full range of conflicts, but the impartial-rule system does no more to settle this problem than our framework does. It does not follow that our principles are inconsistent or that we encounter incompatible moral commitments in embracing them. A strength of our theory is that it calls for and indeed demands balancing and specification, and a problem in Clouser and Gert's account is that it supposes that its "more concrete" rules escape the need for specification. Only a theory that could put enough content in its norms to escape conflicts and dilemmas in all contexts could live up to the Clouser–Gert demand. No theory approximates this ideal.[9]

Experience and sound judgment are indispensable allies in resolving these problems. No one has attained or ever will attain a fully specified system of norms for health care ethics. Thomas Nagel has forcefully argued that an unconnected heap of obligations and values is an ineradicable feature of morality, and W. D. Ross has rightly argued that many philosophers have forced an "architectonic" of unwarranted "simplicity" on ethics.[10] Whereas some critics of Ross's account (and ours) rely on an ideal of systematic unity—at least in moral theory—we regard disunity, conflict, and moral ambiguity as pervasive features of the moral life that are unlikely to be eradicated by a moral theory. Moral theory offers methods such as specification, balancing, and reflective equilibrium to help us deal with these problems, but theories will not eliminate all untidiness, complexity, and conflict.

Regarding the criticism that our principle-based analysis fails to provide a general ethical theory, the criticism is correct, but off target. We do not attempt to construct a general ethical theory and do not claim that our principles mimic, are analogous to, or substitute for the foundational principles in leading classical theories, such as utilitarianism (with its principle of utility) and Kantianism (with its categorical imperative). We expressed a constrained skepticism about this type of foundationalism in Chapter 9. We doubt that such a unified foundation for ethics, beyond explication of the common morality, is possible without distortion of the moral life.[11]

In response to the criticism that the principle of beneficence expresses an ideal, not a moral obligation, we believe that this thesis is incorrect. The claim by Gert et al. implies that one is never morally required (except by role and professional duties) to prevent or remove harm or evil, but only to avoid causing harm or evil. They recognize no requirement to *do* anything, only to *avoid* causing harmful events.[12] We believe that their thesis deeply misreads the commitments of the common morality. The claim that beneficence is never morally required is not even supported within Gert and Clouser's own account of moral obligations. In his book, *Morality: A New Justification of the Moral Rules,* Gert relies on the premise that one is morally obligated to act beneficently under many conditions. He interprets one of his basic rules, "Do your duty," to incorporate many obligations of beneficence. Gert explains his system and its commitments as follows:

> Although duties, in general, go with offices, jobs, roles, etc., there are some duties that seem more general....A person has a duty...because of some special circumstances, for example, his job or his relationships....In any civilized society, if a child collapses in your arms, you have a duty to seek help. You cannot simply lay him out on the ground and walk away. In most civilized societies one has a duty to help when (1) one is in physical proximity to someone in need of help to avoid a serious evil, usually death or serious injury, (2) one is in a unique or close to unique position to provide that help, and (3) it would be relatively cost-free for one to provide that help.[13]

Although Gert maintains that all such requirements are supported by the moral rule "Do your duty," they often appear to be effectively identical to the obligations that follow from what we call beneficence (and we here follow established traditions in ethical theory since the eighteenth century). It therefore cannot be the case that Gert's system lacks obligations of beneficence in our sense of the term, although his theory might be reconstructed to mean only that there is no *general principle* of beneficence, only specific duties of beneficence.[14] To generalize, much in principlism that Clouser and Gert appear to reject is presupposed by Gert's final rule, "Do your duty." It is therefore hard to see how their impartial rule theory provides an alternative to our substantive claims regarding the nature and scope of obligations and the importance of specification.

A reason for preferring our theory to theirs is that some substantive requirements of the common morality can be better expressed in the language of principles than in the language of rules. Consider respect for autonomy, which Gert and his colleagues find as problematic as the principles of justice and beneficence. Their disregard of this principle renders their assessments of some cases convoluted and puzzling. Here is such a case: Following a serious accident, a patient, while still conscious, refuses a blood transfusion on religious grounds; he then falls unconscious, and his physicians believe that he will die unless he receives a transfusion. Gert and Culver argue that the provision of a blood transfusion under these circumstances is paternalistic and wrong because, after the patient regains consciousness following the transfusion, the physicians would violate either the moral rule against deception or the moral rule against causing pain: If they did not tell the patient about the transfusion, they would violate the rule against deception; if they did tell him, they would cause him pain.[15]

Gert and Culver's inattention to the principle of respect for autonomy produces this misleading analysis. They lack the normative resources to argue that the transfusion, in this case, is paternalistic and prima facie wrong because it violates the patient's expressed wishes and choices. Paradoxically, their analysis implies that if the patient had died after the transfusion without regaining consciousness, the physicians would not have acted wrongly because they would have violated no moral rules. Gert's moral rule "Do not deprive of freedom" was originally construed to prohibit blocking a person's opportunities to take action. To address the problems that arise from the blood transfusion case, and similar cases, Gert and his colleagues later came to interpret this moral rule to include the "freedom from being acted upon."[16] This expanded interpretation is reasonable, but their rule, so interpreted, now approximates the principle of respect for autonomy.

BOTTOM-UP MODELS: CASES AND ANALOGY

Many writers in biomedical ethics concentrate on practical decision making rather than on principles or theories. They believe that moral justification proceeds bottom up (inductively) by contrast to top down (deductively). Inductivists, as we call them, argue that we reason from particular instances to general statements or positions. They hold that we use existing social practices, insight-producing novel cases, and comparative case analysis as the starting points from which to make decisions in particular cases and to generalize to norms. Inductivists emphasize an evolving moral life that reflects experience with difficult cases, analogy from prior practice, and exemplary lives and narratives. From this perspective, "inductivism" and "bottom-up models" are broad categories that contain several methodologies that are wary of top-down theories. Pragmatism,[17] particularism,[18] and narrative approaches,[19] as well as some forms of feminism and virtue theory, qualify as such accounts.

Inductivists propose that cases and particular judgments provide warrants to accept moral conclusions independently of general norms. They usually see rules and principles as derivative in the order of knowledge, not primary. That is, the meaning, function, and weight of a principle derive from previous moral struggles and reflection in particular circumstances. For example, physicians once regarded withdrawing life-saving medical technologies from patients as an act of impermissible killing. Progressively, after confronting agonizing cases, they and society came to frame many of these acts as forms of permissible allowing to die and even as morally required acts of acknowledging refusals of treatment. Finally, all specific moral norms arise and are refined over time; they never become more than provisionally secure points in a cultural matrix of guidelines. A society's moral views find their warrant through an embedded moral tradition and a set of procedures that permit and foster new insights and judgments.

Consider an example from the explosion of interest since 1976 in surrogate decision making. A series of cases beginning with the *Quinlan* case challenged medical ethics and the courts to develop a new framework of substantive rules for responsible surrogate decision making about life-sustaining treatments, as well as authority rules regarding who should make those decisions. This framework was created by working through cases analogically, and testing new hypotheses against preexisting norms. Subsequent cases were addressed, in part, by appealing to similarities and dissimilarities to *Quinlan* and related cases. A string of cases with some similar features established the terms of the ethics of surrogate decision making. Even if a rule was not entirely novel in a proposed framework, its content was shaped by problems needing resolution in the cases at hand. Gradually, as we discussed in Chapters 4 and 5, a consensus emerged in the courts and in ethics about a framework for such decision making.

Casuistry: Case-Based Reasoning

Casuistry, an influential version of bottom-up thinking, has revived a model that enjoyed an impressive influence in medieval and early modern philosophy and has refashioned it for modern biomedical ethics.[20] The term *casuistry* refers to the use of case comparison and analogy to reach moral conclusions.[21] Albert Jonsen and Stephen Toulmin, who spearheaded this approach in biomedical ethics, have also criticized our framework of principles.[22]

Casuists are skeptical of rules, rights, and general theories that are divorced from cases, history, precedents, and circumstances. Appropriate moral judgments occur, they say, through an intimate acquaintance with particular situations and the historical record of similar cases. Casuists dispute, in particular, the goal of a tidy, unified theory containing general and universal principles.[23] Although a foundational and absolute principle is conceivable, casuists maintain that moral beliefs and reasoning, in fact, do not assume or stand in need of such a principle.

Casuists do not entirely exclude rules and principles from moral thinking, but they insist that moral judgments often are made when no appeal to principles is possible. For example, we make moral judgments when principles, rules, or rights conflict and no further recourse to a higher principle, rule, or right is available. When principles are interpreted inflexibly, irrespective of the nuances of the case, some casuists see a "tyranny of principles"[24] in which attempts to resolve moral problems suffer from a gridlock of conflicting principles, and moral debate becomes intemperate and interminable. This impasse can often be avoided, Jonsen and Toulmin argue, by focusing on points of shared agreement about cases rather than on principles. The following is their prime example, drawn from their experiences during four years of work with the National Commission for the Protection of Human Subjects of Biomedical and Behavioral Research:

> The one thing [individual commissioners] could not agree on was *why* they agreed.... Instead of securely established universal principles,... giving them intellectual grounding for particular judgments about specific kinds of cases, it was the other way around.
>
> The *locus of certitude* in the commissioners' discussions... lay in a shared perception of what was specifically at stake in particular kinds of human situations.... That could never have been derived from the supposed theoretical certainty of the principles to which individual commissioners appealed in their personal accounts.[25]

Jonsen and Toulmin maintain that casuistical reasoning, not universal principles, forged agreement. That is, the commission functioned successfully by appeal to paradigms and families of cases, despite the diverse principles and theoretical perspectives held by individual commissioners. Although commissioners did often cite moral principles to justify their collective conclusions—and did unanimously endorse the Belmont principles late in the commission's existence[26]—Jonsen and Toulmin argue that these principles were less certain and less central than particular judgments about cases.[27]

A simple example illustrates their claim that moral certitude resides in case judgments rather than in principles or theory: We know (in most cases) that it is morally wrong to introduce significant risks to children in biomedical research. We are sure of the statement, "We should not give this healthy baby the flu in order to test a new decongestant," but we may be unsure which principle controls this judgment or whether some viable theory sanctions the judgment. The casuist holds that we are almost always more certain about particular moral conclusions than we are about *why* they are correct. In this respect, practical knowledge takes priority over theoretical knowledge. Moreover, if a principle or a theory were to instruct us to give the flu to children in order to test drugs (as some versions of utilitarianism might), this outcome would provide us with a good reason for rejecting the principle or theory. Moral certitude, then, is found at the bottom—in the cases and traditions of practical judgment—not at the top in a principle or theoretical judgment.

Casuists decide about new cases by comparing them to paradigmatically right and wrong actions and to similar and acceptable cases (as well as similar and unacceptable cases). Thus, precedent cases and analogical reasoning are paramount in this method. For example, if a new case involves a problem of medical confidentiality, casuists consider analogous cases in which breaches of confidentiality were justified or unjustified to see whether such a breach is justified in the new case. So-called "paradigm cases" become the most enduring and authoritative sources of appeal. For example, the current literature of biomedical ethics constantly invokes cases, such as the *Quinlan* case, the Tuskegee syphilis experiments, the *Cowart* case, and the *Quill* case, not only to illustrate claims, but also to serve as sources of authority for new judgments. Decisions reached about moral rights and wrongs in seminal cases become authoritative for new cases, and they profoundly affect prevailing standards of fairness, negligence, paternalism, and the like.[28]

A similar method appears in case law through the doctrine of precedent. When an appellate court decides a particular case, its judgment is positioned to become authoritative for other courts hearing cases with *similar* facts. Casuists see moral authority similarly: Ethics develops from a social consensus formed around cases. This consensus is then extended to new cases by analogy to the past cases around which the consensus was formed. As similar cases and similar conclusions evolve, a society becomes increasingly confident in its moral conclusions and acknowledges secure generalizations (principles, rules, and the like) in its evolving tradition of ethical reflection. These generalizations are summary statements of a society's developed moral insights about cases.

The Limits of Casuistry

Casuists sometimes overstate the power of their account and understate the value of competing accounts, but a balanced assessment of the role of cases in moral reasoning should remedy these defects.

First, casuists sometimes write as if paradigm cases speak for themselves or inform moral judgment by their facts alone. Clearly they do not. For the casuist to move constructively from case to case, some recognized and morally relevant norm must connect the cases. The norm is not part of the case, but rather a way of interpreting and linking cases. All analogical reasoning requires a connecting norm to indicate that one sequence of events is like or unlike another sequence in relevant respects. The creation or discovery of these norms cannot be achieved merely by analogy. We cannot simply appeal to the fact that one case is similar to another to reach a moral conclusion. We must show that the two cases are similar in and not dissimilar in morally relevant respects. It is not enough to know that certain features of a case are morally significant. We must know *how* they are significant. Such cross-case evaluation seems to require general principles or rules.

Jonsen seems to address this problem by distinguishing descriptive elements in a case from moral maxims that are embedded in the case: "These maxims provide the 'morals' of the story. For most cases of interest, there are several morals, because several maxims seem to conflict. The work of casuistry is to determine *which maxim* should *rule the case* and to what extent."[29] We accept this thesis, which conforms to our views about prima facie principles and rules, as well as analogy. So understood, casuistry presupposes principles, rules, or maxims as essential moral elements *in the case.*

The casuists' "paradigm cases" thus combine both *facts* that can be generalized to other cases (e.g., "The patient refused the recommended treatment") and *settled values* that are generalized (e.g., "Competent patients have a right to refuse treatment"). These settled values are analytically distinct from the facts of particular cases. In casuistical appeals, values and facts are bound together—mutually embedded—and the central values are preserved from one case to the next. The more general the central values or connecting norms, the closer they come to the status of prima facie principles.

Just as other philosophers have a problem with conflicting principles (ostensibly a reason to favor casuistry), so casuists have a problem with conflicting analogies, judgments, and case interpretations. Casuists stress that cases point beyond themselves and evolve into generalizations, but they also may evolve in the wrong way if improperly resolved from the outset. Casuists have no clear methodological resource to prevent a biased development of case-based judgments or an ignoring of morally relevant features of cases. There can be a "tyranny" of the paradigm case just as there can be a tyranny of rigid principles.

These problems lead to questions about the justificatory power of casuistry. How does the *justification* of a moral judgment or choice of a paradigm case occur? The casuists' answer seems to rest on social convention and analogy. However, different analogies and novel cases still might generate competing "right" answers on any given occasion. Without a stable framework of norms, we lack both control on judgment and ways to prevent prejudiced or poorly formulated social conventions.

This criticism is a variant of a much discussed problem about casuistry: Because casuistry works only bottom up, it lacks critical distance from cultural blindness, rash analogy, and tyrannical popular opinion.[30] How is the casuist to identify unjust practices, predisposing bias, and prejudicial use of analogy to avoid one-sided judgments? In casuistry, identification of the morally relevant features of a particular case depends on those who make judgments about cases, and these individuals may operate from very partial perspectives. In this respect, the ethics of casuistry contrasts sharply with a stable system of impartial principles and human rights (although, even in the case of these impartial norms, there are problems of partial perspectives entering in specification and balancing). Even if we are confident that morally mature cultures usually have built-in resources for critical distancing and self-evaluation, these resources do not seem to emerge from the methods of casuistry.

The root of this problem is that casuistry is a method that fails to provide content. It is a vital tool of thought that displays the fundamental importance of case comparison and analogy in moral thinking, but it lacks initial moral premises. It also lacks any substantive ground of "certitude," as Jonsen and Toulmin put it. It is true that we reason by analogy every day, and we are often confident in the conclusions we reach. For example, if we feel better after using a certain medicine, then we feel comfortable in recommending it to other persons, in the expectation that they too will feel better. A logical form is present in all uses of analogy: If some person or thing has one property associated with a second property, and another person or thing also has the first property, we may feel justified in inferring that the second person or thing also has the second property. However, such analogies also often fail: Our friends may not feel better after they take our favored medicine. Analogies never warrant a claim of truth, and we often do not know something by analogy that we think we know. The method of casuistry leaves us with this problem: No matter how many properties one case and another share, our inference to yet another property in the second case may mislead or produce false statements.

These are not reasons for rejecting the casuistical method any more than for rejecting the use of analogy. Both are helpful as long as we have a solid knowledge base that allows us to use them. However, to obtain that knowledge, the casuistical method must be supplemented by norms of moral relevance that incorporate prior judgments of right and wrong conduct.[31] We return to this problem of a proper knowledge base when we come to the subject of "considered judgments" later in this chapter (see pp. 382–87).

Casuists seem to confuse the fact that we often have no need for a general theory in practical ethics (a view with which we have considerable sympathy) with the lack of a need for practical *principles* and their specification. They also conflate certitude about principles with certitude about theory. We believe the general public and the mainstream of moral philosophy have found a "locus of certitude" in universal moral principles, although not in any particular moral theory. We agree that in practical deliberation we often have more certitude about particular cases and conclusions than we do about moral theories, but principles that form the cement of the common morality also enjoy a high level of certitude.

In a later methodological statement, Jonsen describes connections between principles and casuistry:

> Principles, such as respect, beneficence, veracity, and so forth, are invoked necessarily and spontaneously in any serious moral discourse.... Moral terms and arguments are imbedded in every case, usually in the form of maxims or enthymemes. The more general principles are never far from these maxims and enthymemes and are often explicitly invoked. Thus, casuistry is not an alternative to principles, in the sense that one might be able to perform good casuistry without principles. In another sense, casuistry is an alternative to principles: they are alternative scholarly activities.[32]

We agree that the two are complementary, but it is unclear that *alternative* scholarly activities are at work. Prima facie principles of the sort we accept are not vulnerable to the casuists' critique and are not excluded by their methodology. The movement from principles to specified rules is similar to Jonsen's account of casuistical method, which involves tailoring maxims to fit a case through progressive interactions with other relevant cases. Casuists and principlists should be able to agree that when they reflect on cases and policies, they rarely, if ever, have in hand principles that were formulated without reference to experience with cases, or paradigm cases that have no embedded commitment to general norms.

AN INTEGRATED MODEL USING REFLECTIVE EQUILIBRIUM

Accounts from "the top" (principles, rules) and "the bottom" (cases, individual intuitions) both need supplementation. Neither general principles nor paradigm cases without principles can guide the formation of justified moral beliefs. Principles need to be made specific for cases, and case analysis needs illumination from general principles. Some general rules lack an adequate justification without support from more specific considered judgments. There is no fixed order of inference or dependence from general to particular or from particular to general.

Instead of a top-down or bottom-up model, we support a version of a third model, referred to as "reflective equilibrium" (and sometimes as "coherence theory"). John Rawls coined the term *reflective equilibrium* to refer to his

influential statement of this method.[33] He views justification as a reflective testing of our moral beliefs, moral principles, theoretical postulates, and the like to
make them as coherent as possible. Method in ethics properly begins with our
"considered judgments," which are the moral convictions in which we have the
highest confidence and believe to have the least bias. The term *considered judgments* refers to "judgments in which our moral capacities are most likely to be
displayed without distortion." Examples are judgments about the wrongness of
racial discrimination, religious intolerance, and political repression. "Without
distortion" refers to more than correct judgments, which would run the risk
of circular argument. It refers to the conditions under which the judgments
are formed. These considered judgments occur at all levels of generality in
moral thinking, "from those about particular situations and institutions through
broad standards and first principles to formal and abstract conditions on moral
conceptions."[34] Whenever some feature in a moral theory that we hold conflicts
with one or more of our considered judgments (a contingent conflict), we must
modify one or the other to achieve equilibrium.

Even the considered judgments that we accept as landmark fixed points are,
Rawls argues, subject to revision. The goal of reflective equilibrium is to match,
prune, and adjust considered judgments and their specifications to render them
coherent with the premises of our most general moral commitments. We start
with considered judgments of moral rightness and wrongness, and then construct
both a more general and a more specific account that is consistent with these
judgments, rendering the whole as coherent as possible. We then test the resultant guides to action to see if they yield incoherent results. If so, we must go
back and readjust the guides further.

We can never assume a completely stable equilibrium in our moral beliefs.
The pruning and adjusting of beliefs occur continually in light of the goal of
reflective equilibrium. To refer again to the rule "put the patient's interests first,"
we seek in biomedical ethics to make this rule as coherent as possible with other
considered judgments about responsibilities in clinical teaching, to subjects in
the conduct of research, to patients' families, to sponsors of clinical trials, and so
forth. It is a demanding requirement to bring such diverse moral commitments
into coherence and then to test the results against all other moral commitments.
Even the basic rule "put the patient's interests first" is not absolute when we
consider all possible cases. It is an acceptable starting premise—a considered
judgment—but not acceptable as a final conclusion. We are left with a range of
options about how to specify this rule and check it against other norms. Some
problems of reflective equilibrium will always remain because new contingent
conflicts can always arise.

To take an example from the ethics of organ transplantation, imagine
that an institution is attracted to each of two policies: (1) distribute organs by
expected number of years of survival (to maximize the beneficial outcome of

the procedure), and (2) distribute organs by using a waiting list (to give every candidate an equal opportunity). As they stand, these two distributive principles are inconsistent. We can retain both in a defensible theory of fair distribution, but to do so we have to introduce limits on these principles that would render them consistent. We have to explain how to specify and balance our various commitments. These limits and accounts, in turn, have to be made coherent with other principles and rules, such as norms regarding discrimination against the elderly and the role of ability to pay in the allocation of expensive medical procedures. (See our discussion of this subject in Chapter 7.)

All general moral beliefs are indeterminate for some range of cases and require that we eliminate contingent conflicts among the beliefs. Any specification aimed at eliminating a conflict is justified only if there is a maximal coherence of the overall set of relevant beliefs. These beliefs could include empirical beliefs, basic moral beliefs, and previous specifications. This is a version of so-called wide reflective equilibrium.[35] Equilibrium occurs after one evaluates the strengths and weaknesses of all plausible moral judgments, principles, and relevant background theories, incorporating as wide a variety of kinds and levels of legitimate beliefs as possible. To be included are beliefs about particular cases, about rules and principles, about virtue and character, about consequentialist and nonconsequentialist forms of justification, about the moral status of fetuses and experimental animals, about the role of moral sentiments, and so forth.

We emphasize again that there is no reason to expect that the process of revising moral judgments and specifying and balancing principles will come to an end in a perfect equilibrium. The state of reflective equilibrium is an idealization that can never be comprehensively realized, but it is not a utopian vision toward which we cannot make progress. Particular moralities are, from this perspective, continuous works in progress rather than finished products. Moral projects such as developing the most suitable system for organ procurement and distribution are projects frequently in need of adjustment by reflective equilibrium. Virtually any set of theoretical generalizations achieved by this method will fall short of the ideal. We should assume that we face a never-ending search for coherence, for counterexamples to our beliefs, and for novel situations that challenge our moral framework.[36]

Consider, as an example of the threat of incoherence in the search for reflective equilibrium, our support (in Chapter 5, pp. 172–85) of physician-assisted death at a patient's request. In this same chapter we take seriously the slippery-slope arguments in opposition to physician-assisted death. David DeGrazia has greeted with skeptical disbelief our assertion that these two points of view can be rendered consistent. He views our position as a "compromise [that] apparently leads to contradiction."[37] To see how the two views are consistent, we need to return to the distinction that we introduced in Chapter 1 between the justification of *policies* and the justification of *acts*. Public rules or laws sometimes justifiably prohibit conduct that is morally justified in individual cases. Two moral questions about physician-assisted hastening of death need to be distinguished: (1) Are physicians ever morally justified in complying with first-party requests that they assist patients in *acts* of hastened death? (2) Is there an adequate moral basis to justify the *legalization* of physician-assisted hastening of death? We argue in Chapter 5 that there are morally justified *acts* of assisting patients in hastening their deaths, but that once public considerations and consequences external to the private relationship between a physician and a patient are the issue—such as the implications of legalized physician-assisted hastening of death for medical education and medical practice in hospitals and nursing homes—these external considerations may (but also may not) provide good and sufficient moral reasons for prohibiting physicians from engaging in such actions as a matter of public law. We argue that some policies that legalize physician assistance would, under some circumstances, be morally unacceptable. There is no inconsistency in this position on physician-assisted hastening of death.

From the perspective of reflective equilibrium, moral thinking is analogous to the process of evaluating scientific statements such as hypotheses. Science is neither strictly inductivist (involving only observation and experimentation), nor strictly deductivist (using mathematics and a priori premises). Scientists make mutual adjustments among large-scale, abstract theories, specific hypotheses, and concrete experiments to reach the most coherent viewpoint. Justification in ethics is no more deductivist (giving general norms preeminent status) than inductivist (giving experience and analogy preeminent status). Different considerations provide reciprocal support in the attempt to fit moral beliefs into a coherent account. Many particular moralities are reasonably coherent ways to specify the common morality. Normatively, we can demand no more than that agents faithfully specify their considered judgments with an attentive eye to overall coherence. However, proponents of particular moralities can and should continue to ask whether the system is more or less coherent when compared to other particular moralities.

Although justification is a matter of reflective equilibrium in this model, bare coherence never provides a sufficient basis for justification, because the body of substantive judgments and principles that cohere could themselves be morally unsatisfactory. Bare coherence could be nothing more than a system of prejudices, and therefore needs constraint by substantive norms. An example of this problem is the "Pirates' Creed of Ethics or Custom of the Brothers of the Coast."[38] Formed under a democratic confraternity of marauders circa 1640, this creed for pirates is a coherent set of rules governing mutual assistance in emergencies, penalties for prohibited acts, the distribution of spoils, modes of communication, compensation for injury, and "courts of honour" that resolve disputes. This body of substantive rules and principles, although coherent, is a moral outrage. Its appeal to "spoils," the awarding of slaves as compensation for injury, and the like involve immoral activities. But what justifies us in saying this coherent code is an unacceptable code of ethics?

This question points to the importance of starting with considered judgments that are the most well-established moral beliefs, which we here take to be those in the common morality. Once this group is assembled we must cast the net more broadly in interpreting, specifying, and generalizing those convictions. Certain normative views are wrong not merely because they are incoherent; incoherence is not enough. They are wrong because there is no way, when starting from "considered moral judgments" in the common morality, that one could, through reflective equilibrium, wind up with anything like the beliefs in the Pirates' Creed.

The thesis is that reflective equilibrium needs the common morality to supply *initial norms* (foundations), and appropriate *development* of the common morality requires reflective equilibrium (a method of coherence). A warranted approach using reflective equilibrium does not involve the relentless reduction to coherence of any set of beliefs whatever. We start in ethics, as elsewhere, with a particular set of beliefs—the set of considered judgments that are acceptable initially without argumentative support. We cannot justify every moral judgment in terms of another moral judgment without generating an infinite regress or vicious circle of justification in which no judgment is justified. The way to escape this regress is to accept some judgments as justified without dependence on other judgments.

These claims are usually associated with so-called foundationalist moral theories rather than coherentist theories, whereas we have often indicated the vital role of coherence through the process of reflective equilibrium. Coherence theory is generally considered antifoundationalist, whereas common-morality theory appears foundationalist. This is one reason why we do not speak of our account as *coherentism* or a *coherence theory,* but rather speak of coherence through the process of reflective equilibrium. We cannot here engage the tangled issue of whether coherentism is to be preferred to foundationalism, but it is clear that a common morality approach does not sit well with traditional understandings of the coherence theory of justification. The easiest path around this problem, and the one we take, is to accept reflective equilibrium as a basic methodology and to join this model with the common morality approach to considered judgments. In this way, coherence serves as a basic constraint on the specification and balancing of the norms that guide actions. This proposal is fundamentally Rawlsian (whatever its departures from Rawls), and it escapes categorization by labels such as foundationalism and coherentism.[39]

The considered judgments we are recommending typically have a rich history of moral experience that undergirds confidence that they are credible and trustworthy. Considered judgments therefore cannot be simple matters of individual intuition. A moral belief that is used initially and without argumentative support can only serve as an anchor of moral reflection if it survives subsequent testing. This outlook may seem to introduce an unwarranted conservative bias into the account, but this worry is not a problem because of the close connection to reflective equilibrium, which allows—indeed encourages—many sorts of development of moral belief. Almost all criticisms of social practices proceed by appeal to entrenched and well-considered moral judgments, which are extended in new ways. It is not conservative to suggest, as we did in Chapter 3, that the principle of nonmaleficence needs to be extended to give greater protection to animals in biomedical research. This extension would modify social practices, but would not modify norms of nonmaleficence.

To avoid an unduly conservative or parochial basis of belief, it is also advisable to consult a wide body of moral experience to collect points of convergence. Consider an analogy to several eyewitnesses in a courtroom. If sufficient numbers of independent witnesses converge to agreement in recounting the facts of a story, the story gains credibility beyond the credibility of any one individual who tells it. We can eliminate a bias that is detected and set aside stories that do not converge and cannot be made consistent with the main lines of testimony. The greater the coherence in a story that descends from initially credible premises and convergent testimony, the more likely we are to believe it and accept the story as right. The case is similar in moral theory. Depending on one's metaethical account, there may or may not be robust (metaphysical) *facts* corresponding to the right set of moral beliefs. However, on any plausible metaethic, there is some respect in which beliefs can be correct or incorrect. As we increase the number of accounts, establish convergence, eliminate biased observers, and increase coherence, we become increasingly confident that our beliefs are justified and should be accepted. When we find wider and wider confirmation of hypotheses about what should be believed morally, the best explanation of this confirmation is that these hypotheses are the right ones. This does not mean that we should always accept convergent moral conclusions any more than we should always accept the convergent accounts of eyewitnesses. Several factors will be at work in determining whether moral beliefs held by others actually have epistemic legitimacy.

The criteria of a good theory of authoritative beliefs in the model we are defending correspond to the criteria of good theories developed in Chapter 9. The following, then, are basic criteria of a justified set of ethical beliefs: consistency (noncontradiction), coherence with warranted nonmoral beliefs (empirical evidence, well-established scientific theories, and inference from both), comprehensiveness (covering the appropriate territory in the moral domain), absence of bias, argumentative support, and restriction of starting premises to considered judgments (those worthy of belief independent of whether they can be supported by reasons). Any theory or body of beliefs about morality is justified if it satisfies these conditions.

In conclusion, we note a few unresolved problems about the method we have supported in this chapter but that we are not able to address here.[40] First, ambiguity surrounds the precise aim of the method: We might be reflecting on communal policies, constructing a moral philosophy, or improving an individual's set of moral beliefs. The focus might be on judgments, on policies, on cases, or on finding moral truth. Second, it is not always clear how we should attempt to achieve reflective equilibrium, or how to know when we have done so. Third, justification requires that the reasons offered be publicly stated. Public justification is especially important when dealing with rules for constraints on public policy, a common task in biomedical ethics. This publicity condition is incompletely developed in the account we have provided here.[41]

COMMON-MORALITY THEORY[42]

We have argued that justification requires considered judgments, but we have yet to establish in this chapter the nature and source of these judgments. To do so, we reach back to Chapter 1, where we started to develop a theory of the common morality. This shared morality supplies the initial moral content needed in our account of justification and method, or the initial considered judgments. Our starting assumption is that no more basic moral content exists than the collection of rules and general moral judgments that are developed from the four clusters of principles presented in Chapters 4 through 7. Theoretical reflection augments this initial content by specifying the basic principles and making the various specifications as coherent as possible. In this section, we develop the idea that the common morality supplies considered judgments and connect this idea to the prior sections of this chapter.[43]

All common-morality theories share several features: First, they rely on ordinary, shared moral beliefs for their starting content; and they make no appeal to pure reason, rationality, natural law, a special moral sense, or the like. Second, all common-morality theories hold that any ethical theory that cannot be made consistent with these pretheoretical moral values falls under suspicion.[44] Third, all common-morality theories are pluralistic: Two or more nonabsolute (prima facie) principles form the general level of normative statement.[45]

Our common-morality theory does not hold that *customary* moralities qualify as part of the common morality. An important function of the general norms in the common morality is to provide a basis for the evaluation and criticism of groups or communities whose customary moral viewpoints are in some respect deficient. Criticisms of those customs and attitudes are warranted to maintain fidelity to the common morality. Our account unites the common morality with the method of reflective equilibrium delineated earlier. This strategy allows us to rely on the authority of the norms in the common morality, while incorporating tools to refine and correct unclarities and to allow for additional specification of the principles. As ethical reasoning progresses, the insights gathered along the way should form a body of more specific moral guidelines (the set of specifications of the principles). The reason why norms in particular moralities, including customary moralities, often differ is that the abstract starting points in the common morality—the considered judgments—can be developed in different ways to create practical guidelines and procedures with varying degrees of coherence.

Serious questions arise, however, about how to justify particular specifications when *competing* specifications emerge. As we maintained in Chapter 1, different resolutions by specification are often possible, and nothing in our method can ensure that only one specification or only one line of coherent specification will be justifiable. Our view, as previously hinted, is that although specifications and adjustments of moral beliefs beyond the common morality should be guided by considerations of overall coherence, such considerations will not always pick out a unique set of moral beliefs as most justified.

The Limitations of General Ethical Theories

We now consider why the common morality is better suited to play a foundational role in bioethics than the ethical theories examined in Chapter 9.

Many writers in biomedical ethics seem to think that we would rightly have more confidence in our principles and considered judgments if only we could justify them on the basis of a comprehensive ethical theory. However this outlook may have the cart pulling the donkey: We should have more confidence in an ethical theory if it could be shown coherent in a comprehensive way with the norms and considered judgments comprising the common morality. If an ethical theory were to reject any of the four clusters of principles defended in this book, for example, we would have a sound reason for healthy skepticism about the theory, not for skepticism about the principle(s). Our presentation of the principles, together with our attempts to show the consistency of these principles with other aspects of the moral life, such as moral emotions, virtues, and rights, constitutes *the normative account* in this volume. In this theory (if it is a "theory") there is no single unifying principle or concept.

Any moral theory should attempt to capture the pretheoretical moral point of view, and in this regard morality is the anchor of theory. If we could be confident that some abstract moral theory was a better source for codes and policies than the common morality, we could work constructively on practical and policy questions by progressively specifying the norms of that theory. At present, we have no such theory. Advocates of systematic theory may have aspirations of decisively settling applied questions, but they are no better positioned to do so than pluralistic accounts. Proponents of the same type of general theory commonly disagree about its commitments, how to apply it, and how to address specific issues (for which we do not fault them, given our earlier arguments that such disagreement is ineliminable). The general norms and schemes of justification found in philosophical ethical theories are invariably more contestable than the norms in the common morality. We cannot reasonably expect that an inherently contestable moral theory will be better for practical decision making and policy development than the morality that serves as our common heritage.

Nor do we need a general ethical theory to introduce moral reform. Innovation in ethics commonly occurs by interpreting, extending, and constraining norms within the common morality. For example, we have reformed our policies about bringing to market, purchasing, and distributing AIDS drugs. This reevaluation of policy required us to invoke available conceptions of compassion, fair funding, and just distribution, rather than to construct a totally new set of moral norms. "New" norms are creative extensions of old norms and creative constraints on other old norms. Rarely is a moral theory the sole source of social innovation, and when it is, it is only because the theory brings to light a new and compelling way of understanding the common morality and its implications. Rarely, if ever, does the common morality change, a problem to which we turn next.

Moral Change

Because the common morality can and should be progressively made more specific, specified moral norms are certain to be altered over time. It is simply a fact that particular moralities, customary practices, and so-called consensus moralities can and do change; they may even change by a reversal of position on some issues. For example, a code of research ethics might at one time endorse placebo-controlled trials only to reverse itself and condemn such trials at a later time. When relevant circumstances change or new insight is achieved, such revisions are warranted and to be welcomed. Change in *particular moralities* therefore occurs and can be justified and praiseworthy.

A more interesting question is whether the *common morality* changes by a process of either subtraction or addition. Is it possible *in principle* for this morality to change? Such moral change entails that what was not previously morally required (or prohibited) in the common morality is at a later time morally required (or prohibited). Could it come to be the case, morally, that we no longer have to keep our promises, that we can lie and deceive, or that a vice can become a virtue? To the extent that we can envisage circumstances in which human society is better served by substantively changing or abandoning a norm in the common morality, change in the common morality could occur and would seem to be warranted. For example, it is conceivable, however unlikely, that the rule that we are obligated to tell the truth could become so severely dangerous that we might therefore abandon the rule of truth-telling altogether. Whether unlikely or not, the possibility of such a change seems to weaken the idea of a *common* morality, unless it is part of the common morality itself that new circumstances require shifts of belief.

How could we conceivably *justify* such a profound change in basic moral belief? It either would require that one or more moral norms remain unchanged or, at least, would require that the nature of the institution of morality not change. Without some stability of this sort in the moral system, justified moral change is incomprehensible.[46]

Although it cannot be dogmatically asserted that moral norms in the common morality cannot change, it is difficult to construct even a single actual or plausible hypothetical example of a moral principle in the common morality that has been valid only for some limited duration. Nothing suggests that we do now or might in the future handle problems of profound social change by altering norms in the common morality. It is most likely that we will proceed as we always have: As circumstances change, we will find moral reasons for saying that there is a valid *exception* to a particular norm in the common morality. Of course there can be new specifications of basic obligations such as the obligation to tell the truth, which allows for exceptive cases. We have always allowed a rather clear-cut set of exceptions to the rule against killing. Particular moralities have carefully constructed exceptions in cases of war, self-defense, criminal punishment, martyrdom, misadventure, and the like. There is no reason to think that we cannot continue to handle social change through allowing exceptions to one or more stable norms in the common morality. These exceptions are made explicit through new specifications.

However, there is one important respect in which it could be said that moral change in the common morality has occurred and will continue to occur. Even if abstract *principles* do not change, the *scope* of their application does change. That is, to whom many or all of these principles are deemed to apply has changed and we may anticipate still further change. Our arguments in Chapter 3 regarding moral status anticipate this problem: "Who qualifies as belonging to the moral community?" may be the same question as, "Who qualifies for moral status?" It is possible that we might radically alter our understanding of the constituents of the moral community. For example, research animals might be incorporated into the moral community so that research involving animals comes to be conducted under the same principles and rules as research involving human subjects. It is conceivable under these conditions that we would come to the conclusion that these animals are owed equal moral consideration. This would be a momentous change in the scope of individuals covered. It may be unlikely to occur, as with other changes of this magnitude, but we can conceive of the conditions under which such change would occur.

The common morality has arguably already been refined in a conspicuously similar manner by changes in the way slaves, women, people of differing ethnicities, and persons from many groups who were once denied basic rights have come to be acknowledged as owed equal moral consideration. Such changes in the scope of the application of norms constitute major—and actual rather than hypothetical or merely conceivable—changes in moral beliefs and practices. But are the many changes in upgrading the moral status of certain classes of individuals that have taken place in recent centuries changes *in the common morality?* Changes in the way slaves, women, and people of various ethnicities are regarded seem more to be changes in either particular moralities or in ethical and political theories than in the common morality. The most defensible view, we suggest, is that the common morality does not now, and has never in fact, included a provision of equal moral consideration for all individuals or conferred moral status on all individuals. We are confident that empirical investigation of rules determining who should receive equal consideration, who should not be enslaved, and the like would reveal pervasive differences across individuals and societies, even among people who could reasonably be said to be committed to proper moral conduct.

A *theory of* the common morality will remain open to the possibility that the common morality *could* and *should* include rules of equal moral consideration for slaves, women, people of every ethnicity, the great apes, and other parties who are now excluded. This change would be a substantial change in the common morality through an increase of scope. Where we are in the common morality is not necessarily where we should be.[47] It may be possible to justify the claim that rules of equal moral consideration ought to be applied to all persons—not merely to some groups of persons—and that these rules should themselves be a part of the common morality. This change would be one of the addition of a norm—not one of norm-modification or abandonment of a norm.

We can now ask whether we can confidently assert that some societal developments of the shared common morality are more justified than others. For example, can we argue that norms against slave owning are justified by the common morality, whereas norms allowing slave owning are not? The answer is that we can, but not because the common morality has explicit standards of this sort. The justification is that the explicit commitments of the common morality to respect for autonomy, nonmaleficence, and the like contain implicit commitments to norms that prohibit slave owning. Slave owning involves violations of respect for autonomy and nonmaleficence, whether or not slave owning societies recognize this fact. Much the same conclusion can be reached regarding the causation of harm to experimental animals, although in that case the conclusion might not be a prohibition of biomedical research, but only a significant change in the thresholds of harm and safeguards against unnecessary harm.

From this perspective, the common morality reaches out and extends many kinds of moral protections, even if particular cultures have failed to recognize the implicit reach of the common morality. Social customs, including very deep ones, often blindly disregard the welfare of many individuals. This inattentiveness is not permitted by the common morality, and it would be an abuse of common morality to try to justify such practices in its name. Traditions and customs by themselves justify nothing. Justification requires that we take account of all the morally relevant features of a circumstance. Often even basic facts about individuals, such as whether they are autonomous, determine to a significant degree how we must treat them. Although it may have taken centuries to recognize and incorporate the right viewpoint in some societies, enslavement is wrong by its disrespect for autonomy, even if for no other reason. From this perspective, the common morality warrants prohibitions against slavery even if they are not explicit rules in the common morality.

Although we will not further pursue this line of argument, we mark its importance. Among the most momentous changes to occur in the history of moral practice have been changes in the scope of those persons to whom moral norms are applied. A *theory* of the common morality that deprives us of the capacity to criticize and evaluate traditions or communities whose viewpoints are morally unacceptable would be an ineffectual and unacceptable theory.

Three Types of Justification of Universal Common Morality

There are three very different ways in which one might attempt to justify claims about norms in the common morality: (1) empirical justification, (2) normative theoretical justification, and (3) conceptual justification. Each type of justification is discussed in this section. Although we do not provide an argued justification (a large project in each case), we explain each type.

Empirical justification. In Chapter 1 we indicated that the existence of the common morality can conceivably be demonstrated empirically, although many are skeptical of this possibility. Some have interpreted us as holding that "common morality theory is empirical in nature."[48] We are now positioned to explain why this is a nuanced problem and how it is possible to pursue empirical research questions about the existence of the common morality.

First, we have not claimed that the moral norms of all societies are indistinguishable. Only the most general norms are held in common. Moreover, what we now know or could know empirically and whether the propositions that we have advanced about the common morality are falsifiable by scientific investigation are not matters of straightforward empirical inquiry. It would be difficult to design empirical studies without either missing the target (namely, the beliefs of all and only those who are *committed* to morality) or begging the question. The question could be begged either by (1) designing the study so that the only persons tested are those who already have the commitments and beliefs the investigator is testing for (e.g., our four clusters of principles) or (2) designing the study so that all persons are tested whether or not they are seriously committed to moral norms and conduct. The first design risks biasing the study in favor of our hypothesis that a common morality exists. The second design risks biasing the study against our hypothesis.

This problem can in principle be overcome, however difficult in practice. We have defined the *common morality* in terms of "the set of norms shared by all persons committed to morality." Some persons are committed to morality but do not always behave in accordance with their commitments; other persons are not committed to this morality at all.[49] Because persons who are not committed to morality are not within the scope of our argument, they could not appropriately be included as subjects in an empirical study. Some might conclude that we have constructed a circular and self-justifying position. They might say that we are defining the common morality in terms of a certain moral commitment and then allowing only those who accept the norms that we have identified to qualify as persons committed to morality. We appreciate that our position risks stipulating the content of "morality." Nonetheless, we think that this risk can be avoided by careful research design. Here we can provide only a basic explanation of the research that would have to be conducted to support or to falsify our hypothesis.

First, no empirical studies known to us have shown that only some particular cultural moralities accept, whereas others reject, what we have identified as the principles and rules of obligation in the common morality. Empirical investigations of morality typically study differences in the way such rules are embedded and applied in different cultures. These studies *assume* rather than *investigate* the most general standards. They show differences in the *interpretation, specification,* and *balancing* of these standards, but they do not show that any cultures ignore or reject these standards. For example, empirical studies rarely test whether a cultural morality rejects rules against theft, promise-breaking, or killing. Rather, investigators study when theft, promise-breaking, and killing are deemed in these cultures to occur, how cultures handle exceptive cases, and the like. Empirical data show variation in what we have called particular moralities and in the specification, ranking, and balancing of the rules of the common morality, but these data do not provide evidence for or against the hypothesis of a common morality.

Second, the conclusions we reach here about the existence of a common morality—our hypothesis—can be tested empirically. An investigation would include only persons who had already been screened to assure that they are committed to a principle of morality that is reasonable to expect all morally committed persons to accept. We suggest that a reasonable principle to choose would be nonmaleficence, as it is unimaginable that any morally committed person would reject this principle. Nonmaleficence is therefore a reasonable starting point for an investigation. The group of persons to be tested would not be screened in terms of any other general norms that we claim in this book to constitute the common morality. Thus, persons not committed to the principle of nonmaleficence would be excluded from the study, and the purpose of the study would be to determine whether cultural or individual differences emerge in this group over moral norms such as respect for autonomy, beneficence, justice, and related rules such as promise-keeping.

In another research design, subjects might be tested for commitment to all four principles independently. Statistical analysis could then examine how they are correlated. One might be universal, others not. Research design could also test for other principles that might be universal.

Should it turn out that the persons studied do not share the norms that we hypothesize (in this book) to comprise the common morality, then it would have been shown that there is no common morality of the sort we claim, and our particular hypothesis would be falsified.[50] If norms other than the ones we have mentioned were demonstrated to be shared across cultures, this finding would constitute evidence of a common morality, albeit one different from the account we have proposed. Only if no moral norms were found in common across cultures would the general hypothesis that a common morality exists be rejected.

In every well-functioning society norms are in place to eliminate or reduce lying, false promises, causing bodily harm, stealing, fraud, the taking of life, the neglect of children, failures to keep contracts, and the like. A reasonable hypothesis is that these norms are what they are in societies, and not some other set of norms, because they have proven over time that their observance is essential for stability and civilized interaction.

Normative theoretical justification. Whatever is established empirically about universal norms, nothing follows about the normative justifiability of these norms. Even universal agreement does not render norms authoritative. This takes us to the problem of the normative justification of norms in the common morality.

In Chapter 9 we discussed criteria of normative theories and the approach to justification taken by four different types of theory. We showed that different theories take different approaches to the justification of moral norms. Utilitarian, Kantian, rights-based, and communitarian theories, among others, could be employed to provide a theoretical justification of the norms of the common morality. We argued that the action-guiding norms supported in these theories tend to converge to the acceptance of the norms of the common morality. We also discussed earlier in the present chapter Bernard Gert's attempt to justify the common morality in his book *Morality: A New Justification of the Moral Rules.* As Gert has shown, there is no reason why the norms in the common morality cannot be justified by a general ethical theory.

While we will not here attempt to justify moral norms by appeal to any particular general ethical theory, we do not discourage such theoretical endeavors. Indeed, we encourage them.

Conceptual justification. In Chapter 1 we briefly discussed the importance, in metaethics, of conceptual analyses of normative notions such as *right, obligation, virtue, justification, morality,* and *responsibility.* The concept of *morality* is clearly a normative moral notion. It is perhaps less clear, but still a plausible hypothesis, that the concept of morality contains normativity not only in the sense that moralilty necessarily contains *some* action guiding norms, but also in the sense of necessarily containing *specific* moral norms. These norms are privileged norms that are constitutive of morality itself. No system of belief lacking these norms would count as morality, and if someone claimed that a system of belief without those norms is a moral system, we would reject the claim as necessarily false.

From this perspective, certain norms are essential to morality; and certain particular norms that might be called "moral" (such as norms of genocide and norms that refuse to recognize human rights) are necessarily external to and excluded by the concept of morality. The norms internal to morality are the basic points of reference without which we could not get our moral bearings. As we have occasionally said of the four principles that provide the framework norms in this book, they are very general starting points that are fixed by morality. One way of understanding this claim is that these anchoring norms belong conceptually to morality.

Adequate defense of this claim would involve extensive analysis of the concept of morality. It would require an argument that morality is more than simply an institution that serves a certain social function. For example, it would not be enough to argue that morality is the social institution that functions to ameliorate or counteract the tendency for things to go badly in human relationships. Morality would also have to be more than simply taking what some philosophers have called "the moral point of view"—that is, taking a view with a certain moral attitude (such as compassion) and adopting an impartial perspective that sets aside self-interest. Morality would also have to be more than merely using the moral language of *right, responsibility,* and the like. None of these approaches necessarily requires specific moral norms.

The question, then, is whether certain norms are conceptually essential to morality whereas certain norms are excluded from morality. To illustrate the problem and to anticipate the needed argument, consider the moral vices that we mentioned in Chapters 1 and 2—vices such as malevolence, dishonesty, lack of integrity, and cruelty. These character traits seem necessarily excluded from the domain of the morally acceptable. There is no room in the concept of morality to accommodate them. Similarly, acts that cause suffering to others, involve lying, punish the innocent, and the like are excluded. Conversely, rules that prohibit such conduct are constitutive of morality in that a social institution lacking these norms would not be a moral institution.

Extensive argument would be needed to defend these claims; and we will not further pursue the argument here. We note only that the norms that we take to be constitutive of morality include *only* the very general norms that constitute the common morality. These norms do not include what we called, in Chapter 1, the norms of "particular moralities." Accordingly, to restate a conclusion reached in Chapter 1, only a reasonably small set of norms will be constitutive of morality, whereas there are a plural number of particular moralities with a large number of norms.

Problems for Common-Morality Theory

We acknowledge that our theory of the common morality leaves unsettled problems that we would have to address in a more complete account. Three problems are especially worth noting.

Specification and judgment. Do principles, when specified, enable us to reach practical judgments, or are they still too indeterminate to eventuate in judgments? Our theory requires that we specify to escape abstractness, but we also must not overspecify a principle or rule, which then may become too rigid and insensitive to circumstances. Many specified principles and rules will in some contexts encounter this problem of too little or too much specification, and this is one reason why balancing judgments are as important as specification for moral thinking. However, without tighter controls on permissible balancing than common-morality theories usually propose, critics will insist that too much room remains for judgments that are unprincipled and yet sanctioned or permitted by the theory. Can the conditions intended to limit balancing presented in Chapter 1 reduce intuition to an acceptable level? Can the constraints of our proposals about justification be tightened to respond to these concerns?

Coherence in the common morality? We have linked reflective equilibrium to a common-morality theory of normative ethics, but can the common morality itself be made coherent? If one argues, as we do, that a heap of obligations and values unconnected by a first principle comprises the common morality, is there any hope of coherence, short of so radically reconstructing norms that they only vaguely resemble the norms in the common morality? Is our goal of reflective equilibrium more an article of faith than a demonstrable achievement?

Individuals and societies often profoundly disagree regarding which "considered judgments" should form our starting place for reflecting on particular issues, although we have tried to show (using the slavery case) that such deep disagreements do not necessarily indicate that the common morality is indeterminate. Still, it has to be recognized that many controversies involve disagreement over which among the possible initial beliefs may themselves be reasonably claimed to be supported by the common morality and over how to achieve coherence in working from these initial beliefs.

Theory construction. The language of a "common-morality theory" suggests that a philosophical *theory* can be constructed from the common morality. Is there good reason to believe that a theory—not merely an unconnected group of principles and rules—is possible? Perhaps general principles, analyses of the moral virtues, and statements of transnational human rights are all that we should aspire to, rather than a *theory* that conforms to the criteria delineated at the beginning of Chapter 9. Perhaps "moral theory" has been so diluted in meaning in the case of "common-morality theories" that we should abandon the goal of a theory altogether, in favor of a more modest goal.

A related problem is that attempts to bring the common morality into a more coherent unity through specification risk decreasing, rather than increasing, moral agreement in society. That is, a theory can introduce claims that generate disagreements not found in the initial considered judgments; or, as we have often seen in the history of ethics, the theory may turn out to be less clear and reliable for practical decision making than the common morality in its elemental forms (without use of specification).

In part, these problems turn on different expectations for a "theory." Clouser and Gert expect a strong measure of unity and systematic connection among rules, a clear pattern of justification, and a practical decision procedure that flows from a theory, whereas other philosophers are skeptical of one or more of these conditions, and even of the language of "theory."[51] The latter perspective is more congenial to the views we have taken in this book. A common-morality theory will likely not satisfy the full set of criteria we delineated at the beginning of Chapter 9.

CONCLUSION

The model of working "down" by applying theories or principles to cases has attracted many who work in biomedical ethics, but we have rejected this model. Often we have reason to trust our immediate responses to specific cases and the characteristic responses of moral persons more than a theory, principle, or rule. We also have reason to trust norms in the common morality more than norms found in general theories. We have not defended what is sometimes called an "antitheoretical" position; indeed we have encouraged moral theories in defense of the common morality. However, we have argued that general ethical theories should not be expected to yield concrete rules or judgments capable of resolving all contingent moral conflicts.

NOTES

1. U.S. Supreme Court, *United Automobile Workers v. Johnson Controls, Inc.,* slip opinion (Argued October 10, 1990. Decided March 20, 1991).

2. K. Danner Clouser and Bernard Gert, "A Critique of Principlism," *The Journal of Medicine and Philosophy* 15 (April 1990): 219–36. This article, and others that followed it, defend Gert's book, *Morality: A New Justification of the Moral Rules* (New York: Oxford University Press, 1988), versions of which have been published in earlier and later editions under different titles, including *Morality: Its Nature and Justification,* 2nd rev. ed. (New York: Oxford University Press, 2005) and *Common Morality: Deciding What to Do* (New York: Oxford University Press, 2007). Also Gert and Clouser published, with Charles M. Culver, *Bioethics: A Return to Fundamentals* (New York: Oxford University Press, 1997). This book contains a sustained criticism of our views, as does the second edition, entitled *Bioethics: A Systematic Approach* (New York: Oxford University Press, 2006). However, Gert, Culver, and Clouser accept both the language of the common morality and a conception of it very similar to ours: Clouser, "Common Morality as an Alternative to Principlism," *Kennedy Institute of Ethics Journal* 5 (1995): 219–36; and Gert, Culver, and Clouser, "Common Morality versus Specified Principlism: Reply to Richardson," *Journal of Medicine and Philosophy* 25 (2000): 308–22. For critical essays on Gert's theory, see Robert Audi and Walter Sinnott-Armstrong, eds., *Rationality, Rules, and Ideals: Critical Essays on Bernard Gert's Moral Theory* (Lanham, MD: Rowman & Littlefield, 2003).

3. Clouser and Gert, "A Critique of Principlism"; "Morality vs. Principlism," in *Principles of Health Care Ethics,* ed. Raanan Gillon and Ann Lloyd (Chichester, England: Wiley, 1994), pp. 251–66; Gert, Culver, and Clouser, *Bioethics: A Return to Fundamentals,* chap. 4, esp. pp. 74ff.; Gert, Culver, and Clouser, *Bioethics: A Systematic Approach,* chap. 5.

4. Gert, Culver, and Clouser, *Bioethics: A Return to Fundamentals,* pp. 7–8, 31ff, 62, 75–76, 82–88; *Bioethics: A Systematic Approach,* pp. 11–14, 32ff, passim.

5. "A Critique of Principlism," p. 233. Cf. their demand for "a complete system that provides guidance" and "an explicit account of the entire moral system," in Gert and Clouser, "Concerning Principlism and Its Defenders: Reply to Beauchamp and Veatch," in *Building Bioethics: Conversations with Clouser and Friends on Medical Ethics,* ed. Loretta Kopelman (Boston: Kluwer Academic, 1999), pp. 191–93; and their "Common Morality versus Specified Principlism: Reply to Richardson."

6. As we narrow the territory governed by a norm (principle, rule, paradigm case, etc.), the conditions become more specific—for example, making a shift from "all persons" to "all competent patients." As these shifts to the specific occur, it becomes increasingly less likely that the norm will qualify as a principle. For instance, the principle of respect for autonomy applies to all autonomous persons and autonomous actions, whereas a norm of respecting informed refusals by competent patients is, due to its narrowed scope, more plausibly a rule than a principle.

7. Moreover, Gert and associates, like us, appeal to a relatively small number of norms drawn from the common morality. See Gert, Culver, and Clouser, *Bioethics: A Return to Fundamentals,* pp. 16–17, 33–35; and *Bioethics: A Systematic Approach,* pp. 22–23, 34–36.

8. Gert's moral rules can be treated as falling under broader principles. Gert has maintained in private conversation that once principles are interpreted as normative headings under which rules fall, they become unobjectionable, but also expendable. His view is that "if specified principlism develops properly, it will become our account." See Gert, Culver, and Clouser, *Bioethics: A Return to Fundamentals,* p. 90. See also a clarification and partial retraction of their earlier criticism in Gert and Clouser, "Concerning Principlism and Its Defenders: Reply to Beauchamp and Veatch," pp. 190–91.

9. For a proposed method to handle this problem, see Gert, Culver, and Clouser, *Bioethics: A Return to Fundamentals,* pp. 26–31, 36–41, 55–58; *Bioethics: A Systematic Approach,* pp. 27–32, 38–42, 83–87; and "Morality vs. Principlism," pp. 261–63. They propose that a moral rule may be violated only if "an impartial person [would] advocate that violating it be publicly allowed." However, this "solution" is

subject to many competing judgments, and there is no method in their theory for determining how one harm is greater than or outweighs another.

10. Thomas Nagel, *Mortal Questions* (Cambridge: Cambridge University Press, 1979), pp. 128–37; W. D. Ross, *The Right and the Good* (Oxford: Clarendon, 1930; reprinted Indianapolis, IN: Hackett, 1988).

11. See, further, Michael Quante and Andreas Vieth, "Defending Principlism Well Understood," *Journal of Medicine and Philosophy* 27 (2002): 621–49.

12. Gert, Culver, and Clouser, *Bioethics: A Return to Fundamentals,* p. 7; *Bioethics: A Systematic Approach,* pp. 11–13.

13. Gert, *Morality: A New Justification of the Moral Rules,* pp. 154–55.

14. Cf. Gert, Culver, and Clouser, *Bioethics: A Return to Fundamentals,* pp. 62–68; *Bioethics: A Systematic Approach,* pp. 89–93; and the formulation in Gert and Clouser, "Concerning Principlism and Its Defenders: Reply to Beauchamp and Veatch," pp. 190–91. Often, when Clouser and Gert critique our views, it appears that they want to categorize all norms of beneficence as moral ideals, but it would be inconsistent to take this line given their latent commitments to duties of beneficence. These duties appear to be relative to cultures in their theory, though they venture apparently normative judgments that "civilized societies" agree on many duties of beneficence.

15. See Bernard Gert and Charles Culver, "The Justification of Paternalism," *Ethics* 89 (1979): 199–210; for a critique, see James F. Childress, *Who Should Decide? Paternalism in Health Care* (New York: Oxford University Press, 1982), pp. 237–41.

16. See Gert, Culver, and Clouser, *Bioethics: A Return to Fundamentals,* p. 34; *Bioethics: A Systematic Approach,* p. 36.

17. See the comments, formulations, and frameworks in John D. Arras, "Pragmatism in Bioethics: Been There, Done That," *Social Philosophy and Policy* 19 (2002): 29–58; Heike Schmidt-Felzmann, "Pragmatic Principles—Methodological Pragmatism in the Principle-Based Approach to Bioethics," *Journal of Medicine and Philosophy* 28 (2003): 581–96; Henry Richardson, "Beyond Good and Right: Toward a Constructive Ethical Pragmatism," *Philosophy and Public Affairs* 24 (1995): 108–41; Joseph J. Fins, Franklin G. Miller, and Matthew D. Bacchetta, "Clinical Pragmatism: A Method of Moral Problem Solving," *Kennedy Institute of Ethics Journal* 7 (1997): 129–45; and Lynn A. Jansen, "Assessing Clinical Pragmatism," *Kennedy Institute of Ethics Journal* 8 (1998): 23–36.

18. See Alisa L. Carse, "Impartial Principle and Moral Context: Securing a Place for the Particular in Ethical Theory," *Journal of Medicine and Philosophy* 23 (1998): 153–69; Daniel Callahan, "Universalism & Particularism: Fighting to a Draw," *Hastings Center Report* 30 (2000): 37–44; Earl Winkler, "Moral Philosophy and Bioethics: Contextualism vs. the Paradigm Theory," in *Philosophical Perspectives on Bioethics,* ed. L. W. Sumner and Joseph Boyle (Toronto: University of Toronto Press, 1996), pp. 50–78; and Brad Hooker and Margaret Little, eds., *Moral Particularism* (Oxford: Clarendon, 2000).

19. For interpretations, defenses, and critiques of narrative approaches to bioethics, see Hilde Lindemann Nelson, ed., *Stories and Their Limits: Narrative Approaches to Bioethics* (New York: Routledge, 1997). See also Anne Hudson Jones, "Narrative in Medical Ethics," *British Medical Journal* 318 (January 23, 1999): 253–56.

20. See Albert R. Jonsen and Stephen Toulmin, *The Abuse of Casuistry: A History of Moral Reasoning* (Berkeley, CA: University of California Press, 1988); Carson Strong, "Specified Principlism: What Is It, and Does It Really Resolve Cases Better than Casuistry?" *Journal of Medicine and Philosophy* 25 (2000): 323–41 (with a reply by Tom L. Beauchamp) and his "Critiques of Casuistry and Why They Are Mistaken," *Theoretical Medicine and Bioethics* 20 (1999): 395–411; John D. Arras, "Getting Down to

Cases: The Revival of Casuistry in Bioethics," *Journal of Medicine and Philosophy* 16 (1991): 29–51; and James F. Keenan and Thomas Shannon, *The Context of Casuistry* (Washington, DC: Georgetown University Press, 1995).

21. Casuists have had relatively little to say about the nature or definition of a "case," or about the meaning of the term "casuistry," but see Albert R. Jonsen, "Casuistry as Methodology in Clinical Ethics," *Theoretical Medicine* 12 (1991): 297–98; and Albert R. Jonsen, Mark Siegler, and William J. Winslade, *Clinical Ethics,* 6th ed. (New York: McGraw-Hill, 2006).

22. See, for example, Albert R. Jonsen, "Casuistry: An Alternative or Complement to Principles?" *Kennedy Institute of Ethics Journal* 5 (1995), esp. pp. 246–47; "Strong on Specification," *Journal of Medicine and Philosophy* 25 (2000): 348–60; and "Morally Appreciated Circumstances: A Theoretical Problem for Casuistry," in *Philosophical Perspectives on Bioethics,* ed. Sumner and Boyle, pp. 37–49. See also John Arras, "Principles and Particularity: The Roles of Cases in Bioethics," *Indiana Law Journal* 69 (1994): 983–1014.

23. Here are two kinds of claims of a unified theory of the sort casuists disparage. (1) Jeremy Bentham: "From utility then we may denominate a principle, that may serve to preside over and govern...several institutions or combinations of institutions that compose the matter of this science." From *A Fragment on Government,* ed. Burns and Hart (Oxford: Clarendon, 1977), p. 416. (2) Henry Sidgwick: "Utilitarianism may be presented as [a] scientifically complete and systematically reflective form of th[e] regulation of conduct." *Methods of Ethics* (Indianapolis, IN: Hackett, 1981), bk. 4, chap. 3, '1, p. 425.

24. Stephen Toulmin, "The Tyranny of Principles," *Hastings Center Report* 11 (December 1981): 31–39.

25. Jonsen and Toulmin, *Abuse of Casuistry,* pp. 16–19.

26. National Commission for the Protection of Human Subjects of Biomedical and Behavioral Research, *The Belmont Report: Ethical Principles and Guidelines for the Protection of Human Subjects of Research* (Washington, DC: DHEW Publication OS 78–0012, 1978); and see James F. Childress, Eric M. Meslin, and Harold T. Shapiro, eds., *Belmont Revisited: Ethical Principles for Research with Human Subjects* (Washington, DC: Georgetown University Press, 2005).

27. Ibid. See also Toulmin, "The National Commission on Human Experimentation: Procedures and Outcomes," in *Scientific Controversies: Case Studies in the Resolution and Closure of Disputes in Science and Technology,* ed. H. T. Engelhardt, Jr., and A. Caplan (New York: Cambridge University Press, 1987), pp. 599–613; and Jonsen, "American Moralism and the Origin of Bioethics in the United States," *Journal of Medicine and Philosophy* 16 (1991): 113–30.

28. See Arras, "Getting Down to Cases: The Revival of Casuistry in Bioethics," 31–33; Jonsen and Toulmin, *Abuse of Casuistry,* pp. 16–19, 66–67.

29. Jonsen, "Casuistry as Methodology in Clinical Ethics," p. 298.

30. See Cass Sunstein, "On Analogical Reasoning," *Harvard Law Review* 106 (1993): 741–91, esp. 767–78; Loretta M. Kopelman, "Case Method and Casuistry: The Problem of Bias," *Theoretical Medicine* 15 (1994): 21–37; John D. Arras, "Getting Down to Cases"; Kevin Wildes, *Moral Acquaintances: Methodology in Bioethics* (Notre Dame, IN: University of Notre Dame, 2000), chaps. 3–4; Tom Tomlinson, "Casuistry in Medical Ethics: Rehabilitated, or Repeat Offender?" *Theoretical Medicine* 15 (1994): 5–20, esp. 13–14; and Mark G. Kuczewski, *Fragmentation and Consensus: Communitarian and Casuistic Bioethics* (Washington, DC: Georgetown University Press, 1997).

31. See the argument in John Arras, "A Case Approach," in *A Companion to Bioethics,* ed. Helga Kuhse and Peter Singer (Oxford: Blackwell, 1998), pp. 106–13, esp. 112–13.

32. Jonsen, "Casuistry: An Alternative or Complement to Principles?" pp. 246–47.

33. John Rawls, *A Theory of Justice* (Cambridge, MA: Harvard University Press, 1971; rev. ed., 1999), esp. pp. 20ff, 46–50, 579–80 (1999: 17ff, 40–45, 508–09). See also Rawls's comments on reflective equilibrium in his later book, *Political Liberalism* (New York: Columbia University Press, 1996), esp. pp. 8, 381, 384, and 399.

34. John Rawls, "The Independence of Moral Theory," *Proceedings and Addresses of the American Philosophical Association* 48 (1974–75): 8; and, more generally, Rawls, "Outline of a Decision Procedure for Ethics," *Philosophical Review* 60 (1951): 177–97.

35. Norman Daniels, "Wide Reflective Equilibrium and Theory Acceptance in Ethics," *Journal of Philosophy* 76 (1979), pp. 256–82; Daniels, "Wide Reflective Equilibrium in Practice," in L. W. Sumner and J. Boyle, eds., *Philosophical Perspectives on Bioethics* (Toronto: University of Toronto Press, 1996), pp. 96–114; and *Justice and Justification: Reflective Equilibrium in Theory and Practice* (New York: Cambridge University Press, 1996). See also Daniels, "Reflective Equilibrium," *Stanford Encyclopedia of Philosophy* (Online, first published April 28, 2003; accessed August 24, 2007).

36. Compare Rawls, *A Theory of Justice,* pp. 195–201 (1999: 171–76).

37. DeGrazia, "Common Morality, Coherence, and the Principles of Biomedical Ethics," *Kennedy Institute of Ethics Journal* 13 (2003): 219–30, esp. p. 226. On another, perhaps more charitable, interpretation of DeGrazia, he means only that our view leads to incoherence regarding whether we should accept (or at least be concerned about) slippery slopes if physician-assisted suicide were to be legalized. But these worries, too, can be shown coherent.

38. Circa 1640. Published 1974 by Historical Documents Co., available at http://www.jollyrogercayman.com/web%20pages/pirates_creed.htm (accessed August 17, 2007).

39. Rawls himself regarded considered judgments as judgments of individuals and not necessarily ones that are shared convictions. At the same time, Rawls' theory of an overlapping and stable social consensus is presented as an account of shared convictions.

40. For these and other problems, see Michael R. DePaul, *Balance and Refinement: Beyond Coherence Models of Moral Inquiry* (London: Routledge, 1993); M. Holmgren, "The Wide and Narrow of Reflective Equilibrium," *Canadian Journal of Philosophy* 19 (1989): 43–60; and Kai Nielsen, "Relativism and Wide Reflective Equilibrium," *Monist* 76 (1993): 316–32.

41. However, see Rawls's account of public justification fused to reflective equilibrium in *Political Liberalism,* pp. 381–87.

42. Revisions in our theory in this edition have benefited from the criticisms of David DeGrazia, Ronald Lindsay, and Avi Craimer. We have also benefited previously from criticisms and constructive suggestions from Ruth Faden, Norman Daniels, Bernard Gert, Danner Clouser, Albert Jonsen, Earl Winkler, Frank Chessa, and Robert Veatch, among others.

43. Several moral philosophers have built their theories from foundations in the common morality and appeal to principles as their structural basis. See, e.g., William K. Frankena, *Ethics,* 2nd ed. (Englewood Cliffs, NJ: Prentice-Hall, 1973), pp. 4–9, 21–22, 43–56, 113; and *Thinking about Morality* (Ann Arbor: University of Michigan Press, 1980), pp. 26, 34; W. D. Ross, *The Right and the Good,* esp. pp. 19, 41; and Ross, *The Foundations of Ethics* (Oxford: Clarendon Press, 1939), pp. 169–70. Neither philosopher, however, quite captures the right set of basic principles either for general moral theory or for biomedical ethics.

44. On "common values," see Sissela Bok, *Common Values* (Columbia, MO: University of Missouri Press, 1995).

45. H. A. Prichard presented powerful arguments in the common-morality vein to show that all single or absolute-principle theories disintegrate in the face of the diversity in the considered judgments of pretheoretic commonsense morality. See his *Moral Obligation: Essays and Lectures,* ed. W. D. Ross (Oxford: Clarendon, 1949).

46. See Joseph Raz, "Moral Change and Social Relativism," in *Cultural Pluralism and Moral Knowledge,* ed. Ellen Paul, Fred Miller, and Jeffrey Paul (Cambridge: Cambridge University Press, 1994): 139–58.

47. We are indebted in this formulation to Ronald A. Lindsay, "Slaves, Embryos, and Nonhuman Animals: Moral Status and the Limitations of Common Morality Theory," *Kennedy Institute of Ethics Journal* 15 (December 2005): 323–46.

48. Peter Herissone-Kelly, "The Principlist Approach to Bioethics, and Its Stormy Journey Overseas," in *Scratching the Surface of Bioethics,* ed. Matti Hayry and Tuija Takala (Amsterdam: Rodopi, 2003), pp. 65–77. We profited greatly from the criticisms in this article and have attempted to remove some of the unclarities to which the author points.

49. When we say that some persons are not committed to morality, we do not mean that they are not dedicated to a way of life that they consider a moral way of life. Religious fanatics and political zealots have this self-conception even as they act against or neglect the demands of the common morality. In our comments about moral commitment, we do not mean to invoke elitist notions of moral superiority, but we also do not back away from the conclusion that some people are morally better than others, that some people are morally extraordinary, and that some people are morally depraved, even if they do not so view themselves.

50. If the selected group shares the norms, this supports the idea of a common morality, but it is not conclusive. For a conclusive confirmation one would need to investigate all persons committed to a moral way of life, which is not feasible. Thus, there remains an issue of what would constitute sufficient evidence.

51. See Annette Baier, *Postures of the Mind* (Minneapolis: University of Minnesota Press, 1985), pp. 139–41, 206–17, 223–26, 232–37.

INDEX